KU-579-858

Clonskeagh

A Place in History

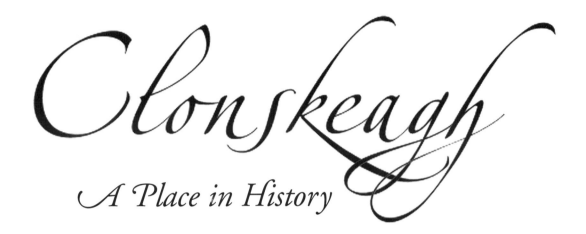

Clonskeagh

A Place in History

MARTIN HOLLAND

Mart Holland

2.9.07

Maurice McCarthy

LINDEN
Publishing Services
DUBLIN IRELAND

Published in 2007 by
LINDEN PUBLISHING • DUBLIN • IRELAND

ISBN 13: 978 1 905487 12 7

This book is typeset by Linden Publishing in 11 on 13 point Adobe Garamond
Designed by SUSAN WAINE
Printed in Ireland by ßETAPRINT LIMITED, DUBLIN

Contents

We acknowledge sponsorship from:

G & T Crampton Ltd
Allied Irish Bank plc

Preface

HOW TO MARK THE FIFTIETH ANNIVERSARY of the dedication of the Catholic church on Bird avenue in Clonskeagh, Dublin – that was the question. One idea floated by Father John Murphy, parish priest, was to have a history of the area written. In a discussion with me as to who might be suitable and willing to undertake the project, I soon discovered that I was myself at the end of his fishing line being slowly reeled in – there was no escape.

The work was challenging and unusual covering as it did a very lengthy time frame, towards the end of which the area changed from being rural to urban. There was also the fact that relatively little had been written about the area in the past. Tackling the problem required the retrieval of as much material relating to the area as it was possible to find but I am in no doubt that much has been missed; that I leave to future historians. What has emerged from the exercise is largely focussed on those people who left some written trace behind them, some famous, some not. Apart from that, other aspects of local life have been touched on such as church, school, culture, industry and sport.

During this work, I received help from various people for which I thank them. In particular I acknowledge the help of following: Fr. John Murphy, Clonskeagh; Dr Charles Smith; Kieran Swords of the County library, Tallaght; Sr Teresa of the Carmelite monastery, Roebuck road; staff at the National Archives, Bishop street; staff of the Research area, Berkeley library, Trinity College, Dublin; Jim Higgins; photographer, Matt Walsh. I am also grateful to those who advised on computer problems and to those who read the text. Any errors that remain are entirely my own responsibility.

SEPTEMBER 2007
Dublin

I

Introduction

THIS STUDY OF THE PLACE of Clonskeagh in history is divided into two parts, one chronological, the other thematic. The first deals with the interaction of certain individuals living in Clonskeagh with important events in Irish, and occasionally, British history; the second with different subjects to a large extent confined within Clonskeagh. Many of the people who are discussed lived but for a limited time in the area; few were natives. This arises from the nature of the place dealt with – in particular for the period from the end of the 18th century up to the early 20th but before the modern suburb emerged. However, no distinction is made between natives and residents; to do so would introduce an unneccessary division.

Similarly with the geographical area itself; it was clear from the start of research into the subject that what is now understood to constitute Clonskeagh was not always the case. Another name in particular was continuously in the frame as research progressed – Roebuck; it was to remain inextricably linked with Clonskeagh throughout. In fact Roebuck featured more prominently in the earlier historical period; Clonskeagh had to wait until modern times to predominate. There are a number of factors which underlie this but the most important of these, from the perspective of an historian, is the availability of source material. The fact that there is more of that available for Roebuck in the early period is undoubtedly due to the presence there of the headquarters of those to whom land in the area had been granted by king Henry II after his arrival in Dublin in 1171. This factor dominated throughout the medieval period with only occasional references to Clonskeagh and in particular to the mill there. However, from about the end of the 18th century Clonskeagh began to emerge from the mists to which the lack of historical source material had consigned it. But before that, evidence is available that ties Roebuck and Clonskeagh together. The most important is the findings of an inquisition [i.e. a sworn inquiry] held in Dublin castle on 3 May 1575 before the Barons of the Exchequer to determine the extent and tenure of the lands of Robert Barnewall, lord Trymleteston, who had died on 7 August 1573. It reported as follows: 'Robert Barnewall, lord Trymleteston & Anne (Amy) Fyane his wife were seised [i.e. in possession of] for life of the manor of Rabo [i.e. Roebuck] divers lands etc in Clonshyaghe *alias* Clonskeagh & the mill of the same, held in chief by knight service, amount unknown.'[1] This, apart from a will made by Robert's father at some date previous to this in which some of his lands were listed as the 'manor of Raboo, Clonskeagh & the mill thereof',[2] is the first record of the name 'Clonskeagh' that it has been possible to find in the historical sources.[3] It is important for a number of reasons. First, it makes quite clear that Clonskeagh (or part of it) was within the manor of Rabo, which, as will be seen in the historical sources, is also called Raboo, Rathbo or Rathbó, Rabowe, Raboge, Rabuck, Rawbuck and later Roebuck.[4] The name Rabo survives to the present day in the place-name Knockrabo where the pronunciation of the ending, 'rabo', the emphasis being on the second syllable, betrays its origin. That Clonskeagh (or a section of it) was part of Rabo fits well with its modern situation largely within the townland of Roebuck, although some of its western parts are in the townland of Farranboley.[5] In fact, according to Ball, Clonskeagh was at one time occasionally called 'Little Rabo'.[6] Secondly, this manor extended as far as the Dodder as the reference to the mill suggests. Finally, it may be possible to detect from the earlier spelling of the name as 'Clonshyaghe' the manner in which it had been pronounced at an earlier period as Irish names were often spelled phonetically by English-speaking officials.

This evidence from the inquisition, of course, still emphasizes the predominance of Roebuck since it is dealing with the extent and tenure of the land of one of the successors of the original grantee who had been given the land by Henry II. It was probably the arrival of a top industrialist of the period, Henry Jackson, in Clonskeagh in the late 18th century to use the waters of the Dodder to power his mills that finally saw Clonskeagh emerge from the obscurity of the

---

1   Margaret C. Griffith, *Calendar of Inquisitions formerly in the Office of the Chief Remembrancer of the Exchequer prepared from the MSS of the Irish Record Commission*, Irish Manuscript Commission (Dublin 1991) 217-18.

2   Ibid. 218 n (2).

3   Ball says that 'Clonskeagh … is mentioned in 1316 as belonging to the owners of Roebuck and then contained a mill' (F.E. Ball, *A history of the county Dublin* (Dublin 1903) vol ii, 77). It has not, however, been possible to find the source upon which this statement is based.

4   As it would be anachronistic to use the modern name when discussing the place in earlier periods, the version in use at any particular time will be used as far as is possible.

5   This can be seen in the Ordnance Survey map of the area.

6   Francis Elrington Ball, *The vicinity of the International Exhibition Dublin: an historical sketch of the Pembroke Township* (Dublin 1907) 12.

historical sources. As well as locating his industrial enterprise there he also built for himself a substantial residence – Clonskeagh castle. This was part of a wider trend which saw mansions of considerable proportions being built around Clonskeagh, stretching out as far as Roebuck castle and beyond. The occupants of these were business and professional people whose work was in the city and who, perhaps initially, retained living quarters also in the city. However, in time these houses were their exclusive dwellings.

It took the compilers of the city directories some time to catch up with this trend and only in 1834 did they include Clonskeagh residents in their lists. Although there was initially some confusion, such as listing Vergemount under Ranelagh, they settled down very quickly to a consistent pattern for a period of time with Clonskeagh a main heading among others in the section devoted to the suburbs of Dublin. Underneath that heading the following sub-headings were listed: Vergemount, Milltown, Roebuck and Bird avenue. Residents close to Clonskeagh bridge appeared immediately under the main heading; they did not require a separate sub-heading. When *Thom's Directory* took over from its predecessor *The Dublin Almanac and General Register of Ireland* around 1848 it included a short description of the area under the main heading before going on to list the names of the residents in areas covered by the sub-heads. The following is the description for 1848:

> CLONSKEAGH, a village in St Mary's, Donnybrook, parish, barony, and county of Dublin, two[7] miles S. from the General Post Office, Dublin, comprising an area of 68 acres. Population, 352, inhabiting 67 houses. It is situated on the river Dodder, and on the road to Enniskerry. It contains two hammer-smith iron works; and a marble saw mill. The neighbourhood is studded with gentlemen's seats and neat villas. *Virgemount* is a pretty range of houses close to the village. *Roebuck,* a district half a mile further on, is covered with elegant mansions and demesnes, the principal of which is the castle of that name, the seat of A B Crofton, esq., which, when originally erected, was strongly fortified, the residence of Lord Trimleston, and occupied by James II and the Duke of Berwick, when encamped in the neighbourhood. *Milltown* is less than half a mile to the right of Clonskeagh, a dilapidated village in St Peter's parish, Uppercross barony, and comprises an area of 185 acres. Population 736, inhabiting 118 houses. It contains a small church as a Chapel of Ease to St Peter's, and a small Catholic Chapel. Its vicinity is adorned with

---

7   *Thom's Directory* continued to state that it was two miles from the GPO until 1862 when it was revised to three miles; it continued with this until Clonskeagh ceased to be included as a separate heading in the directory of 1908.

many pleasing villas and respectable residences, the principal of which are *Milltown-park* and *Fairy-land*. Three omnibuses ply through Clonskeagh from and to Dublin and Dundrum several times a day. The nearest Post Office receivers are Rathmines and Dundrum.

At the end of the 1850s there was a change in approach; the houses listed before that time within the Clonskeagh section but under the sub-heading of Roebuck were now split in two. One of these continued to be listed under Clonskeagh while the rest was given a separate sub-heading of Roebuck under Dundrum. The deciding factor in this split was the postal service. The part of Roebuck that was 'in the delivery of Milltown' remained under the heading of Clonskeagh while that which was 'in the delivery of Dundrum' was now listed under the Dundrum heading. While new sub-headings such as Vergemount hall and St James's terrace were added to Clonskeagh as they came into being the overall division of Roebuck into the part near Clonskeagh and that which was further out continued. The dividing line was approximately where Roebuck road begins today. However, the general description of Roebuck, including the item on its castle which we have seen included in the 1848 directory (above), continued to appear under the heading of Clonskeagh. From 1875 this main heading got an addition; it appeared as Clonskeagh (Pembroke Township) but the sub-headings continued as before until 1907. In the year following that, however, there was a major change; the main heading 'Clonskeagh' disappeared and the places that were hitherto listed under it were now listed in alphabetical order among many other places under the general heading 'Pembroke Urban District'. Shortly thereafter, in 1909, a new heading 'Roebuck' appears for the first time; it had got its own main heading at almost the same time as Clonskeagh, which had one for more than 60 years, lost its. Initially it contained only that part of Roebuck which had previously been listed under Clonskeagh. However, over subsequent years it gained most of the listings (including the growing number of new housing schemes) that were located from the bridge out as far as the dividing line already established; from that line (i.e. approximately the point where Roebuck road now starts) outwards the listings appear under the heading of Dundrum. The part of Clonskeagh on the city side of the bridge was now integrated into the section of the directory entitled 'Dublin street directory (Pembroke district)'.

This lasted until 1965 when another, major and final change occurred; this year Roebuck as a separate heading disappeared along with all other headings in county Dublin. All were now treated as being simply part of Dublin and the various roads and avenues were listed alphabetically. Thus Clonskeagh road (from Sandford road to Bird avenue) is listed immediately after Clonsilla road and Roganstown (Swords) is found immediately after Roebuck road. What had hitherto been treated as being unique places in the county were now subsumed into the city by the compilers of the directory. This does not mean that these places had ceased to exist; it merely reflects the growth of the city and the perception that they were now integral parts of it. Older divisions would, of course, be retained for various purposes such as electoral boundaries. However, when it came to a decision as to what constituted Clonskeagh for the purpose of this study there was no problem in deciding the limits on the city side. On the other (southern) end, where Clonskeagh and Roebuck joined one another in different ways historically, it was decided to include all as far as the end of Roebuck road and not to take in any substantial part of what is now called Goatstown road. On the western side, areas close to where Bird avenue intersects with Dundum road are included, in particular those which are part of the Catholic parish of Clonskeagh. One problem remains; sometimes Roebuck is given as the address of a house that would now clearly be seen to be in Clonskeagh. The approach adopted here is to use the address as currently understood in discussing the house or its occupants. However, when citing from contemporary documents, the address used in them is retained.

Before leaving the discussion of the connection between Clonskeagh and Roebuck, it seems appropriate to state here that both of these places were named while the Irish language still predominated; neither Norse nor Norman had any influence in this process despite the close proximity of their respective power centres. Clonskeagh or its shortened version Clonskea, is the manner in which the original Irish *Cluainsgeach*[8] is now rendered. There are two elements in the name, both of which are quite common in place-names throughout Ireland. The first element '*Cluain*' is variously translated as 'meadow, pasture-land, glade'[9]. This element, spelled either 'clon' or 'cloon', occurs around 1500 times in a list of the names of townlands and towns in Ireland which was compiled in 1861.[10] As well as that, it was quite commonly used as part of the name of ancient ecclesiastical establishments. Clonmacnoise, Clonard, Clonfert and Clondalkin

---

8   Michael Herity (ed), *Ordnance Survey letters: Dublin* (Dublin 2001) 74. Place names of Dublin in this work are taken from manuscripts compiled by John O'Donovan, Eugene Curry and George Petrie as extracted by The O'Rahilly in 1915/16. O'Donovan, in particular, was an expert toponymist (Patricia Boyne, *John O'Donovan (1806-1861): a biography*, Studies in Irish Archaeology and History (Kilkenny 1987) 14).

9   Royal Irish Academy, *Dictionary of the Irish language* (Dublin 1913-76) s.v.

10 William Donnelly, *General alphabetical index to the townlands and towns, parishes, and baronies of Ireland* (Dublin 1861 repr. 1984) 249-74.

spring readily to mind in this context. In fact there are around eighty such examples recorded, some more obscure than others.[11] The second element 'sgeach' (also 'sceach') is translated as 'hawthorn' or 'whitethorn; the latter is sometimes rendered as *sceachgheal*.[12] These thorn–bushes can be seen growing in the wild all over Ireland and, because of that, the word has found its way into a vast number of place-names. Sometimes it stands alone as a place-name but it also occurs as a termination, accompanying some other word. For example: Gortnaskey ('the field of the whitethorn'); Tullynaskeagh and Knochnaskeagh (both 'whitethorn hill') and perhaps better known Lisnaskea in Fermanagh ('fort of the whitethorn'). It is not surprising therefore to find that the place-name Clonskeagh is not unique; there is another Clonskeagh in Mayo, this time spelled a little closer to the original Irish 'Cloonskeagh'.[13] There cannot be any doubt, given that the two elements in the name are both Irish and given their meaning, that the area got its name when Irish was the spoken language there and at a time when the land was as yet largely uncultivated; its origins are therefore very ancient and not in any way influenced by the presence in neighbouring Dublin of the Vikings and, later, the Anglo-Normans. The name most likely antedates their arrival there.

As regards the name Roebuck its origins would also appear to be very ancient. The name has descended in variously related anglicized forms from Rathbó; this can be clearly observed in the historical sources. The first element in that place-name, *Rath*, is very commonly used throughout Ireland and is derived from the Irish word *Ráth* which means 'earthen rampart'. Such ramparts were built to surround living quarters which would, given the pastoral nature of the Irish people during the early period, also have been used to contain animals at certain times. The word therefore took on the meaning, not just of the earthen ramparts themselves, but of the space which they enclosed. That brings us to the second element of the place-name, *bó*. This, of course, is the Irish word for 'cow'. In the context where the word is found here, it is the genitive plural of the word which happens also to be *bó*; it can thus be tentatively translated as 'the enclosure of cows'. The absence of the definite article need not be of concern; other place

---

11   Aubrey Gwynn & R. Neville Hadcock (ed), *Medieval religious houses: Ireland* (Dublin 1988) 421-24. See discussion on this in Alfred P. Smyth, *Celtic Leinster: towards an historical geography of early Irish civilization A.D. 500-1600* (Blackrock, Co. Dublin 1982) 30.

12   The form '*sgeach*' in the place-name '*Cluainsgeach*' is the genitive plural: it is spelled in the same way as the nominative singular.

13   P. W. Joyce, *The origin and history of Irish names of places* (Dublin 1869 repr. 1995) 518-19.

names similarly omit it e.g. *Árdbó* or *Achadbó*. The translation currently used in street names that carry the English name Roebuck is *Reabóg* (e.g. *Plás Reabóige*); this seems to be taken from Raboge which was but one of the stages which existed during the long transition of anglicisation by which Rathbó eventually became Roebuck.

As regards the timescale covered by this study, the early limit to this was easily solved by the availability (in reality, the non-availability) of historical sources. However, the later limit was not as easily determined. The place is a living area and changes are occurring all the time; in fact, in recent years, these changes seem to be accelerating. It was decided, therefore, to limit the later timescale to the third quarter of the 20th century. The reason for this is that the modern suburb as we know it was complete by that time. Subsequent changes are still under way and it is left to future historians to chart them when time gives sufficient perspective to properly assess their import.

The sources available for the early period were quite limited and despite efforts to cast the net as wide as possible it is entirely possible that some have been missed. However, those that are available allow a reasonably continuous, although neccessarily sketchy, picture to be painted at least for the period from the time of the Norman invasion onwards. Of necessity this is centred upon particular individuals. In order to make some sense of the material encountered in relation to these individuals it has been necessary to discuss the political (and it is mostly political) situation in which their activities took place. Their actions or involvements in certain affairs are virtually meaningless unless the contexts in which they occur are explained. On occasion, these contexts require a considerable amount of discussion but to ignore them would be to deprive them of substantial meaning.

Dublin directories are extensively used as a source for the later period. These, it has been discovered where it was possible to test them against other sources, are substantially quite accurate. One point, however, is worth bearing in mind. The dates which are culled from them may on occasion be slightly at variance with the actual date of an event. This is a necessary consequence of the manner in which the directories were compiled. Each directory was published for a particular year and an item in it may have been the result of a survey carried out at some time before publication. A slight problem occurs where details of that entry may have changed in the meantime; this, however, is most likely to have been resolved in the following year's directory which is likely to have noted that change although now with a date that is a little later than that of its occurrence.

While the directories have been extremely useful for the later period, in one particular area they have been of limited value since the information from them is, in the main, confined to the period after 1834. Many of the mansions erected in the general area had already been built at that date so they provide no clues as to who their first occupants were and when they had been built. This information, of course, is available but would require extensive research in the Registry of Deeds, an option that was not pursued; it is open to any future historian to follow this up if desired. A number of items based upon information found in the directories have been footnoted but after some time it was decided that this was no longer necessary since it became clear that it would have been obvious from the text where the material had been sourced; at that point footnoting of such items ceased.

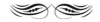

2

The early period – setting the boundaries of Dublin locally

CLONSKEAGH, as it is understood today, is in the unusual position of being comprised of an area which is located within the jurisdiction of two different civic authorities. In some respects this does not have any significant impact upon the lives of its residents today. For example, very few of its people who live south of the Dodder river would now give their address as Clonskeagh, county Dublin. Yet there remain some differences. An obvious one is that, in elections, residents of the two parts vote in different wards or constituencies. Many years ago these differences were much more significant.

The origin of this border within the area goes back, as far as we know, to the arrival of king Henry II in 1171; although there is no evidence, it may even pre-date his arrival as those who take land by conquest often use existing boundaries for their own purposes. Henry celebrated Christmas 1171 in Dublin where he entertained his new Irish subjects in a pavilion specially built for him outside the city walls. He gave a charter to the inhabitants of Dublin in which he granted them the liberties of Bristol. The charter also set the bounds of the municipality which would, from that time forward, be a royal borough under the king's constable; this office would later be superceded by that of the mayor. Six years later, in 1177, Henry granted to his nine year old son John the lordship of Ireland, the intention being that he would, in time, become king of Ireland. When John first came to Ireland in 1185 he confirmed earlier charters granted by his father, including the one which set the boundaries of the municipality of the city of Dublin.[1] Unfortunately this is not clear enough to allow us to identify

---

1   James Lydon, *The making of Ireland from ancient times to the present* (London 1998) 63-8.

Clonskeagh; the relevant section states (as translated from the Latin by Harris): 'on the east and south sides of Dublin, by the pasture-grounds which lead as far as the port of St. Kevin's church, and so along the road as far as Kylmerekargan, and from thence as they are divided from the lands of Donenobroogi [Donnybrook] as far as the Doder, and from the Doder to the sea'.

A number of subsequent extant descriptions of the boundaries still leave this matter unclear. However, due to a practice which later became a regular feature of Dublin civic life, the riding of the franchises, we can fill out, in some detail, where the boundary in the neighbourhood of Clonskeagh was. In an age when there were difficulties in keeping records of where one jurisdiction ended and another began, a custom such as riding the franchises (also called 'perambulating the city liberties') served to preserve the integrity of such boundaries as well as being a regular display to all and sundry of precisely where they were. It was, in fact, a ritual witnessing of these boundaries by a wide variety of people led by the lord mayor and it took place every three years. Should a dispute arise at any time over such a boundary, jurors would have had no difficulties in arriving at an equitable decision on the matter. Although it came to be associated with great festivity, at its core it was a serious business.

A fairly detailed description of the route which the perambulation followed exists for the year 1488 but, unfortunately, there is no specific reference to Clonskeagh. A later version (c. 1766 or shortly before), however, does make such a reference although some of its detail is now difficult to interpret. The description is that given by Harris and the excerpt now given follows the perambulation from the beginning until it has left Clonskeagh:

> They draw up at the custom-house [i.e. the old Custom House, which was located around where the Clarence Hotel now stands], then pass along Essex-street, Temple-bar, and to the east end of Lazer's-hill, from thence to Ring's-end, and so to the low water-mark, where the dart is cast. From thence they cross the strand to the Blackrock †, and so westwards to a Red-house on the east side of Merrion †. From thence through the garden on the back of the Red-house, and across the fields to Simmon's-court; from thence across the fields into the road to Bray, and then southward along the said road to two little cabbins on the south side thereof. From thence they cross the fields into the road to Clanskiagh, opposite to a mill on the river of Donnibrook; from whence they pass along the said road to the bridge of Clanskiagh, and under the east arch thereof, and then to and through the mill of Clanskiagh, and so to Clanskiagh-lane †, and from thence along the said lane to Mill-town road ….

A more modern version of this contains a few extra pieces of information in relation to Clonskeagh. This is included in *The First Report of the Commissioners appointed to inquire into the municipal corporations in Ireland, presented to both Houses of Parliament by command of His Majesty* which was published in 1835. Among these commissioners, incidentally, was a Clonskeagh man, John Richard Corballis, whom we will have opportunity to discuss at a later point. In the report we are told that, in the city Grand Jury room, there is a map of "the boundaries of the county of the city of Dublin, as ascertained by the commissioners of perambulation". It is dated 1807 and, since it was ordered by the Grand Jury and made by the city surveyor, it may be looked upon as an authentic document. It continues 'The limits of the county of the city differ considerably from those of the modern city of Dublin. (Large wealthy parishes) including streets forming continuous portions of the city, and containing nearly a sixth of its entire population, are outside the limits of the corporate jurisdiction, while villages of Donnybrook and Clonskeagh, and part of Black Rock, at a considerable distance from the city are within them'. In a footnote it gives what it calls 'the form of riding the franchises, as printed for the city authorities'. Of this the part that relates to Clonskeagh is now given and may be compared with that given above:

> … along the same [the old road to Bray] till it crosses the present road to Bray, and along by the south-east boundary of the Half-moon Field, to the south corner of the weir in the river Dodder, along the said river to the bridge of Clonskeagh, and under the eastmost arch thereof to the mill of Clonskeagh, and through the said mill.
>
> From thence to the end of a lane*, called Clonskeagh Lane, and along said lane to Milltown Road …[2]

The significance of the asterisk placed beside the word 'lane' will be discussed shortly (note its similarity to the † at the same point in the description by Harris) but for the present it is perhaps worth noting here that the bridge at Clonskeagh referred to is not the one there at present. That bridge was replaced by a new one which, according to a presentment [i.e. a proposal that payment for the new bridge be levied as a county cess – an early form of local tax] made by the Grand Jury for the county of Dublin [i.e. the predecessor in some respects of the present local authority, superceded by the Local Government Act (1898)

---

2   *First Report of the Commissioners appointed to inquire into the corporations in Ireland, presented to both Houses of Parliament by command of His Majesty,* House of Commons 1835 vol xxvii 83-84.

and abolished in 1948] in 1807, was to cost £535-19s-6d.[3] At the point where the bridge is, both then and now, there is a fairly sharp bend in the river Dodder immediately downstream of the bridge while upstream the river has been redirected by channelling it, most likely at the time the new bridge was being built (or later in the century when, apparently, the bridge was rebuilt after being severely damaged in a flood). It is, therefore, quite likely that the old bridge had a somewhat different orientation to that of the present bridge. This would make sense of the reference to an 'east arch' of the bridge; the present bridge has a north-south orientation and has not, therefore, got an 'east arch'; in fact, it has only one arch and one must assume that the old bridge was a hump-backed bridge with two arches like many of those built in the eighteenth century.

It does not, however, explain why the presentment was made to the Grand Jury of the county of Dublin rather than that of the city, since the present bridge [i.e. the bridge for which the presentment was made] is totally within the city boundary. One possible explanation is that the presentment was made to the Grand Jury of the 'the county of the city of Dublin', rather than to that of 'the county of Dublin'; the expression 'county of the city' was quite common at the time as can be seen in the excerpt from the *First Report of the Commissioners ...presented to ... Parliament* given above. Apart from the reference to the east arch it would seem that the boundary as described in the perambulation still remains as can be seen in the Ordinance Survey map (1969) of the area. In this the boundary is shown to lie along the bank of the Dodder as one approaches the bridge along beside Beech Hill road; it then crosses the bridge at its southern end. At the other side, however, it does not continue to lie along the bank of the river; instead it proceeds westward from the bridge along a path south of and at some distance out from the riverbank for about 50 metres before turning sharply in to the centre of the river. From this point westwards the boundary continues along the centre of the river. This piece of land west of the bridge that is within the city boundary probably coincides with the wording of the perambulation when it says that it goes 'to and through the mill of Clanskiagh'. This mill was located south of the river and west of the bridge.

3   Walter Harris, *The history and antiquities of the city of Dublin, from the earliest accounts; compiled from authentick memoirs, offices of record, manuscript collections and other unexceptional vouchers* (Dublin 1766) 133-34; Constantia Maxwell, *Dublin under the Georges*, (Dublin 1956) 268-9; F.E. Ball & Everard Hamilton, *The parish of Taney: a history of Dundrum, near Dublin, and its neighbourhood* (Dublin 1895) 221-22. For the charter (translated) given by John, lord of Ireland, earl of Mortain to the citizens of Dublin on May 15th, 1192 see J. T. Gilbert (ed), *Calendar of ancient records of Dublin in the possession of the Municipal Corporation of that city* (Dublin 1889) vol 1, p2.

Unlike the boundary between the city and the area that now constitutes the county of Dublin, the boundary between the civil parishes of Donnybrook and Taney lies along the centre of the Dodder even on the eastern side of the bridge. This makes it quite clear which part of Clonskeagh is located within one or the other of these civil parishes. While noting the peculiarities of the municipality's boundary just discussed, it can be broadly stated that the parts of Clonskeagh which lie north of the Dodder were under the control of the lord mayor of Dublin while those south of it were within the manor of Rabo (i.e Roebuck, to be discussed shortly) and in modern times are under the administrative control of the local authority of south county Dublin.

One other point worth noting about the information to be gleaned from the perambulation of the city boundaries as it proceeded through the Clonskeagh area is that there were two separate and distinct mills located there at the time. The one beside the bridge, but upstream of it on the south side, is easy to locate; we have noted the boundary going through it. The one downstream can be exactly pinpointed by comparison of the two descriptions given above. The older one states that the boundary crosses 'the fields into the road to Clanskiagh, opposite to a mill on the river of Donnibrook' while the one dated 1807 states that it 'crosses … to the south corner of the weir in the river Dodder'. From this we can see that the mill was at the opposite side of the river to where the weir touches the south side bank. Up to quite recently there was a factory at that location (Smurfits paper works) and one can see the remnants of construction work in the river designed to channel the water for use in the mill. There is also a marker on Beech Hill road at the south side of the weir marking the county boundary.

There is one quite peculiar item included in the description of the 'riding of the franchises as printed for the city authorities' in 1807. At various locations in the description of the perambulation, there is an asterisk inserted with a footnote indicating: 'Where this * appears a Court is called'. One such asterisk appears in the section that pertains to the Clonskeagh area and for convenience it is repeated here:

> under the eastmost arch thereof to the mill of Clonskeagh, and through the said mill. From thence to the end of a lane*, called Clonskeagh Lane, and along said lane to Milltown Road.

Although the 1969 Ordnance Survey map shows the boundary proceeding upstream along the centre of the river after it turns sharply northwards after going through what was once Clonkeagh Mill, this description would suggest that it goes along a lane which could be on either side of the bridge. However, a simpler answer would be that it did in fact go upstream along the centre of the river but those perambulating went along the lane beside the river; this was probably on the north side of the river i.e. on their own side. But what were they doing holding a Court on Clonskeagh Lane? Unfortunately the *First report of the commissioners appointed to inquire into the municipal corporations in Ireland* which contains this information does nothing to enlighten us despite giving a considerable amount of information relating to the different types of Courts held in Dublin at that time. The most likely issues that were decided at such a Court, held in the presence of the lord mayor, were those that were concerned with disputes relating to the boundary in the immediate location; in the medieval period, however, other matters may also have been dealt with there.

3

The medieval manor of Rabo (Roebuck)

I N EARLY TIMES, before the arrival of the Vikings and, later, the Normans, the area of Dublin immediately south of the Liffey was known as Cuala. Here there were two distinguished families: the Uí Briúin Chualann and the Uí Chellaig Chualann.[1] Although it is difficult to be precise about boundaries it is most likely that Clonskeagh was located in the territory of the former. After the arrival of the Normans in Ireland, king Henry II granted Leinster to Strongbow; this was confirmed later by the king's son John to Earl Marshall. However, the king made an exception of Dublin and certain areas near it; they were excluded from this grant. These areas included the part of the present county of Dublin which lies south of the river Liffey. Within this area he granted Rabo (now Roebuck) to Thomas de St Michael.

The king's son, John, later granted it to Robert de St Michael, a brother of Thomas. The granting of land by the king was the very foundation upon which the government of Ireland was to be based under the new dispensation. It was central to the feudal system now being introduced into Ireland for the first time and it would provide the very structure of government, both local and central. That, at least, was the theory; in practice many problems were encountered.[2] One such can be seen in the manor of Rabo. A manor was a parcel of land, of varying acreage, held in the feudal manner by a lord and we know Rabo was held in that way from the inquisition held in Dublin castle in 1575, which we have already met. In this the manner in which lord Trymleston and his wife were in possession of the manor of Rabo (as well as lands and the mill in Clonskeagh) is

---

1   John Ryan, 'Pre-Norman Dublin' in Howard Clarke (ed), *Medieval Dublin: the making of a metropolis* (Dublin 1990) 110-127: 113.

2   A. J. Otway-Ruthven, *A history of medieval Ireland* (2nd ed, London 1980) 102.

clearly stated; they were 'held in chief by knight service'[3] i.e. directly of the king, not of some intermediary.

Problems were obviously encountered as it did not remain long in the possession of the family of the first grantee who had received it in the last quarter of the 12th century; shortly thereafter, in the middle of the 13th, it had passed into the possession of a branch of the famous Norman family of Basset. Again it was to change hands soon afterwards for it is recorded in a charter, drawn up in the 46th year of the reign of king Henry III (1261-62), that David Basset gave to Fromund le Brun 'the whole manor of Rabo' for ever.[4] Fromund was then lord chancellor of Ireland.[5] Many years later, as we shall see, other lord chancellors were resident in Roebuck, as Rabo came to be called. David Basset had also held land nearby as can be seen in a deed which recorded the granting of 'the manor and whole land of Dundrum beside Rabo' by Walter Purcel, senior, lord of Obargy to Hugh de Tachmun, bishop of Meath in 1267. In this, the grant brought with it 'the homage, rents, and services of the heir of John de Rabo, the heirs of David Basset ... and of the other free tenants of the said holding'. Hugh de Tachmun soon granted the same manor to Sir Robert Bagod around the year 1268; this time we find the then the holder of Rabo and chancellor, Fromund le Brun, among the witnesses on the deed.[6]

Why Rabo should have passed through so many hands and so often is not clear. A great amount of source material for this period was lost for ever in the fire which destroyed the record store in the Public Record Office of Ireland in the Four Courts in June 1922 as well as in previous calamities; what has survived are, in general, calendars of the material there. These, however, were meant merely to provide an easy means of access to the originals. We are, thus, dependant upon, at best, abbreviated versions of sources that managed to survive the vicissitudes of time.[7] Given these limitations, we can only glean some items of interest to the activities associated with the manor of Rabo in general and Clonskeagh in particular.

For example, in July 1304 Nigel le Brun, apparently the successor of the earlier mentioned Fromund, was granted by writ of the Privy Seal, 'the free

---

3   Griffith, *Calendar of Inquisitions formerly in the Office of the Chief Remembrancer of the Exchequer*, 217-18.

4   James Mills, 'The Norman settlement in Leinster – The Cantreds near Dublin', *Journal of the Royal Society of Antiquaries of Ireland*, 24 (1894) 161-75: 161, 167.

5   Ball, *History of the county of Dublin*, ii 77.

6   Pembroke Estate Office, *Calendar of ancient deeds and muniments preserved in the Pembroke Estate Office, Dublin* (Dublin 1891) 3-4.

7   Philomena Connolly, *Medieval Record Sources* (Dublin 2002) 9-13.

warren [i.e. the right to keep or hunt various wild animals and birds] in all his demesne lands in Rabo, co. Dublin'. This deed was witnessed by no less than five earls, a member of the royal household and other men of substance, thus illustrating the importance that was attached to such rights.[8] In the following year, Nigel was involved in a dispute with his neighbour in county Meath, William de la Ryuere, over the possession of land. Initially judgement went in favour of le Brun. However, William brought a complaint before the king and gained an annulment of the initial judgement. As a result, le Brun had to give up possession of the land and pay damages arising from the erroneous judgement. The sheriff, who was mandated to collect these damages, testified that le Brun had nothing 'in his bailiwic' [i.e. in county Meath] to meet these charges except a small amount from rent that was not due for some time. However, he said that le Brun had sufficient resources 'in co. Dublin' with the result that the Sheriff of Dublin was commanded to levy the charges. Later in the year 'at the octave of S. Hilary' [28th October] this sheriff reported that he had 'taken of the goods of Nigel [le Brun] at Rathbo [i.e. Roebuck], four stacks of wheat, in which are estimated 50 crannocs, worth each 4s., the crop of 40 acres of wheat'. Apart from '8 marks of rent at Kyllegh' le Brun had no more goods in county Dublin that could be seized.[9] It may be assumed, therefore, that the land of Rathbo at this time was used for tillage. Had it been in pasture one would expect that le Brun would have had cattle and that these would have been commandeered by the sheriff. It is, perhaps, worth noting at this point that the growing of wheat was not a Norman introduction to Ireland. There is a reference to wheat in an eighth-century Irish law-text, *Bretha Déin Chécht,* in which bread-wheat (*cruithnecht)* is considered to be the most prized of the cereals grown in Ireland.[10] It is possible, therefore, that the growing of wheat had a long history in the Clonskeagh/Roebuck area.

It is possible, of course, that le Brun chose tillage rather than pasturage as cattle would have been vulnerable to being stolen. In this regard it should be pointed out that Rathbo was in close proximity to the Dublin and Wicklow mountains where the Gaelic Irish were still dominant, a fact that is clearly

---

8   H.S. Sweetman & G.F. Handcock (ed), *Calendar of documents relating to Ireland preserved in Her Majesty's Public Record Office: 1302-1307* (London 1886) 112 §319.

9   James Mills (ed), *Calendar of the Justiciary Rolls or proceedings in the court of the Justiciar of Ireland preserved in the Public Record Office of Ireland: Edward I* (Dublin 1914) Vol 1, Part 2: 165.

10   Fergus Kelly, *Early Irish farming: a study based mainly on the law-texts of the 7th and 8th centuried AD,* Early Irish Law Series Volume IV, School of Celtic Studies, Dublin Institute of Advanced Studies (Dublin 2000) 219-21.

reflected in the remarkable differences between the two counties of Dublin and Wicklow. The former, Dublin, became the first county in Ireland and the only one constituted before 1200. The latter, Wicklow, did not become a county until 1606, almost the last to become a county apart from Tipperary and the northern counties.[11] The threat to Rathbo from the Gaelic Irish in the mountains can be seen in the findings of a jury which inquired into a case of stolen oxen in the same year that the Sheriff of Dublin had seized le Brun's goods, 1305; the inquiry took place after it had been reported that the oxen were legitimately taken 'upon their common enemies, [and not] of those which were of any Englishman'. It found that the oxen had been driven 'towards the part of Rathbo' with many people following them. There, in 'the manor of Nigel le Brun, their lord, ... [they] maintained themselves ... against very many of the said Irish of Kilpole, who came to attack them'.[12] Some years later, in 1316, when 'Donnyg Obrynne' [Dúnlaing O'Byrne], described as 'a hardened brigand' (*fortis latro*), together with twelve of his associates were killed by William Comyn and his followers, 'keepers of the peace' (*custodes pacis*), their heads were carried into Dublin. In the same year, it was reported that David O'Toole, along with twenty four others, secretly concealed themselves for a whole night 'in the wood of Colyn' (*in bosco de Colyn*) i.e. Cullenswood, now Ranelagh. However, they were found by people from Dublin (including the same William Comyn) who vigorously pursued them for six leagues and killed around seventeen of them while mortally wounding many others.[13] If Ranelagh came under attack from the Gaelic Irish, then it seems fairly clear that Rabo and, indeed, Clonskeagh would similarly have been vulnerable to such attacks and would then have been considered to be part of what was then called 'march land' [i.e. border or frontier territory].

On a broader level, colonial Ireland was, at this time, under some pressure from Gaelic Ireland, a factor which encouraged Scotsman, Edward Bruce, to invade Ireland (1315-18) and even to threaten Dublin.[14] A certain amount of lawlessness prevailed when this invasion occurred and its effects could be felt on the lands which are situated between Dundrum and Dublin. Here lands, which were part of the manor of the archbishop of Dublin (St Sepulchre), were totally devastated. On the lands of Farranboley, which were then part of that manor, the native Irish tenants of the archbishop, harassed both by settlers and their own

---

11 Mary Daly, 'The county in Irish history', in Mary Daly (ed), *County and Town: one hundred years of local government in Ireland,* Lectures on the occasion of the 100th anniversary of the Local Government Ireland Act, 1898 (Dublin 2001) 1-11: 2-3.

12 Mills, *Calendar of the Justiciary Rolls: Edward 1,* 479-80.

13 John T. Gilbert (ed), *Chartularies of St Mary's Abbey,* 2 vols (London 1894) ii 350-52.

14 James Lydon, *The lordship of Ireland in the Middle Ages* (Dublin 2003) 113-14.

countrymen, were driven off. This was before the time when a castle was erected at Dundrum by the Fitzwilliams. At a later stage these lands would be part of the area which was enclosed within the Pale for the purposes of protection.[15] Before that, however, the all-pervading fear of attack by the native Irish had to be taken into account when deeds were drawn up for the conveyancing of land. An example of this for the year 1360 can be found when John de Endredeby and John de Evesham, clerks, drew up a deed which saw 'the manor of Dundrum except the Lytelrabo' demised for 24 years to John Serjaunt, citizen of Dublin. The rent is specified but the following is added 'If the manor be destroyed by rebels against will of lessee he shall be freed of rent until again able to take the profits'.[16]

At a different level the year 1305 was an eventful one at Rathbo for le Brun; in the same year he bought the remaining land held there by the Fitzdermots. These were the descendants of Domhnall MacGiollamocholmóc, who belonged to the East Leinster dynasty which held the territory of Uí Briúin Chualann in pre-Norman times. He was married to Derbforghaill, the daughter of the well-known Diarmait MacMurrough who had gone across the sea to seek help in his attempt to regain his kingship of Leinster. After some equivocation, watching to see how events would turn out, Domhnall decided to accept Strongbow's overlordship and subsequently submitted, along with other Irish leaders, to the English king Henry II during his sojourn in Ireland in 1171-2. This submission had allowed him to hold on to territory but now, in the feudal manner, directly of the king. His family would subsequently become anglicised and changed their surname to Fitzdermot – a name based upon that of his son Diarmait.[17]

The le Brun tenure of Rabo lasted much longer than those who previously held it. In fact, one member of the family even took the name of the area as his surname; Otho de Rabo acted as bailiff for Nigel. However, like its predecessors it too would come to an end. At some date in the third decade of the fifteenth century [i.e. the 1420s] Elizabeth, daughter and heiress of Christopher le Brun of Rabo, married Robert Barnewall, the first baron of Trimblestown. As a result, Rabo came into the possession of this branch of the Barnewall family and would remain so until the beginning of the nineteenth century.[18]

---

15 Ball, *History of county Dublin*, ii 66-67.
16 Pembroke Estate Office, *Calendar of ancient deeds and muniments*, 18-19.
17 Emmett O'Byrne, *War, politics and the Irish of Leinster: 1156-1606* (Dublin 2003) 20-24.
18 Ball, *History of county Dublin*, ii 77.

4

The Barnewalls at Rabo (Roebuck)

WITH THE ACCESSION OF THIS NEW FAMILY, the manor of Rabo would become associated with memorable events in Irish, and indeed English, history. The first of these was the civil war in England, known as 'The War of the Roses' (1450-1461). This involved a violent clash between two rival and powerful royal dynasties, the Lancastrians and the Yorkists, both of which were in direct line of descent from king Edward III (1327-1377). One of the earliest activists in this war was Richard, duke of York. He was appointed lieutenant of Ireland in 1447[1] and, while he was there, Robert Barnewall entered his service (in 1449). In return for this he knighted Robert at some date before 1455.[2] By this time the war was well underway with the Lancastrian king captured by the Yorkists at St Albans on 22 May 1455.[3] Six years later a Yorkist king, Edward IV, was on the throne and Robert Barnewall was created baron of Trimlestown for his services to the House of York. He was also made a member of the Irish Council for life. Trimlestown is a townland some two miles west of Trim in county Meath and Robert was the first Barnewall to be associated with it.[4]

The success of the Yorkists was, however, relatively short-lived. Each of their three kings, Edward IV, Edward V and Richard III, was driven from his throne: Edward IV, only temporarily, the other two permanently – losing their lives in the process. Richard III lost his throne (and his life) at the battle of Bosworth in 1485 not to the Lancastrians but to the first of the Tudors, Henry VII.[5] Although the Yorkists were now in great difficulty and had no support of any real

---

1 Lydon, *Lordship of Ireland*, 188.
2 Stephen B. Barnwall, 'The Barnewall family during the sixteenth and seventeenth centuries', *The Irish Genealogist* 3 (1963) 311.
3 M. H. Keen, *England in the later Middle Ages: a political history* (London 1986) 436-57: 444.
4 Barnwall, 'The Barnewall family', 311.
5 Keen, *England in the later Middle Ages*, 461, 488-89.

consequence in England[6] they still had a following in Ireland. In fact, the Irish administration headed by Gerald ('Garret Mór'), the 8th earl of Kildare, was reluctant to transfer loyalty from the Yorkists to the Tudors. Because of this, a Yorkist pretender to the throne, Lambert Simnel, was actually crowned as 'king Edward VI of England and Ireland' in Christ Church cathedral, Dublin, in 1487,[7] apparently by the archbishop of Dublin.[8] Among those Irish who supported the coronation of Simnel, the Yorkist pretender, was Sir Christopher Barnewall, now 2nd baron and lord of the manor of Rabo. However, he was pardoned by the king in May 1488 after that plot had failed. Although he had sworn an oath of allegiance to the king before his envoy in Dublin, he was, nevertheless, commanded along with twelve other Irish lords to appear before the king himself at Greenwich in 1489 and renew his oath. Later, he sat in the Irish parliament in 1491 and attended, along with lords and gentry of the Pale, a council meeting at Trim in 1493 where ordinances were passed to promote law and order.[9]

In the following year the famous Poynings' Law was passed and with it the independence of the Irish parliament was ended. This greatly curtailed its value as an instrument in the hands of the Great Earl of Kildare when he was restored to the chief governorship of Ireland in 1496. He, nevertheless, went on to grow in strength, reaching a pinnacle in 1504 when, accompanied by an unusual amalgamation of Gaelic and Anglo-Irish lords, he had an impressive victory at Knockdoe in county Galway over Ulick Burke of Clanrickard and Turlough O'Brien of Thomond.[10] Among those who accompanied Kildare on this expedition was Sir Christopher Barnewall, 2nd baron Trimlestown.[11]

His successor, Sir John, 3rd baron, had a distinguished career. Appointed king's serjeant and then solicitor general for Ireland early in his career, he was promoted in 1514 to Second Justice of the Chief Place [i.e. King's Bench (Ire.)], to be held during pleasure, with a salary of 40 marks.[12] By this time Henry VIII

---

6   David R. Cook, *Lancastrians and Yorkists: the Wars of the Roses* (Harlow 1991) 75.

7   Lydon, *Lordship of Ireland*, 213-15; Keen, *England in the later Middle Ages*, 548.

8   Otway-Ruthven, *History of Medieval Ireland*, 403.

9   Barnwall, 'The Barnewall family', 312; Steven G. Ellis, *Tudor Ireland: crown, community and the conflict of cultures 1470-1603* (Harlow 1985) 74.

10 Lydon, *Lordship of Ireland*, 218-20; Art Cosgrove, *Late medieval Ireland, 1370-1541*, (Dublin 1981) 99-103.

11 Barnwall, 'The Barnewall family', 312.

12 Ibid; James Morris (ed), *Calendar of the Patent and Close Rolls of Chancery in Ireland, of the reigns of Henry VIII, Edward VI, Mary, and Elizabeth* (2vols, Dublin 1861-62) i 1.

was on the throne and the Great Earl was dead, succeeded by Garret Óg. Henry's first direct involvement in Irish affairs saw the replacement of Garret Óg by Thomas Howard, earl of Surrey as chief governor of Ireland.[13] During his governorship, Sir John Barnewall was a member of the Irish Council.[14] Surrey's replacement by Piers Butler, 8th earl of Ormond, led to quarrels with Kildare, his great rival. One outcome of this saw the appointment by Kildare in 1524 of Sir John as undertreasurer, thus undermining the office of lord treasureship held by Ormond.[15]

Continuing problems saw Sir William Skeffington appointed as chief governor in 1530 while Kildare, who had been detained at court in England, was allowed home. Problems remained and, once more, Henry was forced to rely on Kildare; he became governor again in 1532. However, having first ignored a summons to England, he was eventually persuaded to travel; he arrived in England in February 1534 having first appointed a deputy in his absence, lord Thomas, his heir – more popularly known as Silken Thomas. Soon thereafter it was decided to reappoint Skeffington as chief governor; this threat to the Kildare position in Ireland contributed, among other things, to Thomas's renunciation of allegiance to the crown on 11 June 1534 and the subsequent full-scale rising. By July, he was laying siege to Dublin castle. It was not until October, however, that Skeffington arrived with a large army to put down the rising. In the meantime, Sir John Barnewall, lord Trimleston, despite being implicated, along with many Palesmen and Gaelic chiefs, in the rising was appointed lord chancellor, with custody of the Great Seal, in August by king Henry. It would appear that he was also made chief governor in the same month and retained that position until the arrival of Skeffington. In this way, Rabo had become associated with the highest political office in colonial Ireland. Sir John's son-in-law Christopher Eustace, however, was not so fortunate; he was outlawed and executed in 1535 for his involvement. The rebellion having been suppressed, Silken Thomas was executed along with his five uncles, at Tyburn in February 1537.[16]

Perhaps because of the disturbed times in which he lived, it is said that the present castle (much altered and restored in the 19th century) at Roebuck was built by the lord Trimleston of this time (the 3rd baron) although it has been argued that it was, in fact, Robert 5th baron Trimleston who built it. This is

---

13 Cosgrove, *Late medieval Ireland*, 109-111.
14 Barnwall, 'The Barnewall family', 312.
15 Cosgrove, *Late medieval Ireland*, 112; Ellis, *Tudor Ireland*, 117.
16 Cosgrove, *Late medieval Ireland*, 113-20; Ellis, *Tudor Ireland*, 119-29, 328; Barnwall, 'The Barnewall family', 313; Morris, *Calendar of Patent and Close Rolls*, i 13.

based upon the grounds that the initials of the 5th baron and his wife Anne (*recte* Amy) Fyan are engraved upon the castle.[17] Robert's father, Patrick 4th baron, succeeded in 1542 but had already been a member of the Irish Council since 1539; he went on to take an active part in the Council until 1560. In 1541 he sat in the parliament which brought about a major change in how the king was styled; heretofore, he was 'lord of Ireland', now he would be 'king of Ireland'. Introduced with much fanfare and celebration, this was a revolution in how Ireland would be governed.[18] Later, during the reign of Elizabeth (August 1560), he was among a group of important people given a commission to govern the English Pale in the absence of the lord lieutenant.[19]

Like his father before him, Robert (5th baron) was a member of the Irish Council – from 1564 to 1572 – and sat in parliament in 1569. He took part in the war against Shane O'Neill and was dispatched to treat with him in 1565. In the same manner as his predecessors, he was much taken up with the affairs of his possessions in Meath. As noted earlier, he was married to Amy Fyan. Her father was Richard Fyan, alderman and lord mayor of Dublin. The marriage took place in 1559 but he did not succeed to the baronetcy until 1563.[20] In the meantime it would appear that he lived at Rabo. Apparently Patrick (4th baron) granted for the use of his son and heir apparent Robert (and his wife Amy) for life the 'manor of Raboo, Clonskeagh & the mill thereof, the mes. & ten. in Clatterston & Cottre farm excepted'. However, there was an obligation on them to make available to Patrick for his life ' out of Raboo, the finding of 6 horses and 5 boys whenever he visits Dublin, & 2a(cres of) hay & 4 loads of underwood p(er) a(nnum) delivered in Dublin, & to Richard Fyane of Dublin 2a(cres of) hay for life out of Raboo, delivered at his house in Dublin'.[21]

Robert died in 1573 but Amy remarried and lived until 1600; she is buried in St Audeon's. The title and the manor of Rabo passed to Robert's brother Peter (the 6th baron) who gave 25 years of service to the English crown, mainly in its efforts against the Gaelic Irish. In 1578 he was among a group nominated Commissioner of the Peace for counties in the Pale. He was knighted in St Patrick's cathedral by the lord justice in 1583. However, his loyalty to the crown did not prevent his being suspected of involvement with Spain at the time of the armada (1588).

---

17 Ball, *History of the county Dublin*, ii 77; a search for this on the building that is there at present failed to find it.
18 Ellis, *Tudor Ireland*, 139-40; Barnwall, 'The Barnewall family', 313.
19 Morris, *Calendar of Patent and Close Rolls*, i 447.
20 Barnwall, 'The Barnewall family', 314.
21 Griffith, *Calendar of Inquisitions*, viii, 218 n (2).

He was succeeded in 1598 by Robert, 7th baron, who at that time was a prisoner, having been captured at the battle of Tyrell's Pass; he did not get possession of his honour until 1609. In the meantime queen Elizabeth had died and James I had come to the throne; it was the end of the Tudors and the beginning of the Stuart sovereignty over Ireland. In 1603 when James I was proclaimed king, Robert, along with other Roman Catholic peers, subscribed. However, two years later he was to give an indication of his stand in relation to the religious policy of the crown. A royal order directed that there should be a strict enforcement of fines on those who did not attend reformed church services. This was resented and a petition against it was organized; Robert signed it. Later, in 1612, a number of Recusant Peers (i.e. those who refused to attend such services), including Robert, protested at the severe treatment meted out to Catholic priests by the government. He sheltered Jesuits at his castle in Trimlestown and when he sat in the parliament of 1615 he was described as 'a busy and violent recusant'. It was probably as a result of the obstinacy of that parliament that the king, in the same year, made an order that the male heirs of several Irish lords, including that of lord Trimleston, were to be educated in England. Nevertheless, Robert was still loyal to the crown; when Charles I acceded in 1625 he vowed his allegiance.

One of his sons, John, entered the Franciscan order on St Patrick's day in 1616 at the college of St Anthony in Louvain. At a later date he held the chair of theology there for eight years. He returned to Ireland in 1620 and was elected Provincial of the Order in 1638 for three years. He assisted in one of the great works of the Franciscans of the time, the writing of 'The Lives of Irish Saints', a project aimed at counteracting negative attitudes towards the Catholic church in Ireland. He set up a convent of nuns in Drogheda in 1639 and was Guardian of the Franciscan House in Dublin in 1645. He also was active in the pursuit of compromise at the Confederation of Kilkenny.

Matthias (Matthew) Barnewall, the 8th baron, succeeded his late grandfather, Robert, in 1639 and took his seat in the House of Lords in 1640. At this time the king, Charles I, was under great pressure from the parliamentarians in England – he would eventually be executed by them in 1649. In Ireland a rebellion, initially led by Sir Phelim O'Neill broke out – the famous Ulster rising of 1641; it claimed to be acting on behalf of the king. This made it easier for conservative Catholics to join in. The harsh reaction to the rising felt by Catholics resulted in most of the lords of the Pale joining the rebels. In December Matthias, along with seven such lords, met with some of the leaders of the rising near Drogheda and a few days later at Tara; the result was a formal alliance between them. He was outlawed in March 1642 and when the parliamentary forces were approaching Meath, he fled to Kilkenny. A council had been called there through the action of archbishop O'Reilly of Armagh. Its first session was in October and Matthias was in attendance. By this stage the king and the parliamentarians were engaged in open warfare in England while, in Ireland, the rebels (now the Confederate army), both Irish and Old English, were on the side of the king although they had their own demands on him which he found impossible to concede. Attempts were made to negotiate these with the king's government in Ireland headed by the earl of Ormonde. It was, inevitably, a complex situation made even more difficult by the arrival of cardinal Rinuccini in 1645. His greatest ally was Owen Roe O'Neill who won a famous battle at Benburb in 1646. Confusion reigned among the Confederates and it was not until the end of 1648 that agreement was reached between Ormonde and the Confederates. A treaty was signed in January 1649; in the same month the king was executed. Although Ormonde struggled on it was too late. In August he was defeated by an army of parliamentarians at Rathmines and at Baggotrath castle (now upper Baggot street); many of his men fled to the hills, apparently by way of Clonskeagh, after the latter. Two weeks later a huge army of men from England landed unopposed in Ringsend led by Oliver Cromwell. That changed the situation in Ireland completely.[22]

As well as being a member of the Supreme Council of the Irish Confederacy Matthias was also a cavalry captain in its army from around 1646 to 1650. His involvement led to an attack on his castle at Trimlestown. It also resulted in the destruction of Roebuck castle. Furthermore he was not included among those who were pardoned in Cromwell's Act of Settlement in 1652. He was transplanted to Connaught in 1656; his lands and the manor of Roebuck, together with Clonskeagh and a mill were taken over by one called Edward Barry but, according to Ball, it would appear that Mr William Nally – said to be the ancestor of the notorious Leonard McNally (he was a Castle informer among the United Irishmen in the 1790s) – was the main occupant of the lands at this time. He may have been living at the ruined Roebuck castle as early as 1654; he is reported to have been living in a house rated as containing two hearths. He died in 1669 and was buried in Donnybrook churchyard; his is one of the oldest

---

22 Barnwall, 'The Barnewall family', 315-320; Aidan Clarke, *The Old English in Ireland, 1625-42* (Dublin 2000) 179-82, see also 287 where lord Trimleston is called 'Matthew' Barnewall, not 'Matthias'. He is similarly called Matthew in the Cromwellian survey by Fleetwood (Simington, *Civil survey,* 261); Morris, *Calendar of Patent and Close Rolls,* ii 11; Charles R. Mayes, 'The early Stuarts and the Irish peerage', *The English Historical Record* 73(1958) 227-251:230; J.C. Beckett, *The making of modern Ireland: 1603-1923* (London 1981) 82-101; Lydon *The making of Ireland,* 180, 186-191; W. St. John Joyce, *The neighourhood of Dublin* (Dublin 1912) 182-190.

tombstones in that graveyard. However, he is not mentioned in either of the two surveys carried out during the Cromwellian period. One, the Fleetwood Survey, reported that the townland of Rabuck, 'by Estimate four ploughlandes', was the property of 'Matthew', lord baron of Trimleston, 'Irish Papist'. It contained 400 acres (12 in meadow, 360 arable, 28 in pasture and no waste); on the premises were one castle, which had been destroyed by the rebels, one garden plot and one mill ('in use worth, in Anno 1640, ten poundes') and 'the Jury value the Buildings at Sixty poundes'. The tithes belonged (apparently as a result of Cromwellian intervention) to the College of Dublin (i.e. Trinity College, Dublin); previously, they had belonged to the archdeacon of Dublin. It concluded 'The premises are Bounded on the East w(i)th Butterstowne; on the South w(i)th Kilmand; on the West w(i)th Dondrom; & on the North w(i)th Simon's Court'. Second, the Down Survey, carried out by Sir William Petty in 1657, reported that the land held in 'Rabuck' by lord Trimleston amounted to 500 acres. William Nally is not mentioned either in the census of 1659 but there is a reference there to a William Manley, gent, – a name not unlike William Nally – being the titulado (i.e. principal person e.g. nobleman, baron etc) of Rabucke and Owenstown.

Cromwell died in 1658 and less than two years later, in May 1660, king Charles II was restored to the throne. With that, Matthias regained most of his lands in Meath and in May 1667 he regained possession of Roebuck castle and lands. However, he did not live long enough to enjoy it; he died in September of the same year.[23]

It would appear that his successor, Robert, 9th baron, did not return immediately to live at Roebuck as the census of 1659, referred to above and taken during the tenure of his predecessor, states that there were 19 people living in 'Rabucke', 2 English and 17 Irish; however, significantly, it does not give the name of any Titulado of Rabucke (although it does give one for the combined lands of Rabucke and Owenstown – William Manley). Furthermore, according to Ball, the castle was still in a ruinous condition in the eighteenth century.[24] Robert was obviously in good grace with the king as he was granted a pension by Charles II

---

23 Barnwall, 'The Barnewall family', 320; Ball, *History of county Dublin,* ii 77-78; Ball & Hamilton, *The parish of Taney,* 15-21; Robert C. Simington (ed), *The Civil Survey A.D. 1654-56: Vol. VII County of Dublin,* Irish Manuscript Commission (Dublin 1945) 261; M.V. Ronan, 'Archbishop Bukeley's Visitation of Dublin, 1630', *Archivium Hibernicum* 8(1941) 56-98: 62, 73; Séamus Pender (ed), *A census of Ireland circa 1659 with supplementary material from the Poll Money Ordinances (1660-1661),* Coimisiún Láimhscríbhinní na h-Éireann (Dublin 1939) v, 381.

24 Ibid. v 381; Ball, *History of county Dublin,* ii 78.

in 1671; this was continued by his brother James II. His landed possessions are given in the Commissions of Grace of James II in 1685; among these is Roebuck, said to have been 505 acres in extent. In 1688 James II was overthrown in England and William and Mary were proclaimed king and queen; in March of the following year he came to Ireland from France. It is said that, on arrival, he lodged at Roebuck castle but some doubt has been cast on that, given the ruinous state of the castle since the time of the Irish Confederacy. It is also said, perhaps more credibly, that he and the duke of Berwick set up camp in the neighbourhood of Roebuck. The Irish parliament was called and met in May and June ('the patriot parliament'); its members were almost entirely Roman Catholics. Robert attended but died shortly afterwards.

He was succeeded by Matthias, the 10th baron Trimleston. He served as a captain of Horse against the Williamite army which landed in Belfast in August 1689. In the following June William arrived in Carrickfergus and shortly thereafter the famous battle of the Boyne took place with victory going to William. Although James left for France within days and William for England in August, the campaign was not over yet. Matthias was promoted to colonel of Foot after the Boyne and was present at the second siege of Limerick. Towards the end of September 1691 Patrick Sarsfield and others entered negotiations to end the siege; while these were under way, Matthias was one of the hostages exchanged to facilitate the talks. Articles, military and civil, were agreed. The civil ones became known as the Treaty of Limerick, the fate of which is well known. The military ones, however, allowed for the release of prisoners and the transportation to France of those who wished to go. These were to become known as the Wild Geese. Among these was Matthias who went to France where he continued in the service of James II. In January 1692 he was appointed lieutenant in the 1st Troop of Horse Guards under the Jacobite duke of Berwick but was killed (aged 21 and unmarried) in September of that year in the battle of Roumont in Flanders.

The success of the Williamites was to have severe consequences for those who fought against them; for example, the estates of around 270 such participants were confiscated amounting to around one million acres. For his part in the wars Matthias was attainted (i.e. his peerage and lands were forfeited and his civil rights impaired). This was the situation which faced his brother, John, who succeeded him; he was referred to as 'John Barnewall, esquire, commonly called lord Trimleston' i.e. the 11th baron. Like his brother, he too had gone to France where was in the service of king James; he was an ensign in his Guards. He did, however, succeed in recovering the Trimleston estates before 1695. He had been indicted for treason but was not actually outlawed. He made efforts to have his title restored but this was rejected by the Privy Council in 1697. He was, however, permitted to return to Ireland in the following year. It would appear that commercial activities resumed at Roebuck soon thereafter. In the early years of the 1700s there was a bleach yard on the lands there; there were also mills in operation at Clonskeagh. Occasionally advertisements would appear looking for a dairyman for the castle farm offering him excellent accommodation. Those seeking the job were asked to apply to lord Trimlestown at his seat near Trim or his Dublin town house in Mary street. Whatever the view the Privy Council might have in relation to the legitimacy of his title John Barnewall had no compunction in using it in these advertisements. He died in 1746 and was buried at Trimlestown.[25]

As the peerage was still forfeited, his first son and heir who succeeded him as 12th baron was referred to as 'Robert Barnewall, commonly called baron Trimlestown'. This is the reason why the Order, which on 29 March 1762 listed those who were members of the Irish House of Lords, omitted his name. In his early years he spent much of his time in France where he worked as a physician before returning to live in Ireland. Although this was the period of the Protestant ascendancy and the penal laws, this does not seem to have prevented him from socialising with the elite of Dublin in the then fashionable New Gardens in Great Britain street beside the Rotunda (i.e. the Rotunda Gardens) as can be seen from the report: 'there was seen the portly figure of lord Trimleston, dressed in scarlet with full powdered wig and black velvet hunting cap'. Nevertheless, there were severe pressures on the Roman Catholic gentry especially in relation to land tenure. The choice faced by them was to convert to the Established Church in Ireland or else see their estates continually subdivided in succeeding generations. This may be the reason why Robert's son and heir, Mathias, conformed to the established religion in January 1763 and when he died in 1767, the next son by his first wife and now his heir, Thomas, conformed quite soon thereafter.[26]

---

25   Barnwall, 'The Barnewall family', 320-21; Ball, *History of the county Dublin*, ii 78; John D'Alton, *The history of the county of Dublin* (Dublin 1838) 810; Beckett, *Making of modern Ireland*, 139-49; John D'Alton, *Illustrations, historical and genealogical, of king James's Irish Army List (1689)* (Dublin 1885 repr 1997) 115-16.

26   Vicary Gibbs (ed), *The complete peerage of England Scotland Ireland Great Britain and the United Kingdom* (1959) vol xii/2 §43; Patrick Fagan, *The second city: portrait of Dublin 1700-1760* (Dublin 1986) 36, 45; S.A. Ossory Fitzpatrick, *Dublin: a historical and topographical account of the city* (Dublin 1907), see chapter vi 'Social life in eighteenth century Dublin'; Tighearnan Mooney & Fiona White 'The Gentry's Winter Season', in David Dickson (ed), *The gorgeous mask: Dublin 1700-1850* (Dublin 1987) 1-16:9; Beckett, *Making of modern Ireland*, 158; Eileen O'Byrne (ed), *The Convert Rolls*, Irish Manuscripts Commission (Dublin 1981) 6.

Robert, in a will made at some point before 1782, had left to his only surviving son by his second marriage, Joseph, the 'manor of Ro[e]buck, and Glanskeagh otherwise Clonskeagh co. Dublin' but Joseph died unmarried in 1782.[27] When Robert died in 1779, Thomas succeeded as the 13th baron.

These were troubled times as the American war was then in progress. Prior to that, however, the eighteenth century was remarkable for the absence of any sustained violence, apart from that of agrarian origin (e.g. the Whiteboys in the 1760s). Since the opening of the magnificent new parliament house in 1729 (now the Bank of Ireland building in College green) most political activity was focussed there; the growing importance of parliament was such that great efforts were made by the executive, headed by the lord lieutenant, to control it. It had to contend with a small, but important, group there who opposed what they saw as English interference. They were commonly referred to as 'patriots' and they were supported by the press, especially by the *Freeman's Journal*. With the outbreak of the American war in 1775 other problems impinged not least those of an economic and military nature. This would lead ultimately to the founding of the Volunteers, a mainly protestant organization which stood ready to repel a potential French invasion but also to assert the rights of Ireland. Thomas (the 13th baron) joined the Volunteers in 1779-80 and the Dublin Volunteers used Roebuck as their camping ground in 1784. Five years later, according to a report in *The Dublin Journal*, 'a duel was fought near Roebuck Castle, in the County of Dublin, by a Mr H. and a Mr P. when after firing a case of pistols, without effect, the affair was amicably adjusted'. Who these men were, what they were dueling about and why they chose the neighbourhood of Roebuck Castle for their duel (many duels at this time were fought in the Phoenix Park) has not been discovered; it is possible that they had some connection with the volunteers. Notwithstanding these events, however, the owner of Roebuck castle, Thomas, had more serious considerations to engage him – the legitimacy of his title. His efforts in this regard were to bear fruit as the King's Bench in Ireland reversed the outlawries and attainders of his antecedents. His subsequent request to have his title restored was approved by both of the Irish Houses of Parliament and received the royal assent; he took his seat in the House of Lords in April 1795. In line with this restoration, Thomas pursued a parallel project; around the year 1790 he rebuilt Roebuck castle, which had remained in a ruin for so long, as his country residence. He fitted out one of the apartments,

---

27 P. Beryl Eustace (ed), *Registry of Deeds, Dublin: Abstracts of Wills*, Irish Manuscripts Commission (3 vols, Dublin 1954-84) ii 301 §611; Gibbs, *Complete peerage*, xii/2 §§ 43, 44.

described as a noble room 50 feet in length, as a theatre. However, he did not live long to enjoy the fruits of his work; he died unmarried in December 1796 aged 60. According to a report in the *Hibernian Magazine* of January 1797 (p95), the remains of lord Trimleston were moved from Kildare street to the county Meath attended by a detachment of the Roebuck Cavalry.[28]

He was succeeded by his cousin Nicholas (the 14th baron) who was, in fact, around nine years older than him. According to a contemporary almanac, his baronetcy was then the second oldest in Ireland; it also recorded that he was a Roman Catholic.[29] When he died in 1813 he was succeeded by John Thomas (the 15th baron) who was born in France; he was a fluent French speaker and was, from at least 1804, a very good friend of Tom Moore, famous for his *Irish Melodies*.[30] However, it would appear that at some point during Nicholas's tenure the immediate connection between the barons of Trimleston and Roebuck castle ceased. Joseph Archer, in his survey of the county Dublin for the Dublin Society published in 1801, under the heading of 'Gentlemen's seats and Improvements' reported "Roebuck, a fine old castle, in good order, the seat of – Crofton Esq; a small demesne and good gardens". From another source we know that the then occupier of Roebuck castle was Mr James Crofton, an official of the Irish Treasury. He modernised the castle. He pulled down part of it and restored the rest. The large apartment which lord Trimleston had made into a theatre he used as a drawing room; it was the only part of the old castle to remain. Later his son, Arthur Burgh Crofton was the occupier. He, like his father, was a commissioner for the construction of Kingstown (now Dún Laoghaire) Harbour. Subsequently the castle was taken over by Mr Edward Perceval Westby when he married Elizabeth Mary Blackburne. She was the daughter of the Right Hon. Francis Blackburne, who had been lord chancellor of Ireland and had lived at Roebuck hall. This, as Ball pointed out, made a reconnection between Roebuck and the Great Seal (held by the lord chancellor) which went back to the thirteenth century when it was held by Fromund le Brun. He might also have pointed out that it was also held by Sir John Barnewall

---

28 Ibid. xii/2 §§43,44; Beckett, *Making of modern Ireland*, 190-92, 212; David Dickson, *New foundations: Ireland 1660-1800* (Dublin 1987) 128, 130-34, 141-49; Ball, *History of county Dublin*, ii 78, 80; D'Alton, *History of county Dublin*, 810; Ball & Hamilton, *Parish of Taney*, 183, 213; *The Dublin Journal* 1789 (Thursday June 4; Thursday August 20 & Saturday September 5).

29 John Watson Stewart's *Almanack* 1809 p 104.

30 Gibbs, *Complete peerage*, xii/2 §44; W.S. Dowden (ed), *The letters of Thomas Moore*, 2 vols. (Oxford 1964) i 81; W.S. Dowden (ed), *The Journal of Thomas Moore*, 6 vols. (Newark 1983-91) i 77, ii 435, 443, 471-72, 507, 586, 588-90; v 1899.

of Roebuck castle who was lord chancellor in the sixteenth century.[31] Although the connection between Roebuck castle and the Trimleston dynasty was severed around the year 1800 it is worth noting that the 18th baron, Charles Aloysius Barnewall, in 1930 married his third wife, Josephine Francesca, daughter of Sir Christopher John Nixon of Roebuck grove in Clonskeagh. He died in 1937 and she in 1945.[32]

---

31 Gibbs, *Complete peerage*, xii/2 §44; Joseph Archer, *Statistical survey of the county Dublin, with observations on the means of improvement; drawn up for the consideration, and by order of The Dublin Society* (Dublin 1801) 102; Ball & Hamilton, *Parish of Taney*, 183; Ball, *History of county Dublin*, ii 88.
32 Gibbs, *Complete peerage*, xii/2 §45.

5

Henry Jackson, Clonskeagh castle and the politics of the 1790s

L ORD TRIMLESTON'S MEMBERSHIP of the Volunteers and their use of Roebuck as a camping ground in 1784 had placed it close to the centre of political activities in Ireland at that time. Shortly thereafter, however, political events in Ireland would take on a much more radical hue and the local connection with this would shift to the other end of Clonskeagh, close to the river Dodder. Disillusioned by, *inter alia*, the lack of real parliamentary reform and influenced by the American War of Independence which broke out in April 1775 and by the French Revolution of July 1789 many opposition politicians became radicalised and politics became polarised. In the autumn of 1791 political societies, entitled the United Irishmen, were founded in Belfast and Dublin with Theobald Wolfe Tone acting as the mainspring. Earlier that year, in March, the first major Dublin edition of Thomas Paine's radical pamphlet, *The Rights of Man (Part I)*, appeared. It soon became a bestseller. This was due mainly to the work of a committee which was set up in April to fundraise in order to facilitate a large-scale print-run. Most of its members were friends of the radical Napper Tandy; among them was one of the foremost of Dublin's businessmen, the ironfounder Henry Jackson. His attachment to the writings of Paine was such that he called Clonskeagh castle, his country residence, Fort Paine.[1] He apparently saw no contradiction in having a castle as a country seat and naming it after Paine. In doing so he gives us an insight into the type of radicalism that was then espoused; these radicals were no levellers.

Jackson, according to himself, started his business in 1766.[2] By the 1780s he was commissioned by the Volunteers to supply them with cannon from his

---

1 David Dickson, 'Paine and Ireland' in David Dickson, Dáire Keogh & Kevin Whelan (ed), *The United Irishmen: republicanism, radicalism and rebellion* (Dublin 1993) 133-50: 133-38.
2 R. B. McDowell, *Historical essays: 1938-2001* (Dublin 2003) 239.

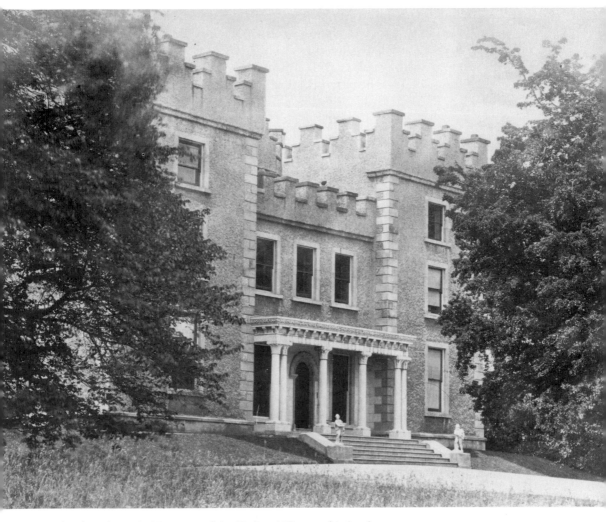

Clonskeagh castle (*Courtesy of the National Library of Ireland*)

foundry, then located at 87 Pill lane.[3] The boring of cannons was very skillful work particularly suited to the manufacture of primitive steam engines. It was around this time that such engines began to emerge. Watt had patented his theory of the steam engine in 1765 but it was not until 1783 that the introduction of the first working rotative steam engine was to herald the beginning of the new

---

3   David A. Wilson, *United Irishmen, United States: immigrant radicals in the early republic* (Dublin 1998) 19; *Wilson's Dublin Directory* 1781.

era of steam.[4] Jackson had the ability to access this new technology; he was the first person ever to erect a steam engine in Dublin. His foundry at 159 Old Church street (the Eagle Foundry) was powered by such an engine. So too were his rolling and slitting mills at 74 Rogerson's quay and his mill for grinding wheat in Phoenix street (here he had, according to Archer, 'one steam engine for corn'). As well as these works, he owned iron-mills at Clonskeagh, close to the bridge over the Dodder and not far from his country residence, Clonskeagh castle. These works, said to have been on a very large scale and costing Jackson £20,000 to build, included 2 iron mills, 1 grinding mill, 1 boring mill and a range of hammers, cylinders, shears, rollers and bellows. Unlike in his other works, these were powered by water turbines; two 12 ft in diameter by 7 ft wide, one 12 ft by 5 ft and another 12 ft by 3 ft. The number of people employed there was considerable. All these industrial activities meant that Jackson was a man of substance; sufficient to allow him the luxury of a country residence at Clonskeagh. Although his ownership of such a property indicates that he was no leveller, his form of radicalism did, nevertheless, manifest itself in his building of quality cottages for his workers in Clonskeagh, this at a time that the landed proprietors were being strongly castigated for the wretched condition of labourers' cottages. Jackson's concern for the welfare of his workers in Clonskeagh is in line with the political philosophy and liberal economic theory which was espoused by the eighteenth century radical who could readily identify with the struggles of the poor but would not in any circumstance accept that they be allowed to form combinations [i.e. the early form of trade unions].[5]

Jackson was a member of the Common Council of Dublin Corporation but in the civic election of 1790 his name, together with those of fellow radicals Napper Tandy and Patrick Ewing, having been submitted by the Commons for selection as sheriffs, was rejected; election as sheriff was an essential step towards becoming an alderman and ultimately lord mayor.[6] In the following year he

---

4   T. S. Ashton, *The Industrial Revolution 1760-1830* (Oxford 1968) 55-57.
5   McDowell, *Historical essays,* 239; *Wilson's Dublin Directory* 1797, 1800; E. Mac Thomáis, 'Dublin 1798', *Dublin Historical Record,* 51/2 (1998) 117-33: 118-19; Archer, *Statistical survey,* 204; Hely Dutton, *Observations on Mr Archer's statistical survey of the county of Dublin* (Dublin 1802) 128-29; D'Alton, *History of the county of Dublin,* 808; James Smyth, 'Dublin's political underground in the 1790s', in Gerard O'Brien (ed), *Parliament, politics and people: essays in eighteenth-century Irish history* (Dublin 1989) 129-48: 133.
6   R. B. McDowell, *Ireland in the age of imperialism and revolution 1760-1801* (Oxford 1979) 345; Jaqueline Hill, 'The politics of Dublin Corporation: 1760-92', Dickson, Keogh & Whelan, *The United Irishmen,* 88-101: 89-90.

joined the newly formed United Irishmen. The founding of this organisation marked the beginning of a decade which would see the transformation of reformative politics into revolution. In 1793, Jackson was the largest contributor to a fund which sought to raise £1000 to pay a fine for the exoneration of Napper Tandy; he subscribed 20 guineas.[7] However, two years later he was identified by the spy, Francis Higgins, as one of the main instigators of a serious and well organised riot in Dublin on the night of the swearing in of Camden, the new lord lieutenant. By this stage, a large number of Dublin's workforce had been politicised and organised. A new force called the Defenders was coming into a closer relationship in the city with the United Irishmen. Although rural in origin and sectarian in purpose, this society was gathering strength among Dublin's working class many of whom had arrived in the city to escape poverty and oppression elsewhere in the country. When the United Irishmen organization was suppressed and forced underground, a meeting was held towards the end of 1794 in Jackson's house in Church street where one of the Sheares brothers proposed that it should be re-organised into 'sections' or 'splits' as they would later be called. As this new form of organisation began to take shape, having more or less incorporated the Defenders, its central core was based in the general area around Church street and Pill lane (this lane, no longer in existence, ran behind the present Four Courts beginning at Church street; it is likely that Jackson started his ironmongery in this lane). According to the government spy, Leonard McNally, reporting in early 1797, most members of the United Irishmen lived in this area; the principal organizer was one Edward Dunn, (he had been imprisoned in 1793 for making seditious statements in a local public house), a clerk at the Church street foundry where most of them were employed. There they were busy making material suitable for battle; shot, pikes, and metal spikes for use against cavalry horses in street fighting. In expectation of help from revolutionary France, Jackson also began to make cannon balls to a specification which would allow their use in French artillery.[8] Although the evidence we have points to all of this activity taking place in his Old Church street foundry, it would be most surprising if some similar work had not also taken place at Jackson's iron-works in Clonskeagh around this time. One writer has stated that pikes were, in fact, made there at that time.[9]

---

7   Jean Agnew (ed), *The Drennan – McTier letters: 1776-1793* (Dublin 1998) 512, letter 423 dated Monday 12 April 1793.
8   Smyth, 'Dublin's political underground in the 1790s', 136-142; Wilson, *United Irishmen, United States*, 25. *Wilson's Dublin Directory 1781* has the following entry 'Henry Jackson, Ironmonger, 87 Pill Lane'.
9   Mac Thomáis, 'Dublin 1798', 118-19.

With General Lake cracking down on the organization in Ulster in 1797, the United Irishmen organization was strongest in Dublin. However, the almost inevitable split now reared its head. Some advocated an immediate rising; others favoured waiting for the expected arrival of the French. Henry Jackson belonged to the faction which believed that the rising should go ahead without waiting for the French. The government, on the other hand, was on high alert; on 12 March 1798, it pounced. Tipped off by an informer, a military detachment surrounded the house and warehouse of Oliver Bond in Bridge street where a meeting of the Leinster Directory of the United Irishmen was taking place. A large number of delegates were arrested including Bond, who incidentally was married to Eleanor, a daughter of Henry Jackson. Lord Edward Fitzgerald escaped but was later fatally wounded during the attempt made to capture him. Jackson himself was arrested in his foundry on that day. Soon after, however, a committee was set up to seek the release of Jackson, Bond and others from prison.[10]

The action of the government in March threw the organisation into confusion before the date it had set for the rising, May 23rd; it was an important factor in the failure of the rising.[11] Executions followed. On 17 July, John McCann, secretary to the Leinster committee and one of Jackson's clerks was tried for treason and executed two days later. However, perhaps reflecting attitudes based on class, the imprisoned leaders avoided such a fate; they made a deal with the government. They were given the option of emigrating to a neutral country of their choice but they first had to give the government all the information they had on contacts made between the United Irishmen and foreign states. It should be remembered that England was at war with revolutionary France at this time. America would have been a possible choice for the prisoners. However, Rufus King, the American minister in London was appalled when he heard about the deal being made; he moved quickly to prevent those being released going to America. In 1799 Henry Jackson sought King's permission to emigrate to the United States and there to re-start his foundry business. Jackson's industrial ability was an obvious attraction. His knowledge of up-to-date technology, together with his considerable capital, would be an asset to America; perhaps sufficient to offset the risks his radical political views would entail. Rufus King thought it over and decided to take that risk; he gave permission for Jackson to enter the United States. It was a decision he would

---

10 Smyth, 'Dublin's political underground in the 1790s', 144; Wilson, *United Irishmen, United States*, 29; Lydon, *The making of Ireland*, 272; Thomas Pakenham, *The year of liberty: the bloody story of the great Irish Rebellion of 1798* (London 1969) 54, 58.
11 Beckett, *Making of modern Ireland*, 262-63.

come to regret. Jackson settled down in Baltimore in 1805.[12]

The America which Jackson and other released prisoners found when they arrived had changed from that which they had admired at the time of the revolution. To their dismay the unity which had then existed had given way to faction or party. Out of this arose two groupings who took different views of how the United States should be ruled; the conservative Federalists and the more radical Republicans. The newly arrived prisoners were naturally attracted to the latter and took an active part in various political activities. Among these was the election for the New York state assembly in 1807. In this the Federalist ticket was headed by the same Rufus King whom we have already met. This provided an opportunity for the ex-prisoners as they were fully aware of the role he had played when he had attempted to prevent their departure for America in 1798. One of them, Thomas Addis Emmet, now created the sensation of the election; he revealed the letter which Rufus King had written to Jackson permitting him to enter the United States. In this King had made disparaging remarks about the Irish. Emmet also bitterly attacked King. As a result, King was blamed for many of the ex-prisoners' woes and even for the execution of Robert Emmet in 1803. King's supporters fought back but he was, nevertheless, defeated to the great joy of the emigré United Irishmen.[13]

It has sometimes been suggested that Jackson was an ancestor of the famous Stonewall Jackson who took a prominent part in the American civil war in the 1860s. However, according to the *Virginia Military Institute Archives* this is not so. It would appear that Stonewall did indeed have an Irish ancestor, but not the United Irishman; his great-grandfather John Jackson was born in Coleraine, co. Derry around 1716 and died in Clarksburg, Harrison county, West Virginia in 1801.[14] Similarly, a report in *Whittock's Guide to Dublin 1846* (p139) has it that Jackson was an ancestor of General Jackson, president of the USA.[15] However, this is an impossibility as the president was born in the backwoods of America to Scots-Irish immigrants in 1767, long before Henry Jackson set foot in the USA. He became a major general during the war against the British in 1812 and served as president during the years 1829 to 1837.

The precise date of Jackson's departure for the United States is not clear. Wilson's *Dublin Directory* lists him as an Iron and Brassfounder at 159 Old Church

---

12   Sir Richard Musgrave, *Memoirs of the Irish rebellion of 1798* (repr. Fort Wayne 1995) 589; Pakenham, *Year o f liberty*, 53; Wilson, *United Irishmen*, 1, 31, 60.

13   George Brown Tindall, *America: a narrative history* (2nd ed, New York & London 1988) volume 1, pp 310-11; Wilson, *United Irishmen, United States*, 64-67.

14   *Virginia Military Institute Archives* [http://www.vmi.edu/archives] January 2006.

15   Cited in Ball & Hamilton, *Parish of Taney*, 144.

street in 1798 and 1799; each year from 1800 to 1805 it lists him as having an Iron, Rolling and Slitting Mills at 74 Rogerson's quay. Thereafter it makes no reference to him. By this time he was probably in America; we have seen above that he was settled in Baltimore in 1805. As for his property in Clonskeagh, it would appear that John Stokes and his brother-in-law William Southwood, who had a property in Kennedy lane, bought it in 1799; they paid £12,000 for it. This covered his country residence, Clonskeagh castle as well as the iron-works. The latter included 2 iron mills, 1 grinding mill and 1 boring mill. It seems likely that business at the works was badly affected in the aftermath of the rising as the new owners re-sold the property shortly thereafter, in 1801. However, things may not have been as clear-cut as that since Archer reports in his *Statistical Survey*, published in 1801 (perhaps compiled in the previous year), under the heading 'State of mills everywhere' and sub-heading 'Clonskeagh'; 'Two iron-work wheels; Jackson and White. Three iron-wheels; Mr. Stokes & Co'. From this it would appear that Jackson had, at least for a time, acquired an associate, Mr White, for some of his works at Clonskeagh while the rest had been sold to Mr Stokes. Whatever the truth of the matter is there can be no doubt that, although there is no known record of it, the effects of all this on the Clonskeagh workforce was not good. Some years later, in 1834, the iron-works were sold by auction to Mr William M'Casky when it was said that there were about ten people employed there. From this it can be gathered that the level of business activity there had declined substantially as the reports from Jackson's time refers to 'numerous' people being then employed and the works being on a 'very great scale'. [16] The subsequent fate of the works is discussed in more detail in Chapter 17 (below).

16   Archer, *Statistical Survey*, 206; D'Alton, *History of the county of Dublin*, 808.

6

Robert Emmet's connection with Clonskeagh

WITH THE FAILURE OF THE 1798 RISING, the English government moved to have the two kingdoms, England and Ireland, brought together in one union; this it believed was the best way to bring Ireland under control and to secure England against a potential threat from the French coming through its backdoor, Ireland. Mainly through bribery and corruption the government managed to gain a majority in the Irish parliament when it resumed in 1800; it ratified the union almost without a whimper of protest. With that, more than 500 years of Irish parliamentary existence was consigned to history. The new United Kingdom of Great Britain and Ireland came into being on 1 January 1801. It made very little or no immediate impact in Ireland. Everything there seemed very quiet; even the threat from France seemed to have evaporated. Then, almost like an aftershock following an earthquake, came Robert Emmet's rebellion. On Saturday 23rd of July 1803 disturbances on Dublin's streets led to the murder of, among others, lord Kilwarden, the chief justice of Ireland. These murders were the result of a rebellion which Emmet had planned but which, when it was put into effect, went seriously wrong.[1] It is not recorded where Emmet was while this plan was being worked upon but it seems very likely that at least part of it was plotted while he resided in the Emmet household which, as will be shown, was located in Clonskeagh.

Robert Emmet was born on 4 March, 1778 at 109/110 St Stephen's green, the seventeenth child of Dr Robert and Elizabeth Emmet. Only four of these children survived early childhood; Robert was the fifth to carry his father's name, all the others having died in infancy. Dr Robert had been appointed state physician in 1770, the year the family had moved to Dublin. This, together with

---

1   Lydon, *The making of Ireland*, 274-79.

income from other medical activity, ensured that he became quite wealthy. Robert junior was educated first at Oswald's school in Dapping court near Golden lane and then at Samuel Whyte's English grammar school in Grafton street. At the latter, he got his first introduction to the art of public speaking, a skill that he would later use to very good effect. It was there also that he made the acquaintance of the poet Thomas Moore. He would renew that acquaintance again later in Trinity College; he entered that college on 7 October 1793 at fifteen years of age. Two years later, at the beginning of his junior sophister year in Trinity, he entered the King's Inns in Dublin with the intention of becoming a barrister. The following year saw him excel academically and, having met all the requirements, was due to graduate with a BA degree at some point in the spring or summer of 1798. While at Trinity he was secretary of one of its four committees of United Irishmen, then a proscribed organisation, and was also a member of its famous Historical Society; in this he displayed his powerful rhetorical skills. It is not clear whether he was expelled from the college or left voluntarily but it would appear that shortly after his brother, Thomas Addis, a leading radical, was arrested along with the Leinster Directory of the United Irishmen on 12 March 1798, he withdrew from the college without having received his BA degree. Tensions were high in the college at the time as attempts were made to expel all students who had radical views. His academic career having thus ended, his career as a revolutionary began; he was just 20 years of age.[2]

During his final year as a student at Trinity College, Emmet's father had retired from his public practice of medicine, sold his house on St Stephen's green and gone to live at his country seat in Clonskeagh.[3] This house was called Casino[4] and is located in grounds at the junction of Dundrum road and Bird avenue; it is now called Mount St Mary's, the property of the Marist Fathers. According to a descendant of Thomas Addis Emmet, in an interview with the Marist Fr Donal Kerr in March 1970, the Emmets first came to Casino around 1770, the year they came to Dublin.[5] It seems that it was they who had the house built and it is more than likely that Robert spent much of his young years there; he certainly lived there around the time that he withdrew from Trinity College.[6] Just two years previously, in 1796, when he was eighteen years old he was one of

---

2   Patrick M. Geoghegan, *Robert Emmet: a life,* (2nd ed, Dublin 2004) 51-2, 56, 65-7, 70-9, 85.

3   Ibid. 62.

4   For most of what follows concerning Casino: Donal Kerr (ed), *Emmet's Casino and the Marists at Milltown* (Dublin 1970) and references therein.

5   Ibid. 7.

6   J. J. Reynolds, *Footprints of Emmet* (Dublin 1903) 48.

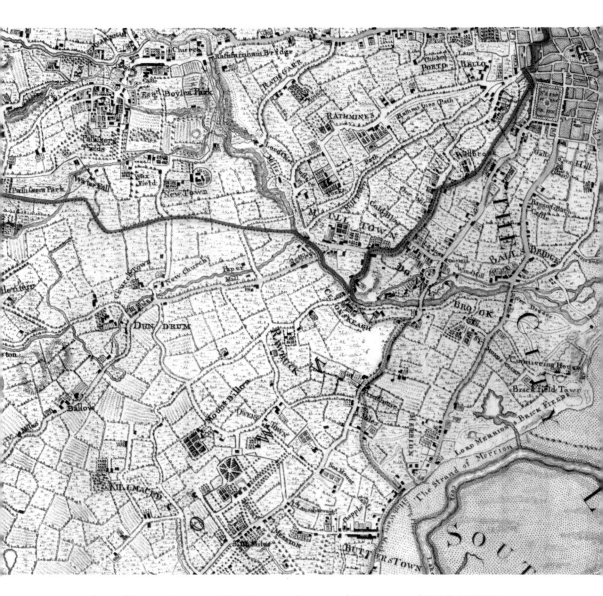

Part of Rocque's map entitled 'An actual survey of the county of Dublin' (1760)

the witnesses when a lease for part of the lands which his father held adjacent to Casino was being renewed.

When it was being leased at a earlier date, the title deed of this piece of land was described in the Registry of deeds (495/50/321029) as 'part of Milltown situate at the corner of the road leading from Milltown to Roebuck [i.e. what is now called Bird avenue], containing two acres, one rood, twenty-nine perches, held for the lives of Frederick, Duke of York, Isaac Gartside, and Thomas Lane, and for the lives for ever thereafter to be added to the lease thereof, dated 5th June, 1790, from Miss Anne Elizabeth Moulds of Kevin street, to Thomas Andrews'. The Registry of deeds also records Dr Emmet's main holding (it is described as 'a large house, garden, and out-offices, and over eight acres of land, known as Casino, Milltown') as well as some others. The most substantial of these is described as 'a plot of ground containing one acre and a half of a rood, bounded on the southern and western sides by Dr Emmet's ground, on the eastern side by ground in the possession of Alderman John Exshaw, and on the northern side by ground in the possession of George Frederick Moulds and Mary Anne Moulds'. This was held under a lease, dated 9 January, 1799, for eighty two years from the 25th March, 1800 and was, therefore, taken by Dr Emmet after he had moved to live full-time at Casino. Two other, less substantial, pieces of land were also acquired at the same time and under the same lease. They are described as follows: (1) 'a piece of ground on the left-hand of the road leading from Dublin to Powerscourt [the Dundrum road], near Milltown, whereon the doorway and part of the wall is built, and which said wall is part of the mearing [boundary] between the ground held by the said George Frederick Moulds and Mary Anne Moulds, and the lands of Casino held by the said Robert Emmet … with the use of the dyke or watercourse between the holdings of the said Robert Emmet and the said George Frederick and Mary Anne Moulds in common, as a passage for the water of said respective premises' and (2) 'that piece or parcel of ground next adjoining the aforesaid doorway and dyke and watercourse, containing in front twenty one feet, in rere ninety eight feet, bounded on west by the garden of the said George Frederick Moulds and Mary Anne Moulds, on the east by the field of the said George Frederick Moulds and Mary Anne Moulds, and on the south by a doorway, dyke, and watercourse aforesaid'.

The existence of a watercourse should make it possible to trace these boundaries should one so desire. The leasing of the pieces of ground that gave access to the watercourse may have been motivated by a need for a supply of water either for the house or garden or both; Dr Emmet is said to have devoted much time to gardening after he had retired to Casino. The family from which these various pieces of land were leased, the Moulds (sometimes spelled Mowlds), had descendants living in Milltown well into the twentieth century according to *Thom's Directory*, one descendant has an address given as 'Bawn house'. As well as that, Donal Kerr records the fact that a local woman, Miss Anne Dowdall, remembered the Moulds sisters living next door to Casino in the early part of the twentieth century.[7]

---

7   Kerr, *Emmet's Casino*, 4, 6.

At the time when Robert Emmet left Trinity College, his brother Thomas Addis was in prison. It was a dangerous time; it was only a matter of weeks before the 1798 rising would commence. Although the rising was originally planned to begin in Dublin that failed to happen; it was, therefore, confined to a limited number of places throughout the country. Because of this, Emmet did not play any part in the fighting. He was, nevertheless, deeply involved with the United Irishmen and his radical views were well known to the government especially from his activities in Trinity College. Despite the fact that he was now living outside Dublin, at Casino, it is almost certain that he could have expected to be arrested at some time. This did not, however, happen although it would seem that he had taken precautions against its eventuality. In 1801, on a visit to Dublin, the poet Robert Southey spoke to a friend of Emmet's and was told by him that Emmet had prepared a hiding place for himself under the study in his father's house and had stayed there for six weeks during the rising. In this hiding place he had enough supplies to support him while there and during the darkness of the night he would emerge on to the grounds to get exercise. This hiding place was probably the same as that which Dr Madden learned about during a visit he made to Casino in 1836. On that visit, he spoke to an old gardener, John Murray, who had worked in the same place from 1803; he also spoke to a man who had been a personal servant of Dr Emmet, Michael Leonard. He was brought to a small room off the kitchen which had once been Robert's bedroom. There he saw a trapdoor over a passage which was said to lead out on to the lawn. Apparently there was a tunnel which emerged from the front of the house, left of the entrance and under the two basement windows; it ran beneath the ground as far as a summer house which was about 50 yards distant from the road [the Dundrum road]. As this summer house had from an early period been prepared as a study it is possible that it was below this structure that the hiding place, referred to by Robert Southey, was excavated; its connection by tunnel with the house and its proximity to the road would seem to be particularly suited as a hiding place and, in the event of a raid on the house, an escape route. In later years, long after the house and grounds had ceased to be the property of the Emmets, the tunnel is said to have been incorporated into a draining system for the land. Later still, a small purpose built vault is said to have been discovered under the ground at some distance from the house. As late as the 1920s, Laurence Patton, one of the first Marist novices at Casino, then renamed Mount St Mary's, found some remaining evidence of these escape routes, both in the main house and in the summer house.[8]

---

8   Ibid. 4, 5; Geoghegan, *Robert Emmet*, 91-2, Reynolds, *Footprints of Emmet*, 49-51; R. R. Madden, *The life and times of Robert Emmet Esq* (Dublin 1847) 97-98.

By the end of the autumn of 1798, after the defeat of the French at Ballinamuck, the rising was finally crushed. Thomas Addis Emmet was, however, still a prisoner, held at Newgate prison where his brother, Robert, visited him regularly. He, along with other state prisoners, came to an agreement with the government that allowed them to emigrate. As this was being discussed by the British authorities it emerged that there was strong opposition to the prisoners going to the United States, especially from Rufus King, the representative of the United States in Britain. This led to great bitterness against King on the part of the prisoners and, as we have already seen, Thomas would at a later time take great pleasure in playing an important role in frustrating the efforts of King to be elected to the New York assembly and later to its governorship. In the meantime, however, restrictions were placed in January 1799 on visits to the prisoners at Newgate prison to the great distress of Dr Emmet; this would become even more distressful two months later when, along with eighteen other state prisoners, he was transferred to Fort George in Scotland. He was destined to remain there for the next three years. Writing to him from Casino on 1 January 1801, his father Dr Emmet expressed his hopes for the future and wrote that 'that thought, my dear Tom, takes in your return and settlement at Casino, which wants but that one circumstance to make it to me a most happy residence'. One can glimpse from this the unhappiness of the Emmet parents at Casino in those turbulent times. His father, in particular, missed his son Tom so much so that he considered selling Casino and moving to England or Wales to be near him. However, his health prevented him from doing so.[9]

By the middle of the year 1800 the Irish House of Commons had passed the bill which enabled the union of Great Britain and Ireland to come into being; Robert Emmet had watched this from the visitors' gallery. As might be expected he was vehemently opposed. Shortly thereafter he was appointed secretary to a group of United Irishmen which was sent on a secret mission to France. Before going there, he visited his brother, Thomas Addis, imprisoned at Fort George in Scotland; afterwards he set out from Yarmouth and eventually reached France in 1801. There he met Napoleon Bonaparte and Talleyrand; plans for invading Ireland were discussed. However, he soon became disillusioned by the French politicians and the old question of whether French aid was necessary to a successful rising in Ireland reared its head once more. Towards the end of that year he heard that his father had put their home, Casino, on the market with an asking price of £2,000. Betraying the sense of disillusionment that was then afflicting him, he welcomed this news and envisaged a scenario where his family

---

9 Geoghegan, *Robert Emmet*, 93-4, 98; Wilson, *United Irishmen, United States*, 64-8; Madden, *Life and times of Robert Emmet*, 12.

would come together on the continent and live out their lives contentedly there. This, however, was no more than fantasy. The cessation of war between France and Britain, signalled by the peace of Amiens in March 1802, reduced even more Emmet's expectation of help from France; he therefore began to intensify his study of military tactics. Not long afterwards he decided to return to Ireland in order to assess the possibility of effecting a rebellion there without the help of the French.[10]

It was late in the year before he arrived back in Ireland. Once there he went to stay with his parents at Casino. By this time his father was quite ill; because of this Emmet did not move very far from the house at any time although he did renew contacts with friends. On 9 December his father died and was buried in St Peter's churchyard in Aungier street. In his will Casino was left to his son Thomas Addis. After financial provisions were made for his wife and other family members Robert received a legacy of around £2,000 in the following March, sufficient to give him financial security. It would, however, be used instead to help the rebellion which he was now planning. Much of this planning, it seems quite reasonable to conclude, would have been carried out while he resided at Casino. By the spring of 1803 the preliminaries were complete; Robert was just 25 years of age and confident of victory in the upcoming rebellion.

As preparations were intensified, weapons of all sorts were being commissioned and stored in various places in Dublin; disaffected people were recruited. Emmet, conscious of security, moved into lodgings in Harold's Cross under an assumed name; the following month, April, he went even further to ground by renting a cottage in Butterfield lane, Rathfarnham not far from the house of the woman he loved, Sarah Curran. There he was visited by the 1798 veteran, Michael Dwyer; he promised to help in the forthcoming venture. So too would his niece, Anne Devlin. According to the plan, Dublin was to rise first; after it was taken, other counties were to follow. However, during early July mistakes and accidents dogged the preparations; government suspicions were aroused but were not acted upon. Even the date set for the commencement of the rebellion, 23 July, was the subject of some confusion. Despite all this, Emmet held firm to this date and the rebellion was set to commence at one hour before midnight. However, a series of accidents and ill luck intervened that evening; despite Emmet's best efforts, the rebellion ended in abysmal failure. Together with some of his men, he fled to Rathfarnham where he encountered Anne Devlin; the next day he sought refuge in the Wicklow hills. [11]

He did not, however, remain long among those hills before returning to

---

10   Geoghegan, *Robert Emmet*, 94-7; 101, 105-09, 112.
11   Ibid. 116-27, 132-34, 144-49, 171-78.

Dublin. This, of course, had to be done with great secrecy. His family home, Casino, is believed to have been closed up since his father's death in the previous year although there is a suggestion that it had been let to a Mr Clibborn (Peter Wilson's *The Dublin Directory* for the year 1802 lists an Edward Clibborn, Linen Merchant, Linenhall, 42 York street). One writer, Mr J Roderick O Flanagan, has stated that this Mr Clibborn accosted Robert Emmet on one occasion as he (Mr Clibborn) was on a watch for intruders. According to this account, Emmet gained entrance to Casino, unbeknownst to the occupants, by using the secret tunnels at some stage after the failure of the rebellion; he was using Casino as a place of refuge while on the run from the authorities. Another account is reported by Madden. He states that a family member continued to live at Casino after the death of Dr Emmet. A man who had been employed there as a gardener, John Murray, told Madden that the house had often been visited by Major Sirr searching for the fugitive Robert Emmet. According to Murray, Sirr was unsuccessful and very disappointed; he is reputed to have said 'the nest is here, but the bird has flown'. Whatever role Casino may have played during Emmet's short period of freedom after the failure of the rebellion it was elsewhere that he was ultimately captured, in Harold's Cross to be precise. His mother had left Casino after the death of her husband; she moved to another house owned by the family in Donnybrook but died while her son was in prison awaiting his trial. With the capture of Emmet, his subsequent trial and execution, a very important phase in the history of Casino ended. It would, nevertheless, retain an interest arising from its association with Emmet because, despite the abysmal failure of his rebellion, his legacy was a powerful source of inspiration to people in the years that followed. Emmet the young revolutionary with his stirring speech from the dock, made on the eve of his execution, became a romantic hero to generations of Irishmen and republicans in particular. Casino would also continue to hold a special place in the hearts of American descendants of Thomas Addis particularly since, as one of them James Emmet remarked to Fr Kerr in 1970, it is one of the few links with the Emmet family that remains in Ireland. [12]

Later owners of Casino have been traced by Fr Kerr. As has already been noted, Casino was left by Dr Emmet to his son Thomas Addis. It was sold on his behalf by his brother-in-law Robert Holmes to a Limerick merchant, James Martin Pike. Some twenty years later it was in the possession of George Stapleton; it was during his tenure that Dr Madden visited Casino as has been noted above. Later, during the 1840s it was held by a solicitor James Dillon

---

12   Kerr, *Emmet's Casino*, 4-7; Reynolds, *Footprints of Emmet*, 49; Madden, *Life and times of Robert Emmet*, 97-8; Geoghegan, *Robert Emmet*, 199-200.

Meldon. He was apparently of Westmeath stock, the family having some property in Galway. According to *Thom's Directory* for 1848 Casino, while in Meldon's possession, had a rateable valuation of £216. The next to hold it was a man of Yorkshire extraction, Michael Errington who was, apparently, a brother of archbishop Errington, coadjutor of cardinal Wiseman of Westminster. After him, in 1872/3, it passed on to a barrister, Henry (later Sir Henry) Harty who was the coroner for south county Dublin. By 1907 its rateable valuation was almost halved; it stood at £114; the valuation it would be assessed at when taken over by the Marist Fathers. But before they took possession it was bought by one other person; a Dublin merchant John C Meyers purchased it in 1915 for his son then fighting in the Great War (1914-18). He died however soon after his return from war; in 1922 Casino was bought the Marists and it is still in their possession today.[13]

---

13   Kerr, *Emmet's Casino*, 6-7.

7

Late 1700s, early 1800s
– other Clonskeagh connections

ALDERMAN JOHN EXSHAW

THROUGH HENRY JACKSON and Robert Emmet, Clonskeagh had a direct connection with the stirring events of both 1798 and 1803; in each case that connection was with the radicals. However, that was not the full story; it also had in its midst an important person who was the obverse of a radical. This man, John Exshaw, was a publisher and bookseller of some note and he was firmly on the government's side. In fact he was on the Board of Aldermen of Dublin Corporation when, at its Michaelmas Assembly held on 19 October 1798, the following was recorded: 'Certain of the Commons, praying to disfranchise Henry Jackson, a freeman of this Corporation, he being deeply concerned in setting on foot the late horrid Rebellion, and having confessed and admitted himself to being a traitor: whereupon it was ordered that the said Henry Jackson be and is hereby disfranchised from all the franchises and liberties of the city of Dublin and that he be henceforth reputed and taken as a foreigner to the said city, and that this order be put under the city seal'. He was also a present on 11 March 1799 when a resolution was passed which stated that anyone who had taken an oath as an United Irishman 'should be deprived of his elective franchise or of any right to vote on any election in any corporation or to be elected to any office therein'.[1] His conservative politics were visible some nine years earlier when he was elected lord mayor of Dublin. On 8 May 1789 at an Assembly of the Corporation he was elected by his fellow aldermen to serve as lord mayor for a year beginning at Michaelmas (29 September) the same year.

---

1   Ball, *History of county Dublin*, ii 80; Lady Gilbert (ed), *Calendar of ancient records of Dublin in the possession of the Municipal Corporation of that city* (Dublin 1911) vol xv, 63, 77-8, 96-7

At the first Assembly of his mayoralty (16 October 1789) it was agreed to present the freedom of the city 'in a gold box not exceeding in value 20 guineas' to John, lord Fitzgibbon, the lord high chancellor of Ireland and to present him with an address complimenting him on his judicial conduct since his appointment to that office in 1789. Strongly authoritarian by nature, Fitzgibbon was adamantly opposed to any concessions being made to Catholics; he was an out and out Castle man. Hugely unpopular with reformers and radicals, who nicknamed him 'Black Jack', he became the very symbol of the power of the Castle. Support for him by the aldermen of the Corporation and its lord mayor, John Exshaw, gives a clear insight into their political stance. As well as the award of freeman of the city, the first Assembly of Exshaw's mayoralty approved the expenditure of £1,200 on a new state coach, made in London, 'for the chief magistrates of this city', the existing coach, called 'the old Berlin', to be disposed of. The new coach, for which this money was approved, still exists; it can be seen in use by the current lord mayor of Dublin on such occasions as the St Patrick's day parade or the opening of the Dublin Horse Show.[2]

During Exshaw's year as lord mayor he resided in the Mansion House; in the same year he also stood for election to the Irish parliament. The city of Dublin was entitled to elect two members of parliament; Exshaw along with Alderman Shankey were put forward for election representing the government interests and the government canvassed strongly on their behalf. Opposing them and representing the Whigs (i.e. an anti-government opposition group) was Henry Grattan and lord Edward Fitzgerald; their canvassing was accompanied by a carnival atmosphere with great crowds taking part. When polling closed the latter were adjudged to have won by a landslide; great celebrations followed. This was an early sign of the radicalism that was to expand during that decade of the 1790s.[3]

During the disturbances that accompanied the rebellion of 1798 Exshaw was said to have covered himself with military glory – on the government side, of course. He was also active on the government side on the night of Emmet's abortive rebellion, 23 July 1803.[4] Exshaw had his country house at Clonskeagh built towards the end of the eighteenth century. His city premises at that time were at 98 Grafton street (1782-1809); prior to that they were at 86 Dame street

---

2   Ibid. vol xiv (Dublin 1909) 112-13, 121-22, 133; Dickson, *New foundations*, 158-62; Hill, 'The politics of Dublin Corporation', 94; Maurice Craig, *Dublin: 1660-1860* (London 1992) 215.

3   *Wilson's Dublin Directory* for 1790; E. A. Coyle, 'County Dublin Elections (1790)', *Dublin Historical Record*, Vol 44, No 2 (1991) 13-24: 14-17.

4   Ball, *History of county Dublin*, ii 80; Geoghegan, *Robert Emmet*, 172-4.

(1774-1782) and later they were at 103 Grafton street (1810-1827).

Born c. 1751, both his father and grandfather before him had been booksellers, printers and publishers. The first record of his business activities is noted in 1774. Two years later he announced that he was continuing the business activities of his father, who had just died. That included the magazine, *Exshaw's Magazine – Gentlemen's and London Magazine.* In May of the same year, he married Miss Wilkinson. On 1 January of the following year he commenced publication of the *English Registry.* On 16 April 1779 he became a freeman of the city by right of birth since his father had been a freeman. Only a few months later, on 6 July, he was nominated to the Common Council and elected sheriff for 1779/80, an extraordinarily rapid promotion. In this latter role, he was commended for his 'spirited conduct' in sending two men to Newgate gaol for drawing swords in a chocolate house. March 1782 saw him elected Alderman while in October 1784 he was elected coroner for the city. In his role as printer and stationer to the Society for Promoting Christian Knowledge and Practice in Ireland he published its *Tract No. 1* in April 1787. Later that year, in October, his wife died. Two years later, as already mentioned, he was elected lord mayor. Commenting on this the *Dublin Chronicle* noted that although he was 'the youngest Chief Magistrate' in the history of Dublin, he had already shown his ability for office since he had for two years been a 'Divisional Magistrate to an institution [i.e. the police] that was confessedly unpopular [he had acted] with judgement, temper, perspicuity and candour.' He is said to have been the publisher of *Hue and Cry,* a police gazette, for which he was received £1,000 a year. Although his printing and publishing business continued throughout his political career, it must nevertheless have been impacted by it.

In 1795, *Exshaw's Magazine –Gentlemen's and London Magazine* ceased publication having first appeared under his father's aegies in 1751. In 1797 as captain, he commanded the 1st regiment of the Royal Dublin Volunteers and was presented by Miss Exshaw with two 'elegent stands of new colours' embroidered by herself. Around the time of the 1798 rising he commanded the 1,000 strong Stephen's green yeomanry and was said to be also 'Adjutant-general to the entire yeomanry forces in the Dublin district'. In 1800 he was once again elected lord mayor on the death of the incumbent. Although not the official printer and stationer to the city, he nevertheless continued to get a substantial amount of business from it. He died in Clonskeagh on 6 January 1827, aged 76; he was buried in the old graveyard in Kevins street although he had been a church-warden at Taney. The location of his house in Clonskeagh has not been pinpointed but it should be noted that, as already indicated, the most substantial of the pieces of the land that Dr Emmet of Casino leased had on its eastern side 'ground in the possession of Alderman John Exshaw'. Going on that basis, his house (or more precisely, the land on which the house was built) was located at some point to the east of the lands presently held by the Marist Fathers. From this evidence it seems most likely that Exshaw's house was that which appears on the Ordnance Survey map of 1837 with the name 'Oak Lawn'; today, that house is called Farranboley house, appropriately enough since it is in the townland of Farranboley. [5]

ALEXANDER JAFFRAY (C.1735-1818)

Another early resident of Clonskeagh/Roebuck, the exact location of whose house has not been located, was one Alexander Jaffray. Ball informs us that he was one of the first to build a villa there at the close of the 18th century. He was a man of considerable substance in the commercial life of Dublin at the time. His city residence was the magnificent Ely house at 8 Ely place, the house which faces directly on to Hume street with a view of St Stephen's green; it is now owned by the Knights of Columbanus. It was built by the marquess of Ely who lived at Rathfarnham castle and its internal decoration was influenced by the work of the famous Adam brothers. Jaffray's business address (referred to as the 'Counting-house' in *Wilson's Dublin Directory* of 1783) was at 19 Eustace street. The same directory describes him as a wholesale merchant 'free of the 6 and 10 per cent in the Custom House'. In the same year (1783) he was also one of the (Merchant) Trustees of the Royal Exchange and was on the Committee of Merchants whose members were Lottery Commissioners. In 1786 his business became known as Jaffray, Fayle and Hautenville of 19 Eustace street, merchants of the Guild of the Holy Trinity and in 1792 simply Jaffrey and Hautenville. These were particularly busy years for Jaffray, perhaps justifying his building a country retreat at Clonskeagh/Roebuck. For it was at this time that he was closely associated with the founding of the Bank of Ireland.

However, earlier in his career he was actively involved in the common pursuit by merchants in Dublin of the interests of trade and therefore their own

---

5 Unknown, *Dublin 18th century printers: list and index* (c. 1930) 10; Robert Munter, *A dictionary of the print trade in Ireland 1550-1775* (New York 1988) 92-93; *Watson's Almanack* for 1781; ibid. 1795; ibid. 1798; G. N. Wright, *An historical guide to ancient and modern Dublin* (2 vols, London 1821) ii 1159; R. R Madden, *The history of Irish periodical literature* (2 vols, London 1867) ii 46; M Pollard, *A dictionary of members of the Dublin book trade, 1550-1800, based on the records of the Guild of St Luke the Evangelist, Dublin* (London 2000) 192-93; Ball & Hamilton, *Parish of Taney*, 110-11; Kerr, *Emmet's Casino*, 6; *National Archives*. Ordnance Survey map no. 105 E 295 – Taney.

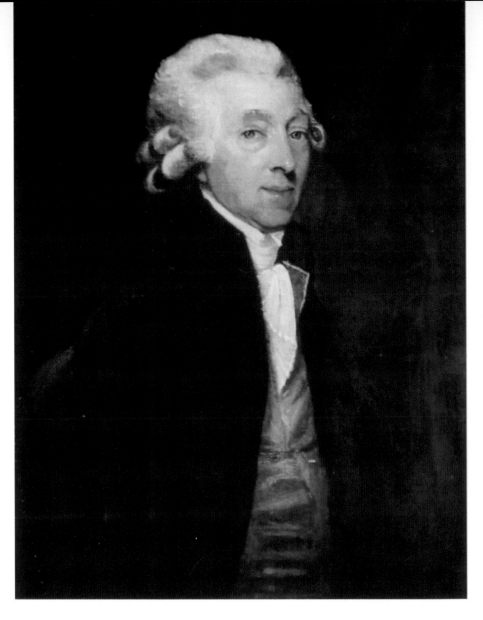

Alexander Jaffray (c. 1735-1818), one-time resident of Clonskeagh: a portrait by Gilbert Stuart, now hanging in the Bank of Ireland, College green (*Photographer: Matt Walsh*)

interests. Perhaps because they lacked political clout despite their growing wealth, the Dublin merchants of the middle years of the 18th century had a tendency towards radical politics. The majority of them were at odds with parliament which was dominated by landed interests and with the Board of Aldermen of Dublin Corporation, a self-perpetuating oligarchy. The result was the foundation in 1761 of the Committee of Merchants, a forerunner of the Chamber of Commerce. According to its own words stated in *The case of the*

Merchants of Dublin, the first published utterance of the Committee, issued in 1768, it was a voluntary society open to all who would share the expenses it incurred with the purpose of defending trade 'against any illegal imposition' and of soliciting 'such laws as might prove beneficial to all'. Among the 21 men on its committee was Alexander Jaffray; he was just over 30 years old at the time. The committee frequently lobbied the lord lieutenant in pursuit of its aims; this was a novel initiative. It organised special meetings of merchants when any specific item arose that threatened to negatively impact upon their interests. Perhaps its most impressive and lasting activity was the building of the Royal Exchange, the outstanding building which faces Parliament street; this, in later years, became the headquarters of the city's Corporation. The Royal Exchange was a symbol of the self-confidence of the merchants of the city at the time and during the 1760s and 1770s, while it was being planned and built, the project saw the Merchants Committee functioning well. In 1766 it started a series of lotteries with which to fund the project and in the following year it nominated trustees in whom the ground on which the Exchange was to be built was vested. Jaffray was directly involved in both of these actions. Soon they were in conflict with the Corporation who wanted to build its own Exchange but they brought their case to the Privy Council in London and won. By the mid-1770s the Exhcange was completed. Thereafter the activity of the Committee slackened and its performance was spasmodic; by 1783 it had been reformulated as the Dublin Chamber of Commerce. Among its initial 219 subscribers was Alexander Jaffray; there too was James Potts who we know was living at Richview in Clonskeagh in the 1790s.

During the 1770s and 1780s there had been much distress in business and elsewhere due to a commercial depression; much of the blame for this was placed on the effects of the restrictions imposed on Irish commerce by the parliament in London. This gave an impetus to the patriotic movement led by Grattan, Flood and Charlemont; they campaigned for the removal of these restrictions. A measure of success was gained when the British parliament, at the end of the decade, removed some of the worst of these and granted a limited free trade to Irish industry. It is against this background, as well as being influenced by the example of the earlier foundation of the Bank of England, that an agitation arose to demand that a national bank be established. Banking in Ireland at that time, apart from one or two exceptions, was insecure and many failures were experienced. As a result the Irish House of Commons was petitioned on 24 February 1780 by prominent people in Dublin for the erection of a public national bank. The petition was well received but it took two years for heads of a bill, required to establish the bank, to be introduced to the Commons. After some debate they were adopted without a division. Although some opposition was afterwards met, the bill was successfully piloted through both houses and received the royal assent on 4 May 1782. According to the Act, the bank was to have £600,000 in capital and commissioners were appointed by the king to receive subscriptions from the public to raise that capital. Alexander Jaffray was one of those commissioners. From 2 August 1782 these subscriptions were accepted by the commissioners and the full £600,000 was achieved by 6 December. Among the original subscribers of capital to the bank who had Clonskeagh connections were Alexander Jaffray (£4,000), James Potts, Richview (he will be discussed in a later chapter) (£2,000), Dr Robert Emmett (already discussed) (£2,000). Stockholders, who intended to vote, had to take various oaths including one which required them to assent to an Act of the Irish parliament entitled *An Act to prevent the Further Growth of Popery*; Catholics, however, were allowed instead to swear allegiance to the king under a special Act and Quakers were permitted to affirm their agreement with the various requirements rather than swear. This was of importance in the case of Alexander Jaffray, who was a Quaker (he was one of the surviving great-grandsons of Robert Barclay of Urie in Scotland, author of the learned *Apology for the people called Quakers*). These concessions to Catholics and Quakers, however, did not apply to those who would be directors of the bank and consequently governor or deputy governor (these were elected from the ranks of the directors). This must have presented a problem to Alexander Jaffray since he became a director on the foundation of the bank and, between 1791-93, its second governor (David La Touche, junior, was its first governor (1783-91); the direct descendant of a Huguenot émigré to Dublin in the 1690s, La Touche may have been responsible for the inclusion of these discriminatory acts in the bank's charter). It is assumed that Jaffray left the Quaker community in order to take up these positions in the bank; his sister was disowned by the Society of Friends because of circumstances surrounding her marriage and there is no further reference to the Jaffray family in the records of the Society. However, in a later obituary in the *Annual Register* (vol. vx, 199) it says that 'when he arrived at the age to form his own decision, he became a member of the Established Church'. If this is so, then he would have no longer been a Quaker at the time the bank was founded since he was nearly fifty years of age at that time and the question of his religion would not have arisen. It must have been because of his being resident in Clonskeagh/Roebuck that, while he was governor of the bank, he became in 1793 a churchwarden of the local church, that at Taney. As well as his own business and his work with the bank, Alexander Jaffray was a Trustee of Simpson's Hospital and a member of the Dublin Society and the Royal Irish Academy. He died in Cheltenham in 1813 without an heir; his portrait still hangs in a corridor of the Bank of Ireland.

The discrimination against Catholics becoming directors lasted until 1829 when, despite the failure of the Catholic Emancipation Act to remove these restrictions, the court of directors of the bank decided to ignore it and the following year, 1830, the first Catholic joined the court. The restrictions were formally lifted by the Bankers (Ireland) Act 1845 and in later years Catholics with close connections to Clonskeagh actually became governors; Sir John Ennis, Bart. (1856-58) and Sir James Power, Bart. (1868-1870). A man, whose family had even longer connections with Clonskeagh/Roebuck, was governor during 1880-1882 – George Kinahan.[6]

THE WINDOW TAX OF 1799 – CLONSKEAGH MEN PROTEST

In October 1817 a controversy arose in the civil parish of Taney, in which Clonskeagh is located. The controversy had its origins in the burden felt by the continuing levying of a tax that was felt to be unjust. Prime movers in the affair were some men with large houses in the Clonskeagh area. But before discussing the details surrounding it, some background on the tax, known as the window tax, must first be given.

The French revolution of 1789 sent shock waves among certain member of society across Europe, not least in Britain and Ireland. Some countries formed protective alliances but the British government held back until the defeat of Prussia by the French in 1792 after which the French went on an expansionist course. The following June, Louis XVI was guillotined and the National Convention declared war on Britain. Early intervention on the continent by the British resulted in defeat; the West Indies also became a theatre of battle. In 1796 the British navy was forced out of the Mediterranean and there were mutinies on some British ships as well as radicals on home ground. The following year saw a financial crisis which forced abandonment of the Gold Standard. The defeat of Napoleon in Egypt in 1798 saw a resurgence of British hopes and in the same year the rebellion in Ireland had been brought under control. All of this cost a lot of money. So in 1799 a new tax was introduced in the Irish parliament in

---

6   Ball, *History of the county Dublin,* ii 80; L M Cullen, *Princes and pirates; the Dublin Chamber of Commerce 1783-1983* (Dublin 1983) 34-9, 45-6, 55; F. G. Hall, *The Bank of Ireland: 1783- 1946* (Dublin 1949) 30-37, 39-43, 402, 493-94, 508-09; T. K. Whittaker, 'Origins and consolidation, 1783-1826', in F. S. L. Lyons (ed), *Bicentenary essays: Bank of Ireland 1783-1983* (Dublin 1983) 11-29: 20; David Dickson & Richard English, 'The La Touche dynasty', in Dickson, *The gorgeous mask* 17-29: 17, 22-23; Craig, *Dublin 1660-1860,* 233; Constantia Maxwell, *Dublin under the Georges* (Dublin 1997) 84; *Wilson's Dublin Directory* 1783, 1786, 1792; Ball & Hamilton, *Parish of Taney,* 120.

College green, the so-called window tax; it was assessed according to the number and size of windows in dwelling-houses.

Not much is recorded about how this was received but since the war against the French was in progress it was, according to subsequent testimony, 'patiently borne (as) a heavy and oppressive tax'. The war continued until 1802 but resumed again in 1803, now called the Napoleonic Wars. The tax continued to be levied. Eventually, with the victory at Waterloo in 1815, the war was over. However, it had been a hugely expensive one both in lives and in money. Proportionally more lives were lost in it than in the 1914-18 war. In money terms it cost more than £1,500 million; this was raised in loans and taxes. After the war ended the window tax continued to be levied and there is no indication of any protest against it in the short term. However, no doubt as the euphoria over the very popular victory over 'little Boney' waned – and especially the part played in it by one of their own Arthur Wellesley, later 1st duke of Wellington – thoughts turned to the tax and how the Act introducing it might be repealed.

In 1817 notices began to appear in Dublin papers of meetings being held in various parishes calling for the Act to be repealed. This was spurred on by a circular letter from Charles Stewart Hawthorne, First Commissioner of Ireland's Excise and Taxes, to the parishes for the purpose of appointing evaluators for a scheme of partial commutating of the tax which he was proposing. By 7 October of that year every parish in the city had met and discussed the topic. On 8 October the *Freeman's Journal* editorialised on the matter. To support its demand that the tax be repealed it quoted from the speech which Mr Isaac Corry, the Irish chancellor of the exchequer, made to the House of Commons in College green on 25 February 1799, part of which it printed in upper case: 'and, upon the return of peace, if it were found grievous or burdensome, it might be taken off by parliament'. After this quote, it commented: 'is there not to be found in these expressions a pledge of a very binding nature'. In another editorial on the following day it pointed out how much the tax had risen between its introduction in 1799 and 1817. It laid out a column in which various examples were given to illustrate this. For example, the tax in 1799 on a dwelling with 30 windows was assessed at £7-8s-5d; in 1817 it was £21-5s-0d.

Quite clearly people were getting agitated about the topic; reports in the papers of people being distrained for non-payment began to appear. One in the *Freeman's Journal* on 16 October 1817 reported that a tax collector called on a Mr Cole of Ormonde quay and demanded payment of the window tax there and then. Mr Cole replied that it was not convenient for him to pay it whereupon the tax man said he should make it convenient, 'adding an oath, which the Society for discountenancing Vice would not be pleased to see in print, that he would remove a competent portion of Mr Cole's goods and chattels'. In this case, the intervention of an important neighbour won for Mr Cole a temporary respite.

It is against this background that a report appeared in the same paper on Monday 13 October 1817 which is headed

WINDOW TAX
PARISH OF TANEY (DUNDRUM).

It stated that on Monday 29 September 1817 'a Vestry was held in the parish church in Taney for the purpose of appointing valuators pursuant to the notice given in Mr Hawthorne's letter. ... The meeting was thinly but respectably attended'. It then reports on a series of resolutions that were proposed but it comments that no one other than the proposer or seconder spoke on the subject. (The seconder, incidentally, was Humphrey Mitchin of Roebuck lodge, off what is now called Goatstown road, high sheriff of Dublin, 1795-96 and whose first wife was Frances, daughter of major Sirr, famed for his arrest of the Leinster committee of the United Irishmen in Oliver Bond's house in 1798.) When the resolutions were handed to the chairman (Rev Mr Ryan, licensed curate in the parish), he suggested that since the meeting was so small and since so few spoke to the topic, the parish should first reflect and he called for a little time to be given to this. The meeting adjourned on the understanding that Rev Mr Ryan would seek some clarifications of Mr Hawthorne's scheme of commutation that had caused some difficulties of understanding.

On the following Monday, 6 October, the Vestry assembled pursuant to the previous adjournment. Unlike the previous week, this time 'the small church was filled with such a large crowd as has been rarely collected in that respectable parish'. The Rev Mr Ryan began the meeting by reading Acts of Vestry of the previous Monday and a letter of clarification which he had received from Mr Hawthorne. Two resolutions were then proposed:

> That the window tax, having been originally proposed to parliament by the Minister of the Crown as a war tax, to subsist during the war and no longer, we claim it as a right from the Crown, now that the war is happily and honourably terminated, to redeem its pledge so solemnly given to the Irish parliament, under the faith of which we have hitherto patiently borne a heavy and oppressive tax.

and

> That relying on the justice of the Crown, and the wisdom of parliament to keep faith with the people, we do reject the proposed commutation, preferring ever to bear those ills we have than to fly to others that we know not of.

Humphrey Minchin, who had been once again the seconder of the motions, then called on Rev Mr Ryan to put a motion before the meeting that a committee and delegates be appointed to prepare a petition against the window tax and to communicate and co-operate with the Dublin parish deputies, for the purpose of petitioning against the measure. Rev Ryan refused saying that he disapproved the principles of the resolutions which had just been passed although he had felt it his duty to put these resolutions to the meeting as they seemed to supply the answers and opinions which Mr Hawthorne had asked for in his letter.

Pressure was, nevertheless, brought on Mr Ryan to put the motion to the meeting by a number of people who held government positions, in particular by George Thompson of the Treasury in Dublin castle and resident of Clonskeagh castle. He was also one of the churchwardens of Taney that year. Others present also pressed Mr Ryan but to no avail. It was asserted that Rev Mr Ryan was under the impression that by giving in to the demands he would expose himself and the petitioners to certain legal penalties under the so-called Convention Act.

At this point, Mr John Power of Roebuck house in Clonskeagh moved that the chairman be directed to quit the chair; the motion was seconded by Mr Moulds. The chairman, however, retorted that he would not resign his chair until the Vestry was regularly adjourned. As he was removing the Vestry books, Mr John Power objected to his doing so and insisted that they should remain in order that the proceedings of a meeting of parishioners which, it was now planned should take place straight away, be entered in them. Rev Ryan then replied that since the Vestry was now over he was the proper keeper of these books and that he would not hand them over.

Despite the absence of the Vestry books the planned meeting did proceed without Rev Mr Ryan. Ball and Hamilton in their work, *The parish of Taney*, written in 1895 and with access to the same Vestry books, note that there was a sheet of paper fastened to the minute book. It states that after the Rev Ryan had left the chair the churchwarden [George Thompson of Clonskeagh castle] was called to act in his place. Although they do not say who called him, it may be assumed that it was done by John Power since it was he who had asked the Rev Ryan to vacate the chair and to leave the Vestry books behind. The meeting, now under the chairmanship of George Thompson, passed two motions:

> Resolved – That the thanks of this meeting be given to the Rev Mr Ryan for his upright and independent conduct in the chair.

and

> Resolved – That the following gentlemen be appointed a committee for the parish to communicate and co-operate with our fellow citizens of the metropolis in petitioning parliament for the repeal of the window tax – viz. Mr

Hime, Mr Dillon, Mr Turbett, Mr Minchin, Mr John Power and Mr McDermott and that these resolutions be published along with the other resolutions of this parish.

These were signed by George Thompson; a vote of thanks was passed to him as 'our churchwarden, for his spirited and proper conduct in the chair' at the end of this extraordinary meeting. The Mr Turbett on the committee, then 27 years old, was resident in Owenstown, just beyond the end of Roebuck road. Also on the committee was a Mr Dillon; he was, most likely, Thomas Dillon of Mount Dillon in Clonskeagh. He and his wife had a stone erected in Taney graveyard to the memory of their infant sons; although there is no date on this it was probably near the date of the birth of their daughter in 1810. Thomas Dillon would have been 39 years old at the time of the meeting we are discussing.

At the end of the sheet of paper which was fastened to the Vestry book, Rev Ryan added a note saying that 'the proceedings mentioned above were not passed at the Vestry, and were inserted thus in this book without my knowledge several days after'. Apart from their appearance in this sheet, they also were published in the *Hibernian Journal* on the Friday after the meeting, 10 October 1817. As this had been requested by the meeting, it must have fallen to George Thompson, who chaired it, to have them so published. The dispute in Taney obviously got the attention of other newspapers which reprinted the item in the *Hibernian Journal.*

However, Rev Mr Ryan did not give up easily. Another meeting of the Vestry to consider the matter was held on the following Monday, 13 October. At this, a vote of thanks to Mr Hawthorne was passed unanimously; also passed unanimously was a resolution: 'That the anonymous publication in the *Hibernian Journal* of the 10th instant (and since republished in other newspapers), purporting to be a statement of the proceedings of our Vestry on Monday last on the subject of said commutation, is an insidious and malignant misrepresentation of the proceedings of this parish on that occasion, calculated to deceive His Majesty's minister in his endeavour to collect the unbiased sense of the people.' It was then resolved that this resolution together with those of the previous Monday's meeting be published in the *Freeman's Journal.* This was recorded under the signature of the Rev Mr Ryan in the Vestry book. The requested publication appeared in the *Freeman's Journal* on 15 October. It included the resolutions held during the regular part of the Vestry meeting of Monday 6 October but also the resolution which was passed when George Thompson had taken the chair. There was a mild rebuke of the publication in the *Hibernian Journal* added but it was not nearly so strong as the resolution passed against it on 13 October which was supposed to be published. When one recalls that this was supposed to be a report of the resolutions passed at the meeting of 13 October it does appear that there was still a difference over the matter. The church notice in the *Freeman's Journal,* it should be noted, appeared over the names of the churchwardens, one of whom was George Thompson, the man at the centre of the controversy that came into the open on 6 October.

There is nothing further known about this controversy in Taney. But the strength of feeling against the tax was obvious. It was probably exacerbated by the fact that the people active on the matter had houses which had a considerable number of windows. The disagreement between Rev Mr Ryan and a number of important parishioners, including at least one of the churchwardens, did not affect Rev Ryan's position in Taney. He remained there as the licensed curate for more than two years after the affair first emerged in September 1817; his successor, Rev Henry Hunt was licensed on 21 July 1820.

An interesting aspect of the controversy was the active part played in the affairs of the Vestry of Taney by John Power, who was a Catholic. Asking the Rev Mr Ryan to vacate the chair of a Vestry, insisting that he leave the Vestry books behind when he was about to leave and, apparently, inviting George Thompson, a churchwarden, to take his place would suggest that when it came to matters of taxation there was no hint of any form of sectarianism in this era known for the prevalence of that particular phenomenon. On the wider front, the controversy continued with parish meetings being held, not only in Dublin but, throughout the country. Eventually, Mr Robert Shaw, the MP for Dublin, moved a motion in the House of Commons (in London; the Irish one had been dissolved in 1801) on 21 April 1818 on the subject but was defeated. That took the heat out of the movement; the measure was not repealed until 1879. [7]

KING GEORGE, MRS FITZHERBERT AND CLONSKEAGH

On a somewhat lighter note, there was an unlikely connection between king George IV, Mrs Fitzherbert and Clonskeagh towards the end of the eighteenth century and well into the nineteenth. At this time rumour was rife in both England and Ireland that the prince of Wales, later to become king George IV, had married Mrs Fitzherbert, a Catholic. There were solid reasons why such a rumour would engage widespread attention at the time; in particular there were

---

7   Juliet Gardiner & Neil Wenborn (ed), *The History Today companion to British history* (London 1995) 323-24, 531-35; *Freeman's Journal* during September – October, 1817; Ball & Hamilton, *The parish of Taney,* 33, 148, 226-28; J B Leslie (compiled) & W J R Wallace (rev. ed. & updated), *Clergy of Dublin and Glendalough: biographical succession lists* (Dublin 2001) 248.

the implications it held for the monarchy. Should it be true, it would mean that the prince would be precluded by the 1701 Act of Settlement from becoming king. That Act stated that a 'Popish Prince' could not be allowed to govern 'this Protestant Kingdom' and if an heir were either to become a Catholic or to marry a Catholic he could not inherit the crown. As well as that there was the Royal Marriage Act of 1772 which meant that all princes and princesses who wished to marry must first get the consent of the ruling monarch. It has to be remembered that there were still many laws on the statute books which greatly disadvantaged Catholics even if these were gradually being repealed; even this level of concession could evoke a very strong popular reaction as the Gordon 'anti-popery' riots of 1780 in London showed.

The behaviour of the prince and Mrs Fitzherbert did nothing to quell the rumour as they were to be seen together in public on numerous occasions. For a long time there was no official denial of the rumour; eventually Charles Fox made a statement in the House of Commons that the rumour was a 'base and scandalous calumny'. This, however, did not stop the rumour, one aspect of which was gaining some currency; in Ireland this had a particular resonance. This was that, not alone did a marriage take place but that, given Mrs Fitzherbert's strong religious conviction, it was a Catholic ceremony conducted by a Catholic priest. The obvious question then arose as to who that Catholic priest was. A number of priests were named by various writers on the subject. In Ireland, lord Cloncurry in his *Personal recollections*, published in Dublin in 1849, stated that it had generally been supposed that it was Abbé Joseph Taylor who conducted the marriage; he was head of the Irish monastery of St Isidore when Cloncurry met him in Rome between 1803 and 1805. This led William J Fitzpatrick to make some inquiries when writing his book, *The Sham Squire*, which was published in 1866. In this the following appears 'We are assured by J. R. Corballis, Esq., QC, a near relation of the Abbé Taylor, and who was closely associated with him at Rome, that he never knew the Abbé to be suspected of having married the prince to Mrs Fitzherbert'.

It is not clear from this statement how close the relationship was between Abbé Taylor and J R Corballis. But is seems most likely that the Abbé was uncle to Corballis on his mother's side. Both her maiden name and her approximate age would suggest that. As Deborah Taylor she had married Richard Corballis in 1791 shortly before they set up residence in Clonskeagh. The prince and Mrs Fitzherbert, we now know, were married in December 1785. It is entirely possible that a brother of Deborah Taylor could have been a priest in 1785. It could, of course, have been her uncle who was the priest in question but, if it was, he would have been quite elderly when he met J R Corballis in Rome at some unknown date much later on. In any case it is certain that the rumour that held

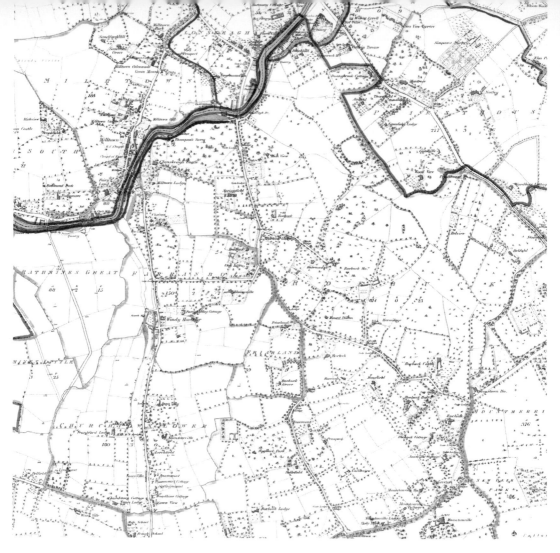

First edition Ordnance Survey map, surveyed 1837, corrected and published 1843

England and Ireland in its grip – Tom Moore's melody 'When first I met thee, warm and young' was based upon it – and lasted well into the nineteenth century, as Cloncurry and Fitzpatrick's books show, was a matter for some detail discussion in at least one household in Clonskeagh at that time. [8]

8   Valerie Irvine, *The King's wife: George VI and Mrs Fitzherbert* (London & New York 2005) 22-23, 33, 41-15, 50-53; Valentine Cloncurry, *Personal recollections of the life and times, with extracts from correspondence of Valentine Lord Cloncurry* (Dublin 1849) 204-06;William John Fitzpatrick, *"The Sham Squire" and the informers of 1798* (Dublin 1866) 215; Danny Parkinson, 'The Corballis/Corbally families of Co Dublin', *Irish Family History: Journal of the Irish Family History Society*, 8 (1992) 84-94: 91; R L Shiel, *Sketches of the Irish bar* (2vols, New York 1854) ii 35.

8

Daniel O'Connell
– local support and opposition

THE RISING OF 1798, the purpose of which was to break the connection of Ireland with England, led rather ironically to an even closer linkage between Ireland and England. And so, on 1 January 1801, the Union of Great Britain and Ireland came into being. With the abolition of the Irish parliament, Ireland was now to be represented in Westminster by twenty eight Irish peers and four bishops in the House of Lords and one hundred MPs in the House of Commons. The transition went smoothly; the impact of the new situation was, in the short term, negligible. The issues which were previously discussed in the Irish parliament were now discussed at Westminster, issues such as Catholic emancipation and parliamentary representation. However, in the longer term, the impact of the Union was to have enormous consequences. The Union would come to be seen by some as the source of many, if not all, of the problems which beset Ireland; others would see it as something which provided a bulwark which would ensure the continuance of their dominance. Out of this divided response to the Union would emerge two disparate groups; those vehemently opposed and those who strongly supported it i.e. the unionists.

Even before the Union came into being, the Catholic question was a matter of contention in the Irish parliament and certain reliefs were conceded to Catholics in 1778 and 1782; in 1793 the right, *inter alia,* to vote was conceded. However, they were still barred from holding certain posts in government and from sitting in parliament. Furthermore, the events of 1798 did nothing to soften the attitudes of those who opposed these concessions. Hopes that the advent of the Union would bring about Catholic emancipation were soon dashed and the wrangle now took place in Westminster rather than in College green. Foremost among the protagonists there was a young barrister, Daniel O'Connell. In 1823 he founded the Catholic Association, dedicated to gain emancipation through constitutional means. This was a novel approach; it sought to involve the Catholic masses by enrolling them as associate members who paid a subscription of one penny a month – the so-called Catholic rent. It was hugely successful in both organization and in the numbers that joined. It brought influence to bear on how the 40 shilling freeholders cast their votes; supporters of emancipation were the direct beneficiaries of this strategy. The climax came with the Clare election of 1828 in which O'Connell himself stood for election. O'Connell's victory was followed by scenes of popular jubilation. The government took fright; this could lead the way to other similar victories and even to violence. The emancipation bill wended its way through parliament and received the royal signature in April 1829.[1]

ANDREW ENNIS AND JOHN POWER, SUPPORTERS OF O'CONNELL

Some days previous to this a meeting was held at 12 Burgh quay where it was decided that 'a deep debt of obligation and gratitude' was owed to O'Connell for the services he had rendered to the cause of civil and religious freedom. A committee was set up to supervise the collection of a Testimonial to O'Connell. Among the treasurers elected, collectively described by the *Dublin Evening Post* as being 'of the very first mercantile rank', was Andrew Ennis, merchant, of 21 Harcourt street and Roebuck (more precisely, as will be argued in Chapter 12, the house that would later be called Wynnstay, Clonskeagh), a baker in North Great George's street and father of Sir John Ennis, baronet, a man whom we have already met when discussing the Bank of Ireland. Also among them was John Power, then residing at Roebuck house in Clonskeagh (this house was later called Roebuck grove); his father, James Power, had founded in 1791 a whiskey distillery which had by 1809 become a limited company under the name of John Power. Its growth was steady until 1823 when laws governing distilleries were changed; thereafter, thanks to that change in the law, it took off and generated great wealth. Already in 1814, John had taken up residence in Roebuck house and developed a friendship with O'Connell. Referring to Power in his correspondence as 'my most respected friend' O'Connell supported his (Power's) son-in-law, Nicholas Fitzsimon, who was elected MP for the King's county (Offaly) in 1832; he also sought to have Power persuaded to stand for election for county Wexford in 1835. In the event Power's son, James, stood and was elected; he was MP for county Wexford in 1835-47 and 1865-68.

The collection of the Testimonial was a great success; it brought in possibly as much as £20,000. It also marked a crucial point in O'Connell's career. Now aged 55 years old, he changed careers. He gave up the bar and with it the substantial income which he was able to generate there – up to £8000 per annum – and

---

1   Gearóid Ó Tuathaigh, *Ireland before the famine 1798 – 1848* (Dublin 1972) 30, 34-36, 43-46, 49-52, 61-73.

concentrated, almost exclusively, on a political career. Because of this it was necessary that he be provided with funds. To this end an annual Tribute was collected for him and again Andrew Ennis and John Power were actively involved, this time as trustees of the fund. This Tribute was also successful; up to £30,000 in the first year and more than £96,000 within the following six years. It allowed him to concentrate on the next political issue which followed emancipation – repeal of the union with Britain. In this too he had support from John Power; O'Connell after all was not advocating a social revolution that would discomfort a wealthy businessman such as Power. There was no contradiction in Power supporting O'Connell while, at the same time, accepting a baronetcy on 18 October 1841; the same applied to John Ennis. Power was also a Justice of the Peace and an Alderman of Dublin. In any case, Power remained true to O'Connell right to the end. Such was the strength of his support for him that he was chosen to lay the foundation stone for the O'Connell monument in Glasnevin in 1854. In the following year, on 25 June 1855, John Power died at Roebuck house and was buried in Dublin's pro-cathedral.

As regards Andrew Ennis it would appear that his residence in Clonskeagh had been inherited by his son John by the mid 1830s and he remained in possession there until the end of the 1840s. While living at Clonskeagh, John Ennis was a director on numerous occasions of the Bank of Ireland (in 1836, 1838, 1840, 1842, 1844, 1846); later, after he had moved from Clonskeagh, he was again a director (1848-79) and was governor from 1856 to 1858. He was for many years a prominent figure in the commercial life of Ireland and has been described as 'one of the merchant princes of Dublin'. At one time he was chairman of the Midland & Great Western Railway. From 1857-65 he was MP for Athlone; he had acquired a country house and a 9000 acre estate at Ballinahown Court, Westmeath. He was created a baronet in 1866. On his death the *Freeman's Journal* referred to him as 'an earnest Catholic and a moderate Liberal, who held aloof from later popular movements'.[2]

---

2   Maurice R. O'Connell (ed), *The correspondence of Daniel O'Connell* (8vols, Dublin 1977-80) iv 41-42, 276-78,476-79; v 2, 132-33,356-59; vii 178-80; viii 161; Ball & Hamilton, *Parish of Taney*, 179; Jim Murray, *Classic Irish whiskey* (London 1997) 190-95; Fergus O'Ferrall, *Daniel O'Connell* (Dublin 1981) 47-49; Denis Gwynn, *Daniel O'Connell* (Oxford 1947) 191-92; Oliver Mac Donagh, *The Emancipist Daniel O'Connell 1830-47* (London 1989) 14-16, 40-41; Ó Tuathaigh, *Ireland before the famine*, 160-64; Frederic Boase (ed), *Modern English biography* (3vols Truro 1891-97) ii 1613; *Pettigrew and Oulton Street Directory* 1835, 1836; *Dublin Almanack* 1840; *Thom's Directory* 1848; (for material on Sir John Ennis, Bart) Hall, *The Bank of Ireland*, 486-87.

FRANCIS BLACKBURNE OF ROEBUCK HALL, OPPONENT OF O'CONNELL

Francis Blackburne, a long-time resident of Roebuck hall and whom we have already met in the context of his daughter's marriage to Edward Perceval Westby of Roebuck castle, had many legal jousts with Daniel O'Connell throughout his carreer. He was born in Great Footstown in county Meath in 1782; his family, which had received threats from the Defenders in the 1790s and, like many others of his class, was affected by the prevailing anxiety which followed the French Revolution of 1789, moved to Dublin. There they lived in Chatham street which, according to his son writing in 1874, 'had then occupants of a different class from those who now inhabit it'. He entered Trinity College in 1798, graduating with distinction in 1803, the year of Robert Emmet's rebellion. Thereafter he had a distinguished legal career being called to the bar in 1805. At this early stage in his career he showed both his potential skill as well as his political orientation in a particular incident which was well noted at the time.

After John Philpot Curran, the famous lawyer who had defended many of the United Irishmen in the 1790s, was appointed by the Whig government as Master of the Rolls in 1806, a meeting of the bar was held to present an address of congratulation to him. It was the year after the young Francis Blackburne had been called to the bar; he could, therefore, attend the meeting. After some of the most eminent and established members of the profession had lauded Curran a great excitement was caused when young Blackburne stood up and spoke with a remarkable coolness and self-possession to oppose the very purpose for which the meeting had been called. Curran was no hero to him and his action at the meeting betrayed a strong conservative, pro-government stance.

He was appointed sergeant in 1826, attorney general in 1830, chief justice in 1846 and chancellor in 1852. His career brought him in contact with the great issues of the time e.g. the Catholic question, the tithe war, O'Connell and the repeal movement, the Young Irelanders. While he was still sergeant, he was seen by Daniel O'Connell, in 1827, as being amongst those whose hold on positions of influence was a serious impediment to the the progress of the Catholic Emancipation Bill. As well as that, Blackburne was considered by O'Connell as being 'excessively overrated', yet despite this he was able, through the position he held, to ensure that there was a succession of partisan judges provided. Despite the opposition of so many influential people, including Blackburne, Emancipation was carried; O'Connell, as a result, was in a position of unrivalled popularity in Ireland in late 1829. He now sought to build on this and bring about further changes in the governance of Ireland; early in 1830 he founded a Society for the Repeal of the Union. This was the start of a long effort to gain

Repeal, seen by the government of the day as most dangerous and therefore to be suppressed. O'Connell, however, used his abundant skills to outwit it often by simple devices such as changing the name of his Society. He used other strategems too.

On one occasion, early in the struggle (January, 1831), he was arrested with a number of political supporters under an Act passed 'for the suppression of dangerous Associations or Assemblies in Ireland'. This time he outwitted it and in the process used Francis Blackburne, now attorney general, to achieve his purpose. On 8 February 1831 O'Connell was served 'notice of trial'; on the following day he got the hearing adjourned for a day by a legal argument. The day after that he wrote to Francis Blackburne stressing the necessity of his attendance in the House of Commons; his duty to his constituents required this. Blackburne was left with no reasonable excuse to refuse the postponment of his trial to the next term which he sought and O'Connell left for London. What Blackburne probably did not realize was that the Proclamation Act, under which O'Connell and his associates were to be tried, was due to expire at the end of the parliamentary session in which O'Connell was now free to attend. As well as that the government in London, then in a precarious position and requiring his support for the passage of the controversial Reform Bill, used this expiry date as an excuse to drop the charges. O'Connell and associates had escaped with the unwitting help of Blackburne.

Some months later, in November 1831, O'Connell would show his contempt for Blackburne by describing him as 'a vile Tory attorney-general' and express the opinion that the connection between Ireland and England would have to be maintained by armed force unless, among others, 'the attorney-general [Blackburne] (is) cashiered'. The following month, in an angry outburst against the administration of earl Grey, the prime minister, O'Connell outlined the many ways in which he saw him driving the Irish people to depair; one of these was the appointment of 'a dogged, pertinacious Orangeman, Mr Blackburne, (as) attorney general'. In the following year Blackburne started proceedings against two Dublin papers, the *Pilot* and the *Freeman's Journal* over the publication of a letter by O'Connell in which he criticized the finding of a jury in a case related to the Tithe agitation (tithes were a taxation which had to be paid by people of all denominations to the clergy of the Established Church); he dropped the case when he came to the conclusion that O'Connell might be well able to sustain his accusation of murder against the authorities who had shot four people during the agitation.

However, O'Connell did not have it all his own way; Blackburne did on occasion have his successes. On one such occasion when he had successfully prosecuted O'Connell and his associates the chief secretary in lord Anglesey's administration, Edward Stanley, wrote to him expressing his appreciation of Blackburne's skill as attorney general:

> 'My best thanks and congratulations on your great and triumphant success. Nothing could have been better or more successfully managed; and we certainly owe it much to your exertion and decision that we have O'Connell so far at our mercy as we have'.

Lord Anglesey was equally appreciative of Blackburne's ability; he said that he had more confidence in him than in any public man with whom he had ever acted.

Unsurprisingly O'Connell's animosity towards Blackburne continued through 1833. In July of that year, he wrote 'All we want is to get rid of Blackburne, and much practical work would be done. If Anglesey [the lord lieutenant] was not such an egregious ninny, we could easily get rid of that scoundrel. If anything could tempt me to join the ministry, it would be to cashier Anglesey and to turn out Blackburne. But I remember the story of the horse and the man, and nobody shall ride me even to get rid of the enemies of Ireland because, if I were once in harness, I could not be free to work for Ireland alone again'. When a vacancy occurred on the King's Bench in 1834 O'Connell suggested that the government could use the opportunity offered to 'easily disembarrass themselves' by promoting Blackburne to a seat in the Common Pleas, made available by a transfer from it to fill the vacancy on the King's Bench. In a letter to James Abercromby, a minister in the cabinet of the Whig prime minister, William Lamb, 2nd viscount Melbourne, he wrote 'If you appoint Blackburne, you take out of the office of attorney general the most decided Orange Tory that ever filled that office. If he refuses to accept the situation you may dismiss him without reproach. Reproach or no reproach, you ought to discontinue him as attorney general. It is impossible for you to conciliate Ireland whilst he is the leading law officer of the crown'. Despite the fact that Abercromby gave a great deal of support to O'Connell's proposal when passing on the letter to Melbourne, nothing happened; Blackburne remained in office although O'Connell, reacting to incorrect news that Blackbourne had been replaced, characterized him as having been 'the mainstay of Orangeism at the Castle'. Given this degree of animosity that O'Connell held towards Blackburne (which most certainly would have been reciprocated), it is not surprising that Blackburne would play such an important role in undoing O'Connell when the opportunity presented itself.

In 1832, O'Connell made repeal of the Union the main ground on which he fought the elections of that year. He was returned for Dublin city himself and was accompanied to parliament by some 40 supporters from other constituencies. However, it was not until April 1834 that he brought up the question formally in the House of Commons. Its defeat was absolute; by 538 votes to 38 the house resolved to maintain the union. Despite this, he continued to exert his political energies entirely for repeal apart from a short period when he co-operated with the Whig government (the Whigs were the predecessors of the Liberal party). With the return of the Tory government in the early 1840s, he renewed his campaign, his popular appeal having been dented by his dalliance with the Whigs. His skill in presenting his case for repeal won over many influential people who previously had been cool to the idea. As well as that the romantic propaganda put out by a group of young enthusiastic journalists in the newspaper, *The Nation* (it began publication in October, 1842), gained for him much popular support.

But above all, it was O'Connell himself who whipped up so much approval for his stance when he addressed a series of so-called Monster Meetings throughout the country. As he progressed around the country the crowds who flocked to them grew ever larger. Although his language at these meetings was strong, even inflammatory, there was never any disorder attending them. The government was very concerned while conservative elements in Ireland called for suppression of the movement. The momentum gained by O'Connell at these meetings was to come to a head at Clontarf on 8 October 1843. Although he had already had a very successful meeting, full of historical resonance, at Tara the choice of Clontarf was deliberate. It was the scene of the famous battle of 1014 in which Brian Boru was believed to have expelled the foreigner from Ireland. However, on this occasion the government would act and, in doing so, it was following the counsel of Blackburne. The meeting at Clontarf was to be the greatest of them all; crowds flocked to it from all over the country. Irish exiles in Britain came home to attend it. One can almost sense the excitement engendered in anticipation of the meeting. However, the enthusiasm of the organizers led them into the use of careless language, language that had military overtones. This was the opportunity Blackburne and the government wanted; it gave them ground on which to proclaim the meeting illegal. O'Connell did not resist; he called the meeting off. Although some of his more moderate supporters agreed with him there was huge disappointment among the large number of people who had been greatly impressed by O'Connell's defiance of the government. His loss of prestige was temporarily halted by his arrest along with eight others two days later and by their being charged with sedition. O'Connell won an appeal to the House of Lords and was released six months later to the great joy of many people; the archbishop of Dublin presided at a solemn *Te Deum* in the pro-cathedral in thanksgiving for his release. However, his Repeal movement was in effect over to be succeeded by a group known as Young Ireland. These, as will be shown later, were also to meet Francis Blackburne in circumstances where he would show his strong disapproval of their activities, for it was he who presided over the political trials of 1848.

Early in his legal career however, apart from his intervention at the celebrations for John Philpot Curran, he avoided overt political involvement. This together with his reputation for efficiency won him business from solicitors across the political spectrum, both Catholic and Protestant. He was so successful at this stage in keeping his political views to himself that when he was appointed sergeant (i.e. a legal officer following in precedence the attorney general and solicitor general) Daniel O'Connell welcomed the appointment as he believed that Blackburne actually favoured Catholic Emancipation. That situation, however, did not last; he soon showed his strong political views, both conservative and unionist. All this became manifest later on when he robustly opposed the Repeal Movement. Similarly in the case of the Established Church; he strongly favoured the retention of its constitutional position.

In 1827, the year after he was appointed sergeant, he moved from Chatham street to Clonskeagh to take up residence at Roebuck hall; he also maintained a city address at 34 Merrion square. Roebuck hall, during his residence there, won an accolade from an observer at the time. Writing in 1838 about the roads in the Roebuck area 'thickly bordered with villas' he went on to say 'The beauty of these avenues is, however, overshadowed by the high walls topped with thick hedges, the closed, tall wooden gates and concealed gate-houses, that give the whole a sombre unsocial appearance, Mr. Blackburne's villa opening the only exception to the remark'.

There was also another, rather unexpected, side to Francis Blackburne's character: he was an excellent singer and had a strong affection for good singing. Writing about him, a contemporary author (1854) had this to say 'It creates no little surprise ... when hearing on a sudden a peculiarly rich and sweet voice breathing in delightful tones one of Moore's ... melodies they ... find in the musician no other than the grave and solemn person whom they might have seen ... in controversy with the Master of the Rolls'. It is not surprising then that he was closely involved with the musical life of Dublin. At various times, he was vice-president of the Anacreontic Society. This was founded in 1740 for the practice and cultivation of instrumental music; members were confined to amateurs and election by ballot. He was also vice-president of the Philharmonic Society of Dublin and president of the Society of the Antient Concert Hall, Great Brunswick street (now Pearse street). The former focussed on instrumental and vocal music; the latter on choral compositions of the ancient masters.

Despite his strong conservative political views and loyal support for the government he was apparently compelled to resign his position as lord chancellor in March 1869, a resignation he considered 'a harsh and cruel return for his abnegation of self, and for the sacrafices he so cheerfully made'. As a result, he refused a baronetcy. In the year before he was appointed lord chancellor, he left Clonskeagh and bought Rathfarnham castle. He died on 17 September, 1867, aged 84 and is buried in Mount Jerome.[3]

Contrary to the views which O'Connell held of him, the notice of his death in the *Irish Catholic Chronicle,* on Saturday, 21 September 1867 was quite kind to him. Among other things it stated: 'During his long and honoured life he took a most prominent part in public life... he was one of a great race of lawyers, who, like the Irish wolf dog, are now almost extinct. ... in the trials for offences under the Insurrection Act ... though there was a cry of "no mercy" then, as there is now, he disregarded it, and discharged his duty without undue severity. ... he did not fail to impress the gentry with the necessity of curbing their passions, and dealing mercifully and kindly with the people. ... At his suggestion, one of the most notorious of the magistrates was deprived of the commission of the peace. ... His taste for music was exquisite. In his more youthful days he sang with a sweetness and a pathos which Moore said gave an additional charm to the Irish melodies. ... with Francis Blackburne ... has passed away the last of a race of lawyers and advocates unsurpassed by any bar in the world'. This obituary was, of course, written many years after the heat generated by the battle for Catholic Emancipation had dissipated and long after the death of its main protagonist, Daniel O'Connell.

3   Edward Blackburne, *Life of the Right Hon. Francis Blackburne, late Lord Chancellor of Ireland* (London 1874); O'Connell (ed), *Correspondence of Daniel O'Connell,* iii 312-14; iv 258 n1, 271, 365- 66, 375-77, 446-48; v 54, 155, 164, 178-82; James Casey, *The Irish law officers: roles and responsibilities of the Attorney General and the Director of Public Prosecutions* (Dublin 1996) 23; Beckett, *The making of modern Ireland,* 313-14, 326-27; Ó Tuathaigh, *Ireland before the famine,* 160-168, 190; *Thom's Directory* of Dublin for 1848; Lydon, *The making of Ireland,* 295-96; Alfred Webb, *A compendium of Irish biography comprising sketches of distinguished Irishmen and of eminent persons connected with Ireland by office or by their writing* (Dublin 1878) 23; *The Post Office Dublin City and Country Directory* for 1851; D'Alton, *History of the county Dublin,* 809; Shiel, *Sketches of the Irish bar,* i 173 n, ii 127-34.

9

Post-emancipation politics – the Corballis input

WHILE THE ACHIEVMENT of Catholic Emancipation in 1829 was of major significance for Catholics, particularly those who were in a position to reap the benefits it offered, there were other important advances made by Catholics around this time; in these too, we find the involvement of personnel from Clonskeagh, in particular John Richard Corballis. Descended from a Catholic family, which had lost much of its patrimony due to the Penal laws but saw a recovery of its fortunes during the eighteenth century, the first member of this family to settle in Clonskeagh was John Richard's father, Richard. Born in 1769 and later a prominent businessman with a base in Upper Mount street in Dublin – among other things during his lifetime he was a member of the Court of Directors of the Grand Canal Company and a director of the Hibernian Joint Stock Banking Company – he took up residence in Clonskeagh in the latter part of the eighteenth century. His first move was apparently to Roebuck hall but in 1793 he purchased Rosemount which, like many of the houses of the Georgian period, was built by a speculative builder. An early indication of his close association with the Catholic church was his decision, in 1807, to send his son John Richard, then eleven years old, as a boarder to the fairly recently opened Royal College of St Patrick in Maynooth (the college had a section for lay students until it was closed down in 1817). He was also a good friend of Daniel O'Connell.

VISITORS TO CLONSKEAGH: O'CONNELL AND ARCHBISHOP MURRAY

On two separate occasions but on dates that were close to one another, O'Connell visited Richard Corballis and dined with him at Rosemount. On Monday 2 June, 1823 in a letter to his wife, who was then at Tours in France,

O'Connell wrote 'I dined yesterday in the country at Mr Corballis' (house). Edward Connor [third son of James and Betsey Connor, Tralee, nephew of O'Connell's wife and an attorney] went with me. We had Doctor Murray [new Catholic archbishop of Dublin; his predecessor, Dr Thomas Troy, had died the previous month on May 11] there and altogether a very pleasant party. Their place is very much to my taste.' Three weeks later, in another letter to his wife, he wrote 'On Sunday [22 June] I went to Mr Corballis. My brother James and Maurice dined with me there. Rick [his wife Mary O'Connell's brother Rickard O'Connell] and Edward Connor dined here [Merrion square]'.

It would appear that there were moves afoot some short while later, in 1824, to get a Catholic church built at a place convenient to where the O'Connells lived in Merrion square. We can see this in yet another letter, this time written by Mary O'Connell on 19 & 20 February 1824, from Southampton, to her husband in Merrion square 'I hope you may succeed about the Chapel but when I left Dublin, [upper] Mount street close to us was the street spoken of for the Chapel, the ground to be given *gratis* by Mr Corballis, to whom all that street belongs. Even in Pembroke street the chapel would be a great convenience to us. Such a one as that we could have a pew to ourselves [in]'. (An interesting sidelight to the information contained in this letter is the fact that in the same year that it was written, 1824, a new church belonging to the Established Church was consecrated on an island site in upper Mount street, the church of St Stephens, commonly known as the Pepper Canister church.)

RICHARD CORBALLIS AND THE CATHOLIC CHURCH

As well as giving an insight into the intimacy of Richard Corballis's connection with O'Connell these letters also indicate his generosity towards the church. Much later, in 1835, he would be seen to be high in the list of contributors to a fund for erecting a new Catholic church near Upper Baggot street, a position that was also held by another resident of Clonskeagh, John Power; the church that was ultimately built was St Mary's, Haddington road. This was an era when the building of Catholic churches was gaining momentum as parishes were being divided and re-aligned. But perhaps the clearest indication we have of Richard Corballis's close association with the Catholic church is to be found in a letter written by his son to his friend Anthony Blake after his father's death, c.1847. In this we read that Richard Corballis had been a close friend of the then Catholic archbishop of Dublin, Dr Daniel Murray, for many years; in fact, they had met at Rosemount in Clonskeagh on many occasions during the course of almost the whole of the previous fifty years (we have noted one of these occasions above in O'Connell's letter of 2 June 1823). He had also attended him in his last illness and stayed on in his house for some time after his death, saying mass for him there on two successive days thereafter.[1]

In fact the friendship between Murray and Richard Corballis went back to the early days of the century. It is believed that it was Murray who had influenced Corballis to send his daughters to be educated at the Institute of the Virgin Mary in York, otherwise known as the Bar Convent. Although this convent had turned down Murray's invitation to set up an Institute similar to that at York in Dublin, it had nevertheless played an important role in preparing outstanding women such as Frances (Teresa) Ball, Mary Aikenhead and Catherine Walsh as they set out to found new religious orders in Dublin. It was around the time that they were present in York that the Corballis sisters arrived for their education. It is perhaps not too surprising to note that, subsequently, three of these sisters became nuns. Margaret (1800-35) became the first person to enter the newly founded Loreto convent at Rathfarham in 1824; her name in religion was Catherine. She was followed a short time later by her sister Elizabeth (1801-39); she entered in 1825 and took the name Gonzaga. It is no coincidence that they chose the Loreto in Rathfarnham since it was founded, along with two other women, by Frances (Teresa) Ball and their father, Richard, had been an advisor to Ball; he had provided her with financial support in the years immediately prior to the founding of Loreto, Rathfarnham, when she had set up an orphanage in Harold's Cross, an area of the city where he had most likely lived earlier in his life. Ball's initiatives did not end in Rathfarnham; she was later responsible for the founding of nine establishments in Ireland and sent members of her convent to carry on her work in many countries abroad. The third of Richard Corballis's daughters – Anna Maria – did not, however, follow the same route; after failed attempts to join the Cistercians and the Carmelites, she joined the Presentation Convent in Bagnelstown in 1850. Under her religious name, Mother Charles, she went on to found the Presentation convent in Mountmellick, co Laois, in 1854; in this she was greatly helped by an inheritance

---

1   Danny Parkinson, 'The Corballis/Corbally families of Co Dublin', *Irish Family History: Journal of the Irish Family History Society*, vol 8, 1992: 84-94; *Wilson's Dublin Directory* for the year 1831; *Watson's or the Gentleman's and Citizen's Almanack* for 1830; Donal A Kerr, *Peel, priests and politics: Sir Robert Peel's administration and the Roman Catholic church in Ireland, 1841-1846* (Oxford 1982) 230; O'Connell, *Correspondence of Daniel O'Connell*, ii 318, 481, 490, 492; iii 39; Craig, *Dublin: 1660-1860*, 294; N. Donnelly, *History of Dublin parishes* (2vols, Dublin 1912) i 41; Donal Kerr, 'Dublin's forgotten archbishop: Daniel Murray, 1786-1852', in James Kelly & Dáire Keogh (ed), *History of the Catholic diocese of Dublin* (Dublin 2000) 247-67: 263.

left to her by her father, £1,000 initially and, thereafter, £440 annually. The latter payment was continued by her brother John Richard after her father's death.

RICHARD CORBALLIS'S DAUGHTER MARIA

It has been surmised that Richard's fourth daughter may have died young as nothing had been discovered about her. But it is clear from the will of her brother, John Richard, made in 1860 that she was very much alive at that time (he refers to 'both of my sisters' and it is known that the two Loreto sisters were dead at that time). Furthermore it seems reasonably clear that she was then living in Clonskeagh and would continue to live there until 1877. In 1847 *Thom's Directory* lists Richard Corballis as living at Rosemount. However, in the following year it lists his son, John Richard. Then in the next year's edition, a new entry is found; Miss Corballis living at Roebuck lodge. It is most likely that Miss Corballis (her first name appears in Griffith's Valuation as Maria) had been living at Rosemount with her father until his death. However, since his son John Richard then took up residence there after that death, his sister moved out and took up residence in nearby Roebuck lodge. Like a number of house names in the area at the time, this name was used by three different houses. Fortunately it is possible to decipher which of them was the one into which she moved. For two years prior to her taking up residence one of them was vacant; this would appear to be the one into which she moved. While there, another house with the same name, Roebuck lodge, was occupied by James Digges Latouche and later captain Frederick Charles Cross; this, however, was further out in Roebuck off the Goatstown road. In 1862 Miss Corballis is listed as living in 'The Cottage'. The possibility that she changed residence can be discounted as there is fairly clear evidence that she merely changed the name of the house. Roebuck lodge occupied by her in 1861 had a valuation of £46, the same as 'The Cottage' occupied by her in 1862. Furthermore, in his will, dated 1860, her brother John Richard refers to the Cottage and we discover that he actually owned it. She would continue to live there until 1877. Later, as we will see, it was in this house that Isaac Butt died. The house continues to bear this name to this day. [2]

---

2 Séamus Enright, 'Women and Catholic life in Dublin, 1766-1852' in Kelly & Keogh (ed), *History of the Catholic diocese of Dublin*, 268-93:284-86; Parkinson, 'The Corballis/Corbally families of Co Dublin', 91-93; Will and four Codicils of John Richard Corballis: Private sources at the National Archives – small private collections 999/658 13; *Dublin Almanac* 1843-45; *Thom's Directory* 1847-1878; First Ordnance Survey Map of Taney parish (1837) in *National Archives*. OS/105 E 295.

RICHARD CORBALLIS'S TWO SONS

As well as his four daughters, Richard Corballis had two sons; of one nothing has been discovered. By contrast, the other John Richard was to feature prominently in public affairs especially in the second quarter of the nineteenth century. He was perhaps even closer to the Catholic archbishop of Dublin, Dr Murray, than his father had been especially in political affairs in which the church found itself. John Richard was born in 1796, most likely at Rosemount, in Clonskeagh, where he got his earliest education from a private tutor; this was followed, as already mentioned, by a number of years as a boarder in the lay section of Maynooth College. Subsequently he entered Trinity College where he became a student of science winning the highest honor there in the process; he gained a BA in 1816. Since 1794 Catholics had been permitted to enter Trinity College. Afterwards he turned to legal studies. First he gained an LL B and later he was called to the bar of the King's Inns, Dublin, during Michaelmas term in 1820. Later still he attained an LL D in Trinity College in 1832 and became a Queen's Counsel on 17 August 1841.

JOHN RICHARD CORBALLIS PROPOSES DR MURRAY FOR MEMBERSHIP OF RDS

It is most likely, however, that it was due to his interest in science that he was elected on to one of the standing committees of the Royal Dublin Society (RDS), the committee for Natural Philosophy. An event associated with his membership of the RDS serves to highlight his closeness to archbishop Murray. In the summer of 1836, the recently founded British Association for the Advancement of Science was expected to hold its annual meeting in Dublin. This was an important event for Dublin. The Association, founded in York in 1831 'to give a stronger impulse and a more systematic direction to scientific inquiry', had a policy of holding its annual meetings in different towns and cities throughout the United Kingdom; it attracted to these meetings the leading scientists of the day and stimulated the foundation of a variety of scientific societies in the cities that it visited. A number of events were planned to mark the event in Dublin. Among these it was suggested that a local man of some eminence would enrol in the Association while it was in Dublin; this man was Dr Murray. However, the rules of the Association required that applicants for membership should first be a member of a local scientific or literary society; because of this it was decided that archbishop Murray should seek admission to the RDS. John Richard Corballis gave notice that he would propose him for membership, seconded by Dr Sandes, a senior fellow of Trinity College. The proposal was rejected in the ensuing ballot; this was followed by an outcry leading even to discussion in both houses of parliament. Members who had not attended the ballot suggested that a new ballot be held and Corballis informed Dr Murray. In a letter to Corballis, Dr Muray turned down the suggestion declaring himself to be upset at having caused disagreement among the members of the RDS; he signed the letter 'with affectionate regard, my dear Corballis, most faithfully yours, D. Murray'. The letter was later inserted into the minutes of the Society.[3]

JOHN RICHARD CORBALLIS – A COMMISIONER INVESTIGATING MUNICIPAL COPORATIONS

Shortly before this episode, Corballis was involved in a project of a totally different kind. On 20 July 1833 the king gave his consent to a request from the House of Commons that a commission be set up to inquire into the state of municipal corporations in Ireland; Corballis was one of the commissioners appointed to carry out this task, being described along with the other commissioners in the formal language of the King's Commission as 'our trusty, and well-beloved … John R. Corballis'. The inquiry sought by the House of Commons was a prerequisite to the much needed reform of these corporations. Electoral reform at a national level had been passed into law the previous year, the famous and controversial Reform Act of 1832; the part of which applied to Ireland was called The Representation of the People (Ireland) Act of 1832. This had increased the number of MPs returned from Ireland to 105 and extended the franchise to 92,000 people; fairly minimal reform when one remembers that there were around 8 million people in Ireland at the time and the property qualifications required for voting were such as to restrict the privilege to people of wealth, whether Catholic or Protestant.

The newly appointed commission, six Catholics and six Protestants, worked very methodically at their task. They took as the basis of their inquiry all the cities, towns and boroughs which had returned members to the old Irish

---

Boase, *Modern English biography,* i 717; *Watson's or the Gentleman's and Citizen's Almanack* for 1830; *The Post Office Annual Directory* for 1832; William Meagher, *Notices on the life and character of his Grace, Most Rev Daniel Murray, late archbishop of Dublin as contained in the commemorative oration pronounced in the Church of the Conception, Dublin on the occasion of his Grace's Month's Mind* (Dublin 1853) 69-70; British Association for the Advancement of Science [http://www.net/the-ba/AbouttheBA/HistoryoftheBA/_BriefHistory2.htm] July 2006. (A short history of the Association is available on this website).

parliament in College green; a total of 117 which they divided into what they called six circuits. Two commissioners were allotted to each while 'the Corporation of the City of Dublin with its numerous members and dependencies was made a distinct subject of investigation' and was reserved for the full commission. Corballis, along with Maziere Brady, was allocated the Western circuit. This consisted of counties Clare, Galway, Galway Town [Galway town along with seven other towns and cities were at the time styled county of town or city e.g. county of Dublin city], Kerry, Limerick, Limerick City, Longford, Mayo and Roscommon along with the towns Ardfert, Askeaton, Athenry, Castlebar, Dingle, Ennis, Galway, Lanesborough, Limerick, Roscommon, Tralee, Tuam and Tulske. At all locations hearings were held in public under oath and were quite thorough. The commissioners presented their first report to the Houses of Parliament in 1835. To say the least, they were not impressed with what they found. Most of the corporations which had survived the pruning that had been carried out at the time of the Union, around sixty-eight, were in various states of disorder. Many provided no service at all to the local community; some were even harmful to it while corruption was rife. Mercantile privileges, patronage and local justice were widely dispensed on a sectarian basis. Most were closed, self-perpetuating oligarchies almost exclusively Protestant. It was an area which was totally untouched by Catholic Emancipation which had quite recently been introduced. As well as that, control over the corporations was almost totally in Tory hands thus giving them an extra advantage in parliamentary representation. As Daniel O'Connell was, at that particular time, in alliance with the Whig government, the report presented him and the government with an opportunity as well as an incentive to bring about change in the civic governance of Ireland.

However, this was to prove difficult; entrenched interests resisted strongly. In contrast to its English equivalent, which passed without much difficulty in 1835, the Irish bill had a much rougher passage through parliament. The Tories fought it in the Commons with a delaying tactic and in the Lords, where they dominated, even more fiercely. It took four sessions to get it on to the statute books. By then, in 1840, its effectiveness had been much reduced although it did retain the proposal that corporations or councils be elected but with much reduced powers. Also, the bar was set much higher for the franchisee in Ireland, £10 householders as against £5 in England. Similarly, there was a higher property qualification to be met by those standing for election in Ireland.

Despite its weakness, the Municipal Corporations (Ireland) Act did provide some form of gains for Catholics, since some of them were for the first time enfranchised as well as being able to stand for office. The most immediate result could be seen in the election of members of Dublin Corporation in 1841.

Preparations for this election were made with extraordinary thoroughness since the newly enfranchised did not trust those who were in charge of the elections. One rule, in particular, caused much activity. This rule stated that only those who had paid all their taxes could vote and many Catholics had, for a number of years, refused to pay tithes since these went to the clergy of the Established Church. Efforts to pay these tithes were now put in place; various church vestries were pressed to supply information on what was due so as to ensure that voters would be accepted on the lists being prepared. Lack of trust also meant that Daniel O'Connell stood in two different wards to minimize the chances of his election being deemed, by some ruse, to be invalid. In the event, he was elected lord mayor; the first Catholic to hold this office since the time of James II and, before him, the Reformation. Although his election was enormously popular among Catholics, the office he had been elected to was much reduced in significance. What was dubbed 'the Orange monopoly' had been broken but much of the power it had held was not won by those who had so long opposed them; instead, it had gone to central government. Although the commissioners, who had shown up the inefficiency and corruption of the old corporations, had played their part in bringing about reform, it is quite likely that a man of John Richard Corballis's stature would, while welcoming O'Connell's election, have been well aware of the deficiencies in the newly defined office to which he had been elected.[4]

JOHN RICHARD CORBALLIS – A COMMISSIONER OF NATIONAL EDUCATION

A few years after Corballis had finished his work on the Commission of Inquiry into Municipal Corporations he became a commissioner of National Education. In doing so, he became engaged in one of the most controversial activities that plagued early 19th century Ireland. He was not the only person with Clonskeagh connections who became involved; as will be seen, a number of others did as

---

4   *First report of the commissioners appointed to inquire into the municipal corporations in Ireland,* House of Commons 1835 vol. xxvii pp.v-vi, 1-3; Alan J Ward, *The Irish constitutional tradition: responsible government and modern Ireland 1782-1992* (Dublin 1994) 40; Desmond Roche, *Local government in Ireland,* Institute of Public Administration (Dublin 1982) 31-35; Oliver McDonagh, 'Ideas and institutions, 1830-45', in W. E. Vaughan (ed), *A new history of Ireland,* V, *Ireland under the Union,1 1801-70* (Oxford 1989) 193-217: 215-21; Beckett, *The making of modern Ireland,* 322; Martin Holland; 'The election of Daniel O'Connell as Lord Mayor of Dublin, 1841' (unpublished essay).

well. Prior to introduction of a system for national education in 1831 by the chief secretary, Edward Stanley, it was illegal, at least in theory, to provide Catholic education for the poor; only hedge-schools were available. There were, of course, Protestant charter schools but because of proselytizing they were resented by Catholic clergy; they were also becoming an embarrassment to the government. More acceptable were the schools of the Kildare Place Society founded in 1811 but in the 1820s it began to move away from its neutrality in matters relating to religion. A way forward was proposed in a report by a select committee of the House of Commons; this was accepable to Catholics but strongly rejected by Protestant interests. Politically there were divisions too; the lord lieutenant, lord Anglesey, favoured it but his chief secretary Stanley, opposed. Anthony Blake, a friend of J R Corballis, was on Anglesey's side while Rev Dr James Henthorn Todd, later of Vergemount house, strongly opposed the separation of secular and religious instruction inherent in the report.

Eventually Stanley was won over and in late 1831 the new system was introduced, not by act of parliament but by instructions issued by Stanley. Although much was devolved to local initiative, these instructions ensured that there would be central control administered by commissioners appointed by the lord lieutenant. The use of commissioners to administer certain aspects of government would become a notable feature during the rest of the 19th century; they were drawn from various sectors to inspire confidence. In this instance, the government would channel funds towards education through commissioners rather than as hitherto through various societies dominated by Protestants. Initially seven in number, they were increased to nine in 1838 and in June of that year Corballis was appointed a commissioner. Also appointed was Alexander MacDonnell, an Anglican and personal friend of Corballis (he was a Trustee of Corballis's marriage settlement and witnessed codicils to his will).

Initial reaction of most Presbyterians to the new system was very negative but, in time, money problems meant that contact was made with the commissioners and at a conference, attended by Corballis, concessions were made which had the effect of moving the system towards denominationalism. Many Presbyterians then joined the system. The move towards denominationalism was reinforced by the refusal of most of the Established Church to take part leaving the schools in the south predominantly Catholic. One prominent member of the Established Church, archbishop Whately (who, incidentally, was a resident of Roebuck for a time around 1862) did join and was appointed a commissioner; he was vehemently opposed, however, by a fellow churchman, Rev Dr Todd, on grounds already stated. Catholic reaction was to cautiously welcome it but soon doubts were raised, mainly by archbishop MacHale of Tuam. Shortly thereafter a very public row emerged between him and archbishop Murray of Dublin, a commissioner, and it was widely aired in contemporary newspapers. Corballis was likely to have been an advisor to Murray at this time. Inevitably the issue was referred to Rome but it took a neutral stance; each bishop was to decide for himself.

The most delicate subject that the commissioners had to deal with was religious instruction. Up to 1840 this was given separately for members of each denomination attending. However, in that year the commission with only three members in attendance (Whately, Corballis and Blake) approved the use of religious books for the instruction of all except those children whose parents disapproved. All seemed well during the 1840s but a dispute arose in 1852 after archbishop Whately discovered the the books were not used at the Clonmel Model school (Model schools served as the commission's teacher training schools). The dispute centred on the interpretation of the 1840 ruling. At this point a new and familiar figure entered, lord chancellor Francis Blackburne who was now a commissioner. The new Catholic archbishop of Dublin, Paul Cullen also entered the fray. Much arguement and many meetings followed; the result was that the books were withdrawn but, if used, were to be confined to the time allocated for religious education. Soon Whately and Blackburne resigned; Corballis had already resigned in 1849. During his time on the commission the number of schools in operation and children on their rolls increased from 1,384 and 169,548 respectively, to 4,321 and 480,623. The commission in the second half of the century was weaker but the national system itself would continue to grow and prosper although it moved even further from its original intention of integrated secular education towards denominationalism.[5]

---

5   Donald H. Akenson, *The Irish education experiment: the National System of Education in the nineteenth century* (London & Toronto 1970) 1-2, 85-93, 102-12, 117-19, 126-30, 140, 162-4, 177-212, 227-30, 247-49; idem, 'Pre-university education, 1782-1870' in W. E. Vaughan (ed), *A new history of Ireland V Ireland under the Union, I 1801-70* (Oxford 1989) 523-37: 523-24, 526; John Coolahan, *Irish education: history and structure,* Institute of Public Administration, Dublin (Dublin 1981) 12-19; William John Fitzpatrick, *The Life, Times, and Contemporaries of Lord Cloncurry* (Dublin 1855) 577; Cloncurry, *Personal recollections,* 389-93, esp. 390; Private Sources at the National Archives: Small private accessions 999/658 13 Copy: Will and four Codicils of John Richard Corballis; Kerr, *Peel, priests and politics,* 136-40; G. O. Simms, 'James Henthorn Todd', *Hermathena: a Dublin University review,* 109 (1969) 5-23: 8-9; *Thom's Directory* for 1848, 1862; P.C. Barry, 'The Holy See and the Irish National Schools', *Irish Ecclesiastical Record* 5th ser. Vol. xcii (1959) 90-105: 98 n.1; Fitzpatrick, *"The Sham Squire",* 215 footnote.

JOHN RICHARD CORBALLIS − A COMMISSIONER FOR CHARITABLE DONATIONS AND BEQUESTS

In yet another controversy of the time Corballis backed archbishop Murray and, this time, he found himself opposing Daniel O'Connell on certain aspects of it. It centred on the Catholic response to one of the reforms introduced by the prime minister, Robert Peel, in 1844. After the humiliating collapse of O'Connell's great efforts to marshal the people behind the demand for Repeal in December 1843, Peel opted for concessions rather than coercion in the hope of defusing the movement for repeal. The first of these was a bill entitled 'Charitable Donations and Bequests for Roman Catholic Ministers (Ireland) Bill' introduced to parliament on 18 June 1844. The second was a bill to improve the financial situation of the Royal College of St Patrick in Maynooth, introduced in 1845. Corballis was involved in the controversy surrounding both of these but especially the former as he became a commissioner on the board which it set up. Innocuous as this may appear, the Charitable Donations Act created great controversy among Catholics and was strongly opposed from the outset by O'Connell and archbishop MacHale of Tuam.

The board, set up by the act, replaced that of 1800 which was almost exclusively Protestant; it now consisted of five Catholics and five Protestants with three other *ex officio* members. Its functions differed from the old one in that it did not have the discretionary powers which had allowed the old board to divert bequests to other charities of its own choosing where the original charity had failed, a function which had made Catholics very chary of making bequests. However, it was specifically laid down that it was still illegal to make bequests to any religious order. Although an improvement from the Catholic perpespective, it fell short of a bill that had been unsuccessfully introduced by O'Connell, in co-operation with the Catholic hierarchy, in March 1844 according to which bishops, not commissioners, would be allowed to hold bequests. Unacceptable to the government as it would put them on a par with bishops of the Established Church, Peel nevertheless decided that three of the commissioners should be bishops.

From the government's perspective the timing of the bill was unfortunate; with O'Connell in jail, many Catholics were in no mood to be conciliated and reaction was negative. Peel, therefore, introduced some amendments but one of them actually increased opposition; death-bed bequests of land were invalidated. A legal opinion from the incarcerated O'Connell, however, was seized upon by MacHale. To Murray's chagrin, he met with like-minded bishops in Dublin; bishops throughout the country were circulated seeking their signature to a protest against the bill. After O'Connell's release from jail was celebrated by Murray with a *Te*

Deum in the pro-cathedral Peel made some concessions on the death-bed bequest issue as he feared Murray would decamp to the Repealers. Murray then agreed to seek out bishops who would become commissioners. However, the *Freemen's Journal* at that point published the protest that MacHale had been organising; it had the signatures of half of the bishops of Ireland attached. But it also brought a new issue to the fore; the illegality of bequests made to religious orders (in origin, one of the Penal laws). As well as that, it spoke of the bill seeking to divide the hierarchy by the government choosing certain bishops -'ministerial favourites' – as commissioners. Although shaken by this protest, Murray was not swayed by it. He feared that rejection of the bill would prevent the emergence of further reforms, especially those related to Maynooth and a university for laymen.

With the hierarchy openly divided on the issue, it inevitably went to Rome where British diplomats were busy in its favour but the rector of the Irish College, Paul Cullen, vehemently against it. At home the newspapers were abuzz with letters, some sprinkled with vitriol, mostly in opposition to the bill. The bishops were still divided at their annual meeting in November but Murray managed to get some bishops from the minority to agree to become commissioners. O'Connell now entered the fray as he feared that the division of the hierarchy would be detrimental to his own political agenda. He addressed many meetings on the subject. Passions were so high that one of Murray's chosen bishops backed out under pressure; this was announced triumphantly by O'Connell. Murray responded by getting another bishop to take his place; he did however get the proposed location of board meetings removed from the Castle and the taint associated with it.

The problem over bequests to religious orders remained. A legal opinion their superiors got from O'Connell disturbed them greatly and they appealed to Murray. He got a reassurance from the lord lieutenant that an amendment would be introduced if O'Connell's opinion was found to stand up and saw to it that this was given publicity in the press. Meetings and agitation continued; in one the president, James Sheridan, declared 'He [Anthony Blake] is, I understand to be joined by Sir Patrick Bellew and Mr Corballis so that we shall have an anointed trio to carry into execution the dark designs of this hellish bill'. At another, O'Connell attacked the lay commissioners accusing them of efforts to secure patronage.

Concerned by this agitation, the government rushed the official publication of the names of the commissioners before it was legal to do so (on 17 December 1844). In the event Corballis was not on this list; he did, however, accept the appointment a short while later. With the official announcement of the commissioners O'Connell's agitation had failed. He admitted as much when he declared at a final meeting on 19 December 'Yes, I acknowledge we are defeated and the

Castle hacks have triumphed'. Afterwards he went home to Kerry; Christmas beckoned.

What could have been a relatively minor government reform effort had, in the event, blossomed into a full scale row that saw senior members of the Catholic church violently disagree with one another in public; had seen the most important Catholic politician of the time take one side and John R Corballis of Clonskeagh clearly on the other side. Whether he had any direct clash with O'Connell on the subject is not clear but it may be significant that in reports of O'Connell's speeches at protest meetings where he touches on the subject of possible members of the board he does not make any reference to him by name. Whatever is the case, it seems clear that Corballis took the responsibilities that went with his appointment seriously. In the report of the Board of Charitable Bequests for 1846, dated 3 July 1846, Corballis is recorded as having a higher attendance rate than all the other commissioners at board meetings in that year.[6]

It is, perhaps, opportune at this point to note that Corballis was not the only man with Clonskeagh connections to become a commissioner; Sir James Power held such a position from 1865 to his death in 1877. He was born 6 December 1800 the son of John Power, the whiskey distiller, who was created a baronet in 1841 while he lived at Roebuck house, Clonskeagh. Although his place of birth is given, somewhat surprisingly, as Johns lane distillery it is clear that he would have spent most of his early adulthood, if not childhood, in Clonskeagh. He succeeded to his father's title when the latter died at Roebuck house on 25 June 1855. Sir John Ennis who had lived in Clonskeagh until the late 1840s also became a commissioner; he retained that position until death in August 1878.[7]

JOHN RICHARD CORBALLIS AND THE MAYNOOTH ACT (1845)

With the success of the first of his reform efforts successfully underway, Peel moved in 1845 on the second, the improvement of the situation regarding the financing of the Royal College of St Patrick, Maynooth. In this too Corballis would become involved, not as a government appointee but as a counsel to the Trustees of the college. Concerned about the exposure of student priests to the

---

6   Ó Tuathaigh, *Ireland before the famine*, 190-93; Beckett, *The making of modern Ireland*, 328-29; Kerr, *Peel, priests and politics*, 122-24, 128, 133-34, 140-43,147,154, 164,175-91; William J Walsh, 'The law in its relations to religious interests: IX. The Board of Charitable Donations and Bequests in Ireland', *Irish Ecclesiastical Record* 3rd ser. Vol 16 (1895) 875-94, 971-996; *Freeman's Journal* November 15, 1844 to December 20, 1844; *Thom's Directory* 1848.
7   Boase, *Modern English biography,* ii 993, 1613.

'contagion' of revolutionary France, the Irish parliament had formally approved the setting up of Maynooth college in 1796 and provided it with an annual grant of £8,000. This grant was to become the focus of bitter attacks especially during the evangelical revival of the 1830s; they were spurred on by the perceived connection between Maynooth-trained priests and O'Connell. Some concession to Catholic bishops, Peel believed, was necessary to break this connection; an increase in the grant to the financially strapped college would admirably meet this aim since this had often been sought by the bishops. Getting the measure on the statute books was difficult, however, given that the proposal was to increase an already unpopular grant almost threefold; this became apparent on the first reading of the bill on 3 April 1845. Peel, however, was determined to press ahead, even allowing the impression to gain currency that he might be forced to resign over it so as to force reluctant members of his own party to vote in favour of the bill. His determination can be seen in the following exchange of letters between him and queen Victoria after the defeat at the first reading; they are of special interest because of the reference in one of them to Anthony Blake, archbishop Murray and John R Corballis.

From the queen

April 9, 1845
We are very anxious to hear the effect which has been produced by the Maynooth Bill in Ireland. The queen anxiously hopes Sir Robert does not feel uneasy about the result of the debate. The measure is so great and good a one, that people must open their eyes and will not oppose it.

To the queen

April 9, 1845
Sir Robert Peel moves on Friday next that the [Maynooth] Bill be read a second time. ...

(He) humbly assures your majesty that he will do all he can do with honour to ensure the success of the measure which could not be defeated, after once being proposed by a government, without very serious evil.

Sir Robert Peel had an interview this morning with Mr Blake, who showed him two letters, one from archbishop Murray, the other from Mr Corballis, an eminent Roman Catholic barrister, each expressing entire satisfaction with the measure, and with the tone and spirit in which it was introduced, each expressing a confident expectation that it would be received with very great feeling by the Roman Catholic body, lay and ecclesiastical.

Your majesty may be interested by seeing the manner in which Mr O'Connell spoke of the measure, and he therefore encloses a report of the speech at Conciliation Hall [the headquarters of the Repeal movement].

Anthony Blake, who was so crucial to the consultation process with the bishops while the bill was being formulated, continued to be of assistance while it was making its way through parliament. It would appear that the defeat at the first reading spurred him into action. He, together with Murray and Corballis, acted in concert to bolster Peel's resolve and to help the bill survive. Unlike previous government measures the Catholic hierarchy was united behind it; it was even praised by the redoubtable MacHale. It also had the support of O'Connell as the speech in the Conciliation hall which Peel sent to the queen shows. It is possible that the letters were consciously written from two different perspectives; Murray representing the bishops' point of view and Corballis that of the laity. That could be the reason why Peel made reference to the expectation that the measure would be warmly greeted 'by the Roman Catholic body, lay and ecclesiastical'. Although there was a great deal of bitter protest outside of parliament it was what happened inside that mattered. There the debate was also bitter though, as in many parliamentary debates, party matters extraneous to the bill came into play. Although Peel's own party was split at the second reading, the measure passed comfortably with the support of the Whigs and Liberals; much the same happened at the third reading. Queen Victoria writing to Peel expressing her pleasure at the success of the third reading went on to say 'We were most enthusiastically received last night in the theatre and outside, and not one 'No Popery' observation was to be heard'. Her apprehension over the possibility of such a slogan being shouted at her is an indication of the religious tension aroused in England by the passing of the Maynooth Bill; she gave it the royal assent on 30 June 1845.[8]

JOHN RICHARD CORBALLIS AND THE 'GODLESS COLLEGE' CONTROVERSY

Even before that assent had been given, Peel had introduced another bill to parliament that marked the beginning of yet another controversy in Ireland that saw the Irish Catholic bishops clash with the government and disagree among themselves. It was a controversy that would rumble on throughout the rest of the century and into the twentieth; in its earliest stage, an action of John Corballis would play an important role. That bill, introduced on 9 May and passed into

---

8   Ó Tuathaigh, *Ireland before the famine*, 15, 28, 46-7; Beckett, *The making of modern Ireland*, 329; *Thom's Directory* for 1848; Kerr, *Peel, priests and politics*, 225-31, 248-54, 259-61, 269-73, 280-87; Charles Stuart Parker (ed), *Sir Robert Peel from his private papers* (3vols, London 1891-99) iii 173-76.

law during the summer as the Provincial Colleges Act, sought to provide a system of university education in Ireland that would be acceptable to Catholics. New colleges were to be built in Cork, Galway and Belfast and they were to be non-denominational although facilities for the pastoral care of students could be provided by private endowment; Dublin already had Trinity College which, despite its Established Church ethos, allowed Catholic students to attend since 1794. These new colleges were modelled on the University College, London which favoured a more secular and utilitarian form of education, an approach which gained for it the title of 'Godless college'; this name O'Connell also applied to the new colleges. From the very outset, they were denounced by a number of Catholic bishops especially archbishop MacHale who wanted a separate system for Catholics. However, among others, the Catholic archbishops of Dublin and Armagh were prepared to go along with the new scheme, despite its imperfections; the latter even tried to have the Belfast college relocated in Armagh. The division emerged quite quickly and MacHale, along with archbishop Slattery of Cashel, engaged the assistance of Paul Cullen, rector of the Irish College in Rome, who was also against the system, to gain papal approval for their stand. Papal rescripts (i.e. official papal pronouncements) followed in 1847, 1848 and 1850 which declared the colleges harmful to religion and suggested that a Catholic University be set up.

The group of bishops prepared to accept the system suffered a major blow when archbishop Crolly of Armagh died of cholera in April 1849 and was replaced by Paul Cullen; this left archbishop Murray of Dublin, now around 82 years old, as the main figure among that diminished group. By this stage the colleges were ready to take in students and soon thereafter they were restructured as constituent colleges of the Queen's University in Ireland. Meanwhile Cullen had settled into his new role as Primate of All Ireland; in May 1850 he called an episcopal synod to meet in Thurles during the following August. It was almost inevitable, given the division of opinion on the topic among the bishops, that the university question would be high on the agenda of the synod when it met. In fact it was while the synod was in session that the news emerged that the government's decision to grant the colleges University status had been given the royal assent. The synod was proceeding in a business-like manner until it came to the question of the university; straightaway the different opinions were voiced. Archbishop Murray led one side of the debate saying that, while he respected the papal rescripts, he would nevertheless do nothing that would be contrary to his conscience; he would not oppose the rescripts but neither would he put their demands into effect. One of these required a bishop to impose a penalty on any of his clerics who took up an office in the colleges. A vote on this issue found 13 take Murray's side but 14 opposed. This was an indication of the strength of the side which opposed the relevant issues in the papal rescripts; the other side, of course, viewed them as obstinate.

Nevertheless, the majority had decided the issue; among other things, the synod condemned the colleges and resolved to set up a Catholic university. It could not make its decisions public until they were approved by Rome; it did, however, issue a pastoral letter five days after the closing of the synod in which it implied that the synod had unanimously condemned the colleges. Meanwhile, those who had been defeated on the issue were not idle; thirteen bishops signed a petition which they submitted to Rome to put their side of the arguement to pope Pius IX. But they did more than that; they made it known in public that there was not unanimity on the issue despite what the pastoral of 14 September said. There had been some leaks to the press during the synod, the sessions of which were held in private but a few weeks after it was over this was done in a more dramatic and open fashion; an exchange of letters between archbishop Murray and John Corballis was published in the *Dublin Evening Post* on 1 October 1850. It appeared there as follows:

Important Correspondence

The following letter will be perused with deep, and, we will add, with grateful interest by every true man in Ireland – nay, by every woman, too – and we do not restrict the interest to any sect or party. That MR CORBALLIS took the right and manly course, in addressing his archbishop there can be no second opinion. As a Catholic and as a father, he was bound to .do so under the circumstances. The reply of archbishop Murray is most important; but we hasten to lay the correspondence before the public:-

Rosemount, Roebuck 1 Oct. 1850

"MY DEAR CONWAY – As the enclosed Correspondence relates to a matter of such general interest, perhaps you will have the kindness to insert it to your paper this evening. Believe me, Your's very sincerely, "JOHN R.CORBALLIS"

[COPY]

Rosemount, Roebuck 30th Sept. 1850

My dear Lord,

May I respectfully ask your grace as well for my own information as for that of some other Roman Catholics of your diocese who have sons either in Trinity College, or in the course of preparation for it, or for the newly established Queen's Colleges, how we are to understand the late synodical address on the subject of these colleges? Are we thereby actually prohibited from sending our children to these colleges? And, if so, how far is such a provision actually binding on us *in foro conscientiæ* [in the exercise of our conscience]? To many of us it appears altogether inexplicable, that after petitioning, in the days of persecution, for admission into Trinity College, after being permitted, with tacit sanction of your grace, and your eminent predecessors and colleagues of the Church of Ireland for upwards of half a century, to receive our education there, and seeing that one of the members of that synod, most distinguished for rank, is actually a graduate of the University, it does appear strange that in the year 1850, education in Trinity College, or even in any of the colleges recently established on such liberal footing as regards us should be unequivocally condemned, and that without one reason being assigned for this sudden change, or any provision in the meantime being made for affording a suitable education to our children. I need not say that this subject is of intense interest to the Roman Catholic gentry of your grace's diocese as well as to the Roman Catholic middle classes of Ireland generally, and I therefore, my dear Lord, take the liberty of entreating such an answer from your grace as I may make known to the numerous persons who have spoken to me upon it; and which if it do not calm our apprehensions, at least may guide our future course of action on this all important point.

> *I am, my dear Lord, with the sincerest*
> *respect and affection, your grace's most*
> *obedient servant* John R Corballis

[COPY]

1 Mountjoy-square, 1 October, 1850

"MY DEAR FRIEND – I have received your interesting letter, and I need not, I hope, assure you, that I participate fully in the deep anxiety which you so justly feel: but I must pray you not to press me to enter at the moment, into details on the painful subject to which you allude. I may, however, mention that a petition signed by thirteen bishops, has, probably 'ere this, reached Rome, supplicating our most holy father, Pius IX, to refuse his sanction to certain proposals on points yet undecided, relative to the subject of academical education. To the decision to be given thereon, whatever it may be (though I still venture to hope that it will be favourable to the petitioners) those prelates will be found to be among the first to most reverently submit; but, in the meantime I am not aware that there is amongst them one who would wish to extend the provisions of the pontifical rescripts, already issued on that subject, beyond the strict letter of the Holy See has prescribed.

> *I have the honour to remain, my dear friend,*
> *your's most faithfully,* + D. Murray

A number of points arise from this remarkable correspondence. First it is very clear that it was published with the prior knowledge and consent of Dr Murray; Corballis had written that he wished to make Murray's answer known 'to ... numerous persons'. Second, it was carried out in great haste. Corballis's letter was written on 30 September and Murray's reply on the following day; Corballis received it that same day and forwarded it to the *Dublin Evening Post* which published it that evening. The motive behind the publication would appear to be a reaction to the pastoral letter, or synodical address as Corballis called it, which spoke of the synod unanimously condemning the new colleges. It was now made public that thirteen bishops did not agree with this; furthermore, they had sent a petition to Rome in an attempt to get the pope to refuse to sanction the resolutions of the synod. It is a measure of the depth of division concerning the new colleges that then existed among the Irish bishops that the archbishop of Dublin would publicly advise one of the most prominent laymen in his diocese not to press him on the subject of whether laymen should obey the pronouncement of a national synod of bishops; in the meantime the advice was to abide within a strict literal interpretation of the pre-synod papal rescripts.

One of the more immediate results of the publication of this correspondence was to make more urgent the task which the majority of bishops at the synod had agreed should be done, the founding of a Catholic university. Corballis had stressed in his letter that it was strange that education in Trinity College or in any of the new colleges should be condemned while no provision was 'in the meantime being made for affording a suitable education for our children'. A committee of four archbishops and four bishops was set up by the synod to look into the possibility of establishing a Catholic university. Now in early October this committee was broadened to include priests and laymen; the new committee met for the first time in Dublin on 17 October with the main focus being on raising enough funds to set up such a university. At that meeting Murray proved to be stubbornly against the whole idea; not alone did he refuse to contribute any funds to it, he would not even agree to be included among the archbishops in whose names money contributed would be received. It was the only meeting which Murray attended. In a letter to his successor as Rector of the Irish College in Rome, Dr Kirby, archbishop Cullen wrote about that first meeting: 'You see with what difficulties we have to contend. There is a real conspiracy to render Protestant or unbelieving the education of the Catholic youth, and what is deplorable is that Catholic bishops are among those who promote the views of our enemies. They are encouraging atheistic schools, and are themselves opposing any institution truly Catholic'. In the event, however, preparations for setting up the university went ahead; fund raising in Ireland, England and the United States raised £30,000 in 1851 and, in November of the same year, John Henry Newman, a distinguished Oxford scholar and recent convert to catholicism was appointed its rector. On 3 November 1854 it was formally opened at 86 St Stephen's green, Dublin. By that stage, however, Dr Murray was dead and his long-time opponent in relation to the necessity of a Catholic university, Dr Cullen had replaced him as archbishop of Dublin; he had been translated from Armagh shortly after Dr Murray's death on 2 February 1852. With that move, Corballis's questions which had been left open in Murray's reply were finally answered. Furthermore it is somewhat ironic that the successor, however indirectly, of the college that Murray and Corballis had opposed- UCD – would one day incorporate Corballis's home and grounds into its new campus at Belfield.[9]

9   F.S.L. Lyons, *Ireland since the famine* (London 1989) 94-96; Beckett, *The making of modern Ireland,* 330-331' Ó Tuathaigh, *Ireland before the famine,* 193-94; Coolahan, *Irish education: history and structure,* 113-19; Kerr, 'Dublin's forgotten archbishop', 259-60; *Dublin Evening Post* 1 October 1850; Gillian M Doherty 'The Synod of Thurles, 1850' [http://multitext.ucc.ie/d/The_Synod_of_Thurles_1850] May, 2006; Tomás O'Riordan 'Cullen, "Letter on the Catholic University to Dr Tobias Kirby" [http://multitext.ucc.ie/d/Cullen_Letter_on_the_Catholic_University_to_Dr_Tobias_Kirby] May, 2006; Ian Kerr, *John Henry Newman: a biography* (Oxford 1988) 376-77.

10

Later 19th century: Isaac Butt,
Fenians and others

QUEEN VICTORIA DRIVES THROUGH CLONSKEAGH

EARLY IN THE SECOND HALF of the nineteenth century Dublin played host to a great exhibition, funded largely by the railway magnate, William Dargan. Queen Victoria came to open it and, to mark his contribution, she called on Dargan at his house in Mount Anville. The Dublin *Evening Mail* of 31 August 1853 paints a picture of what the people of Clonskeagh would have seen as she passed their way. The following is an excerpt:

> Her majesty proceeded at a quarter to five o'clock to visit William Dargan ...
> – two chariots, each drawn by four splendid bays, driven by postilions wearing
> Royal livery and attended by five outriders, drove round to the principal
> entrance of the Viceregal Lodge. Her majesty, prince Albert, the prince of
> Wales, prince Alfred, and the countess of St German's entered the first carriage.
> ... Lord lieutenant ... the second... . In a barouche were the officers of the staff
> in attendance ... . The route taken was along the quays ... Grafton street ...
> Leeson street, Donnybrook road by Clonskeagh and on by Roebuck to Mount
> Anville. ... (the) party arrived at half-past five ... . After more than a half hour
> ... the party ... took leave ... of Mr and Mrs Dargan. In returning (they)
> proceeded at a rapid pace by the route leading through Kilmainham to the
> Park, and arrived at the Lodge shortly after 7 o'clock'.[1]

POLITICAL SITUATION

Emancipation had won Irish Catholics the right to be elected to a seat in the Westminster parliament. The result was the emergence of a new and radical political grouping there led by O'Connell. Initial alliance with the Whig

---

1   Ball and Hamilton, *Parish of Taney,* 166-67.

government achieved some reforms but on the return of the Tories to government reforms were out of the question so demands for repeal of the Union came to the fore. The Repeal Association was re-invigorated; in 1843 monster meetings were held throughout the country which culminated in O'Connell being imprisoned. Four years later he was dead; his efforts to achieve repeal by constitutional means a failure. A more militant approach was advocated by a new movement, the Young Irelanders. This, however, ended disastrously in 1848 in an abortive rebellion in Ballingarry, county Tipperary. The leaders, William Smith O'Brien and Thomas Francis Meagher, were charged with sedition; chief justice Blackburne, who then resided at Roebuck hall, presided not very impartially at the trial. Among those who defended them was a young lawyer, Isaac Butt.[2]

ISAAC BUTT

Early in his career, Butt had been an arch conservative and supporter of the Protestant ascendancy, which he felt to be under threat from O'Connell's repeal activities. His work, however, in defending the Young Irelanders and, later, the Fenians encouraged him to reflect deeply on the problems which gave rise to these movements. He came to believe that the solution might lie in a form of federalism in which Ireland would have a separate but subordinate parliament within the Union. This, he believed, would be the best way to secure the Protestant position in Ireland. From such thinking grew what would later be called the Home Rule movement.[3] Butt was first elected to parliament in 1852 where he witnessed, at first hand, the neglect of Irish issues. After some time spent in England, he returned to Ireland where he gained a reputation for his defence of Fenians. As well as that he helped to organise the Amnesty Association which sought the release of Fenian prisoners. This was to gain some success; a government commission which was set up, as a result, saw the release of some Fenians including O'Donovan Rossa. In 1870, a meeting organized by Butt led to the foundation of the Home Government Association. It was superceded three years later by the Home Rule League which was better organized.

In this, Butt was helped by a Roebuck man, George Kinahan. (His home had been built by one of the family in the 18th century – a substantial house, it was called Roebuck park.) This superior organisation soon paid dividends; Home Rulers increased their seats to 59 in the general elections of 1874. Butt, however,

---

2 Lydon, *The making of Ireland*, 290-96, 300, 310; Ball, *History of the county Dublin*, ii 80; Terence de Vere White, *The road of excess* (Dublin 1945) 138.

3 Lydon, *The making of Ireland*, 310; Lyons, *Ireland since the famine*, 147.

was unable to capitalise on this; the House of Commons simply ignored his attempts to bring Irish issues to its attention. It did, however, pay attention to a small group of Home Rule MPs with a new tactic; they started a campaign of obstruction when non-Irish issues were being discussed, a campaign which exploited the procedures of the house. This small group of obstructionists was soon to be joined by Charles Stewart Parnell who was elected for the first time at the Meath by-election of 1875.[4]

Butt abhorred the strategy of this group but the failure of his own policy, which was essentially one of conciliation and gradualism, resulted in a diminution of his authority. This led ultimately to a fraught meeting of the Home Rule League in February 1879 where he faced what was, in effect, a motion of no confidence. Although he won the vote narrowly it was, in fact, the end of the road politically for him. The way was now clear for the rise of Parnell; he was elected leader of the Home Rule party in May 1880. To add to Butt's woes, he was now a very sick man. A friend who visited him some time later at his home in North Great George's street tells of his condition; he had a stroke and it appeared that death was imminent. Two doctors, who attended, disagreed as to how he should be treated. Finally, it was agreed that a change of air would be of benefit to him. His daughter, Elizabeth, who was married to a solicitor, Thomas Colquhoun, lived at that time in 'The Cottage' in Clonskeagh. As their house was in the country and on high ground it was decided that he should be brought there. And so, he was brought in his carriage to 'The Cottage' where he died some days later on 5 May 1879. There was some discussion about a public funeral for him but his family decided against it. Despite this, there was a substantial gathering, which included Parnell and other members of the Irish Party, when his coffin, which had been brought from Clonskeagh, was put on to a train to be brought for burial in Stranorlar in county Donegal. His daughter, Elizabeth, and her husband did not remain long at 'The Cottage'; in 1881 their residence is given as 69 Upper Leeson street. 'The Cottage' now became the residence of the Misses Colquhoun who, it is reasonable to assume, were related to Elizabeth's husband, Thomas. However, they too moved soon after to 70 Waterloo road; in 1886 Edward Holland is listed as residing at 'The Cottage'.

In the year of Butt's death, a new bridge was finally, and after much debate, built on the seaward side of the old Carlisle bridge (now O'Connell bridge); it was named after Butt, a testament to the high regard in which he was then held.

---

4   Joseph Lee, *The modernisation of Irish society 1848-1918* (Dublin 1973) 62-64; Lydon, *The making of Ireland*, 310; Hall, *The Bank of Ireland*, 478-9, 495; *Thom's Directory* 1870, 1878.

This bridge had a metal span in the centre which could swivel on a pier at its middle to allow boats to sail up river to berth at Burgh quay and Eden quay. However, when the Loopline railway bridge was built downriver in 1888-90, the possibility of sailing up as far as these quays had disappeared; the swivel action of the central span of Butt bridge was no longer needed. Its narrowness, however, (it was only 5.6 metres wide) was a hindrance to the easy flow of traffic. A new wider bridge was built and opened in 1932. Suggestions made at that time to rename the bridge were rejected; Butt's memory was still honoured over fifty years after his death.[5]

The enhancing of Butt's reputation through his defence of Fenians reminds us of a small, but significant, connection between that movement and Clonskeagh. In 1868 a new military appointment was made by the government; major general Cunynghame CB was appointed to the command of the military in the Dublin area, an appointment specifically related to the Fenian rising of 1867. He took up residence in Mount Dillon, on Roebuck road, for the duration of his stay. While residing there he was knighted and as major general Sir Arthur A T Cunynghame, KCB he remained at Mount Dillon until 1872. His duties in relation to the Fenians, however, did not prove to be onerous; the rising which took place early in 1867 was quickly crushed. There was some activity in his area of command (Dublin), in particular the affray which took place at Tallaght but, in the event, this did not prove to be of major significance. One item of local interest was a raid carried out on the Constabulary Barracks at Stepaside on the morning of 6th March in the same year (this was the morning after the day designated for the rising). A Clonskeagh man, Terence Kelly, was one of the armed group which carried out that raid. He was arrested and returned for trial. According to a report in the *Irish Catholic Chronicle* on Saturday 12 October, 1867, he was however discharged on entering security to appear and stand trial whenever the crown should so wish. There is no further record of Terence Kelly; however, there was a Kelly family in Clonskeagh at the time of Griffith's valuation, c1851, as it records the name John Kelly who would have had property with an annual rentable valuation of at least £5. Nothing else could be found out about Fenian activity in the Clonskeagh area but given the fact that Kelly's activity took place in Stepaside it seems possible that there was a Fenian 'circle' in the general area. At the end of major general Sir Arthur A T Cunynghame's stay in Mount Dillon he left to take up command of British troops in South Africa.

---

5   Lyons, *Ireland since the famine*, 154-58; Lydon, *The making of Ireland*, 312-13; White, *The road of excess*, 376-79; *Thom's Directory* 1879 – 1886; J. W. de Courcy, *The Liffey in Dublin* (Dublin 1996) 58-60.

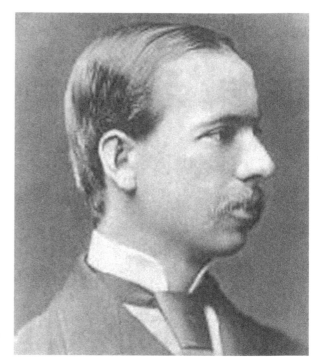

Warren Richard Colvin
Wynne of Wynnstay,
Clonskeagh road
*(with permission: from the
John Young Collection)*

His tour of duty there lasted until 1 March 1878, only months before captain Warren Richard Colvin Wynne, son of captain John Wynne of Wynnstay, Clonskeagh road, took up command of the 2nd field company of the Royal Engineers in Natal in December of the same year; he would go on to play an important part in the Zulu War which was then about to break out.[6]

In the year of Butt's death, 1879, Parnell sailed to America to seek the support of the Fenian organization there, Clann na Gael; in the same year the Irish National Land League was founded with Michael Davitt its main driving force. This marked the beginning of 'The Land War', a successful mass-movement which eventually brought about the end of the dominance of the landlords and saw the transfer of land ownership to those who were hitherto insecure tenants. As a result, Parnell's star shone brighter than ever. He imposed discipline on the

6   Dublin directories; Lee, *The modernisation of Irish society*, 53-59; Captain Warren Wynne is discussed in more detail in Chapter 12 where his parent's home, Wynnstay on the Clonskeagh road; is dealt with; for Cunynghame: website: http://www.geocities.com/layedwyer/cunyghame.htm; Boase, *Modern English biography*, i 788-89.

Irish Party at Westminster and succeeded in having a Home Rule bill introduced by prime minister Gladstone only to see it defeated by conservative elements in parliament.

However, a catastrophe awaited; in 1890 he was cited as co-respondent in a divorce case involving a member of his party and his wife, captain William Henry and Katherine O'Shea. The brother of the latter, incidentally, was married in 1867 to a Clonskeagh woman, hon. Mary Paulina Southwell (born 1841 probably at Mount Dillon as her parents were living there at that time); her husband was field marshal Sir (Henry) Evelyn Wood, GCB, GCMG, VC. The O'Shea divorce and the citation of Parnell was cleverly manipulated for political gain against the background of Victorian mores and the Irish Party split over the issue; within a year Parnell was dead, aged only 45 years, and greatly mourned by many Irish people. The split and the accompanying bickering in the party greatly reduced the impact that the party could make at Westminster. Nevertheless, Gladstone did introduce another Home Rule bill in 1893 but it was, once again, defeated; it was now a virtually lost cause especially since Gladstone resigned in 1894 and a new government dominated by Conservatives and Unionists was elected in 1895; it retained power for the next ten years.[7]

---

7   Lydon, *The making of Ireland*, 314-17; Ian F W Beckett, 'Women and patronage in the late Victorian army', in *History* 85 (2000) 463-480: 474.

II

The 20th century

I N 1900 QUEEN VICTORIA visited Dublin once more and a few interesting observations were made by a niece of John R Corballis of Clonskeagh; she was then a nun with the Sisters of Charity in Gardiner street. Writing to her brother on 8 April 1900 she had this to say: 'The queen's visit has made a great stir in the city and I think will do great good in every way. The feeling of disloyalty among the lower classes is astounding. The children positively refused "queen's breakfast", "queen's sweets" or to go to the Park to see the Procession if they were made sing "God save the queen".[1] Britain at this time was at the height of empire and was engaged in increasing and consolidating its hold on African territories especially South Africa, important because of its position on the sea route to India. Its imperial aspirations were, of course, backed by military force not all of which was successful. Indeed one of the setbacks of this period occurred early in the so-called Zulu War of 1879 during which a man with strong Clonskeagh connections, captain Warren Richard Colvin Wynne RE (whom we have already met), lost his life as a result of a fever contracted during the conflict. We have also met another man involved in this war from an early stage – colonel (later field marshal) Sir Evelyn Wood. He, however, survived the early set-back and eventually the Zulus were defeated. That war was a precursor to another much more serious set of wars – the Boer Wars.

The first of these – fought in February 1881 – resulted in defeat for the British army. Negotiations followed and Wood concluded a convention, disliked by queen Victoria, with the Boers the following April as a result of which the Transvaal regained its independence with the British retaining only nominal sovereignty. This, of course, resolved nothing as the underlying tensions caused by the expansionary policy of Britain remained. The discovery of gold in the Transvaal in 1886 merely added to the existing tensions exascerbated as they later were by the attempt by Cecil Rhodes to overthrow its government. Subsequent demands on that government, refused by president Kruger, provided the excuse

---

1   Papers of John Woulfe Flanagan: National Archives of Ireland, Private Sources 1189/14/9.

for the second Boer War; this ultimately led to the absorption of the Boer republics into the British empire in 1902. Before the second war had begun, a thirty-two year old Irishman, John MacBride, born in Westport, county Mayo had arrived in South Africa seeking to find work. Back in Ireland, he had been a member of the Irish Republican Brotherhood. Reflecting his strongly held political views he was instrumental in the setting up of an Irish Brigade in South Africa which fought on the side of the Boers against the British.

Directly related to the growing importance of the print media at the time, an intense interest was generated in the twists and turns of the war back in England and in Ireland. In England to this day an Afrikaan word 'kop', used to denote a high bank of terracing at a football stadium, derives from this interest. There was intense interest in Ireland too; the triumphal gateway into St Stephen's green at the top of Grafton street was built as a memorial to the Dublin Fusiliers who fought with the British in that war. Not all Irishmen who sided with the British at the time were impressed with their performance however. Richard J Corballis of Rosemount in Clonskeagh apparently had a close interest in its course. Some of his nephews fought in it. He was also in correspondence with his cousin, captain James Corballis, while the latter was engaged in the war. He expressed his opinion in a fortright manner in a letter to his nephew, a reporter for *The Times* of London, in July 1900: 'The British generalship (including lord Roberts) and the subordinate officers seem to an outsider, *bad*'. He was, however, proud of the Distinction gained by the 2nd Dublin Fusiliers. Roberts, incidentally, had been commander-in-chief of the forces in Ireland a few years earlier in 1895 and this could have coloured the opinion expressed; in fact he particularly criticised Roberts by underlining 'including lord Roberts'.

Many in Ireland were opposed to the British in their conduct of this war; their opposing view was held with the same amount of sincerity as those who supported them. An Irish Transvaal Committee was set up to support the Irish Brigade in South Africa referred to above. As a result MacBride became a hero back in Ireland. After the disbandment of the Irish Brigade, MacBride arrived in Paris; he could not return to Ireland as he would have been arrested for his South African activities. In Paris he met two of the stalwarts of the Irish Transvaal Committee, Arthur Griffith and Maud Gonne; he married the latter in 1903.[2]

---

2   'Engineers in the Zulu War 1879' [http://www.remuseum.org.uk/campaign/rem _zuluwar79.htm]: this is the website of the British army's Royal Engineers; Gardiner & Wenborn, *The History Today Companion to British History,* 89, 658, 838; Beckett, 'Women and patronage in the late Victorian army', 474; Keith Feiling, *A history of England* (London 1966) 1013-1022; Papers of John Woulfe Flanagan: National Archives of Ireland, Private Sources 1189/14/9; Anthony J Jordan, *Seán MacBride* (Dublin 1993) 10-11.

Years later, after the execution of MacBride following the 1916 rising, Maud Gonne now known as Madame Maud Gonne MacBride would return to Ireland and a few years after that would take up residence in Clonskeagh.

The onset of the Great War in 1914 saw a substantial number of young Irish people join up for service in Europe. Inevitably a lot of these were from Dublin including Clonskeagh and many of these never returned. The following three people are but a sample of some the latter. Their names and details have been taken from the *Dublin City & County Book of Honour* published in 2004 by a special committee set up to recognize their sacrifice:

> MICHAEL DELANEY. Private. Born Donnybrook [i.e. parish of] Dublin. Resided Clonskeagh, Co Dublin. Enlisted Dublin 5/23692 Royal Dublin Fusiliers, "D" Company, 8th Battalion. Killed in action, France & Flanders, 1st April 1916. Special memorial 10. Bois-Carre Military Cemetery, Haisnes, Pas de Calais, France.
>
> RICHARD CARTON. Private. Born Windy Arbour, Dublin. Enlisted Dublin. 26628. Royal Inniskilling Fusiliers, 8th Battalion. Formerly 19817, Royal Dublin Fusiliers. Killed in action, France & Flanders, 1st March 1917. M.69. Kemmel Chateau Military Cemetery, Heuvelland, West-Vlaanderen, Belgium.
>
> WILLIAM RICHARD JOHN. Private. Born Clonskea[gh], Dublin. Royal Dublin Fusiliers, 7th Battalion. Killed in action, Balkans, 23rd September, 1916. Dorian Memorial, Greece.

It has not been possible to find very much written about the impact the 1916 rising had on Clonskeagh. The Clonskeagh tram would, of course, have been halted for some time given that it travelled from Nelson's Pillar in Sackville street (now O'Connell street) – the very epicentre of the rising. Also, as we will note in Chapter 15, the Masonic Orphan Boys' School (in Richview, Clonskeagh) is known to have encountered problems in having bread delivered at the time; that being so, it seems likely that other such interuptions in the daily lives of the people in general were experienced. There were some military officers living in Clonskeagh at the time (e.g. captain Thomas Wade Thompson, DL, Clonskeagh castle; col. H C de la M Hill, East Kent regiment, Roebuck house) but it is not clear whether they had any active involvement; they may of course have been retired. One person then living in Clonskeagh did pass on some of his recollections of the impact that the rising had on the area: Cecil Harmsworth King, later the owner of the Mirror Group of Newspapers and a director of the Bank of England. He wrote that even where they lived, Roebuck hall just off the Roebuck road, which was four miles from the GPO they 'could hear the rattle of machine-guns getting nearer and nearer, while the gardens and fields were sprinkled with burnt paper and ashes from burning buildings.' King ventured 'as far as our little church [St Thomas at the junction of Foster avenue and

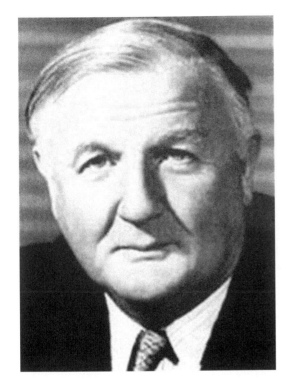

Cecil Harmsworth King of Roebuck hall: one-time owner of the Mirror Group of Newspapers and director of the Bank of England

Stillorgan road] to watch military reinforcements marching into Dublin'. These, he wrote, were Sherwood Forresters who marched without protection and were later ambushed suffering substantial losses. He also stood on the roof of Mount Anville convent and 'watched 4.7 inch naval shells bursting in O'Connell street'. Later with his father he drove around the centre of the city to observe the damage that had been caused.[3]

In much the same way as the 1916 rising, the war of independence does not appear to have seen any activity associated with it happen in the Clonskeagh area. However, it was different with the events that followed the ending of that war. The disagreements which came in the heel of the Anglo-Irish Treaty of December 1921 led to a split among those who had hitherto fought together for independence. Some of those involved peripherally, although very publicly, in that split would soon afterwards take up residence in Clonskeagh where their house would become a focal point for much political activity in subsequent years – Mrs Despard and Madame Maud Gonne MacBride. Another person, more

3   Cecil H King, *Strictly personal: some memoirs of Cecil H King* (London 1969) 35.

centrally but perhaps less publicly involved and very decisively on the other side of the split, would a short while later also reside in Clonskeagh – Hugh Kennedy, the first chief justice of the Irish Free State.

MRS DESPARD AND MAUD GONNE MACBRIDE IN ROEBUCK HOUSE

Under the terms of the treaty, a provisional government took over pending a general election when the people would decide. In the meantime, the Dáil narrowly approved the treaty but did nothing to assuage the growing bitterness. This led to the outbreak of a civil war after the elections of 16 June and the assassination of field marshal Sir Henry Wilson in London less than a week later, dramatically indicated by the shelling of the Four Courts early on 28 June by government forces. Inside, among the opponents of the government, was Seán MacBride, the son of Maud Gonne.

In 1921, during the period of the truce before the treaty, Maud had assisted escaped prisoners at her large house at 73 St Stephen's Green which she shared with Mrs Despard, a woman considerably her senior in age. Although Mrs Despard, then 77 years old, had been for a long time active in radical politics in England – she was a leading suffragette and socialist – and had supported Home Rule for Ireland she had, unlike Maud Gonne, held back from full outspoken support for republicanism in Ireland during the period before the Treaty. The reason for this is that her brother, field marshal lord French, had been lord lieutenant in Ireland since 11 May 1918. Only when that situation was resolved, with the advent of the provisional government taking over, did she fully espouse the republican cause.[4]

Between the Dáil debate on the Treaty and the outbreak of the civil war the following June positions were rapidly polarising. During this period Maud Gonne's position was ambiguous; she was in Paris, having been sent there apparently by Arthur Griffith on a diplomatic mission, when the shelling of the Four Courts took place. On hearing this she rushed back to Dublin but it is not clear whether she knew at this stage that her young son Seán was one of those who was inside. According to her own claims, on her return and at the prompting of the lord mayor, she set up a peace committee consisting of prominent women activists including Mrs Despard to try and negotiate peace between the two opposing groups. This failed and fighting continued for a short time in Dublin before government forces brought it under their control. Some of those wounded on the republican side were treated in the house on St Stephen's green which Maud

---

4   Lydon, *Making of Ireland*, 354-58; Margaret Ward, *Maud Gonne: a life* (London 1993) 128; Jordan, *Seán MacBride*, 19; Margaret Mulvihill, *Charlotte Despard: a biography* (London 1989) 1, 135-37.

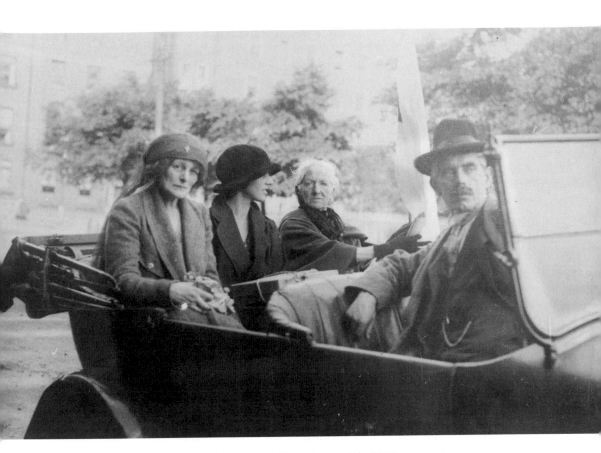

Maud Gonne MacBride (first on left) on Red Cross duty, 4 July 1922
(*Courtesy of the National Library of Ireland*)

Gonne shared with Mrs Despard. Shortly thereafter both of these ladies began, or more properly speaking, resumed their support for those in prison for their political activities. At a meeting in the Mansion House the Women's Prisoners' Defence League (WPDL), later nicknamed 'The Mothers', was formally established with Mrs Despard as president and Maud as secretary; the latter's son, Seán, and son-in-law, Francis Stuart, were then in Mountjoy prison. Concern for the welfare of political prisoners was to almost dominate these ladies' lives for a number of years to come. Maud's initial neutral or, at least, ambigious attitude towards the Treaty and subsequent provisional government had shifted; she was now very much on the anti-Treaty side.[5]

---

5   Ward, *Maud Gonne*, 132-35; Mulvihill, *Charlotte Despard*, 142-44.

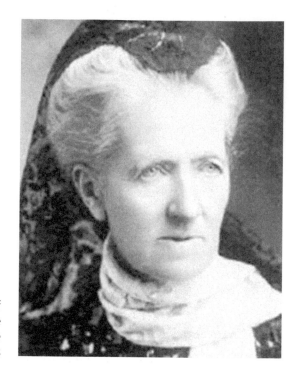

Charlotte Despard: co-owner of
Roebuck house with Madame
Maud Gonne MacBride in the
1920s

Long before the shelling of the Four Courts and the outbreak of the civil war
plans were afoot to leave the house in St Stephen's green and move to Roebuck
house in Clonskeagh. Many years later, Maud Gonne's son, Seán MacBride,
made a list of the documents associated with the Title to Roebuck house. One
of these documents, dated 8 June 1922, is entitled 'Conveyance col. Henry
Fulton to Mrs Charlotte Despard and Maud Gonne MacBride'.[6] That
Conveyance document was prepared at the end of a process whereby a house
suitable to their needs was first located and then purchased. How long that
process lasted is not clear but it certainly took some time; hence the decision to
move from St Stephen's green was taken a considerable period before the 8 June
1922 and was not the result of the outbreak of the civil war.

With their new base at Roebuck house, then only twenty minutes from
Dublin by car, 'The Mothers' carried out an extensive and varied series of

---

6   I would like to thank Caitriona Lawlor for allowing me to see the original
    handwritten list and for giving me a photocopy of this list that had subsequently
    been typed.

activities on behalf of political prisoners. They protested outside prisons, processed through the streets holding banners aloft, held impromptu meetings at street corners, wrote letters incessantly to the press – in fact they tried every method of protest and propaganda they could think of to bring their views on the plight of prisoners into public consciousness. They became a very familiar sight on the Dublin streets in the 1920s, looking quite theatrical in their long floating clothes, one very tall and regal, the other less so. The ever-witty Dubliners nicknamed them 'Maud Gonne Mad and Mrs Desperate'.

They were, however, a thorn in the side of the government. Roebuck house experienced the first of many raids by government forces and in 1923 WPDL was made illegal. Maud was imprisoned but released after one night in Mountjoy; she nevertheless used her experience there to further her propaganda for prisoners. Later that year (1923) a number of women prisoners went on hunger strike and Maud set about organising support for them so as to put pressure on the government. The government reacted; Maud and other prominent women were incarcerated, this time in Kilmainham. They quickly joined the hunger strike that the women, about whom they had been protesting, had already initiated. Mrs Despard took up her position outside the jail where she remained in protest, day and night, for the twenty days which Maud Gonne was on hunger strike. Eventually when the order for release came, Maud was taken, on a stretcher, and in an ambulance requisitioned by Mrs Despard, to Roebuck house where she recuperated. A few weeks later the civil war effectively came to an end when the order was given to dump arms and to cease fire.

Although protests about political prisoners would continue to be central to the activities of the two women in Roebuck house, they soon embarked on another project which was concerned with the plight of released prisoners at a time of great economic deprivation. Some of these were given temporary refuge at Roebuck house where there was much comings and goings in the latter half of 1923. However, an attempt was then made to do something of a more permanent nature that would provide employment for some of them and their family members; something akin to a cottage industry was set up primarily in the outhouses attached to Roebuck house. At first a bakery was considered but it was then decided to start a jam factory instead. Begun in 1924 it was established as a properly registered company – Roebuck Jam Co. Ltd., Clonskea, Co. Dublin. As well as the jam factory which seems to have been primarily Mrs Despard's responsibility – although Kid Bulfin, Seán MacBride's wife, did play a major part in running it – Maud Gonne set up a small industry making floral decorations using shells and twigs as well as other items such as table decorations.

The jam factory involved much more than merely making the jam; it meant also growing the fruit used to make the jam although it would appear that at

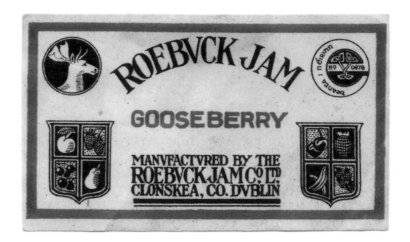

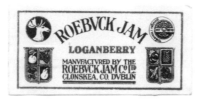
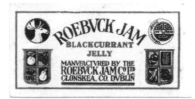

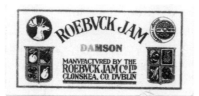
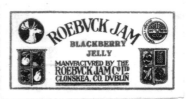

Labels from jam factory operated by Madame Maud Gonne MacBride and Mrs Charlotte Despard at Roebuck house in the 1920s

least some fruit pulp was imported from Belgium or Holland to supplement that which was grown in the fields attached to Roebuck house. It is known that there were three such fields since there are records of their being leased to people living in large houses nearby in 1864 and again in 1883. Of course tending the fruit produced in these fields also provided employment. All this had to be paid for and the sale of the jam and the other items was as heavily promoted as possible. Advertisements were placed in the republican paper, *An Phoblacht,* exhorting the readers to buy their 100% Irish made goods. The jam, they were told in a way that has a very modern resonance, was pure and had no chemicals added; it was good for your health. Other methods to promote sales were also taken including direct calls on various grocery shops.

However, despite valiant efforts the industry proved to be a failure although it did give some employment at a time when it was much needed. Although ailing from 1927 it was not sold off until around 1930. Maud's work, which employed a few young women in the house, did continue for a little longer. She had made great efforts to promote her products, selling them herself at various locations which held Christmas and Easter fairs. She did manage to sell her products, especially to better-off republican supporters, but it was never enough. In any case the problems of unemployment, especially for ex-prisoners, were always going to be beyond her and Mrs Despard's ability to effectively resolve but at least they tried.

The stock market crash of 1929 and the widespread economic depression which followed made matters even worse in Ireland. Around this time Mrs Despard was turning more towards communism although it did not interfere with her attending mass regularly in Donnybrook church. James Connolly's son, Roddy, an executive member of the new Workers' Party of Ireland, was a regular caller at Roebuck house. In 1930, aged 86 years, Mrs Despard visited Russia. The following year, according to her own account, Roebuck house was raided twelve times, the largest number of raids in one year it had experienced. Although Maud had some socialist tendencies – she was on the executive of the Irish Labour Defence League and was involved with other such groups– she was never as radical as Mrs Despard in this area. These differences probably played some part, although it is not clear precisely what part, in Mrs Despard's decision to leave Roebuck house and move into central Dublin. She sold her share of Roebuck house to Maud. The document of which finalised the sale 'Release and Conveyance Charlotte Despard to Maud Gonne MacBride' is dated 10 January 1934. By that date a new government under Eamonn de Valera had come into power after the 1932 elections in the run-up to which Maud Gonne had campaigned vigourously against the incumbent government. DeValera's victory resulted in the release of prisoners as promised and both Maud and Mrs Despard were on the platform in College green when they were greeted. However, it was not long before the welcome they gave to the new government began to ebb away.[7]

---

7 Ward, *Maud Gonne*, 135-47, 155-61; Mulvihill, *Charlotte Despard*, 144-48, 154-58, 169-79; Nancy Cardozo, *Maud Gonne* (New York 1990) 362-63; Caitriona Lawlor, *Seán MacBride: That day's struggle, a memoir 1904-1951* (Dublin 2005) 103; for Release and Conveyance document, see previous footnote.

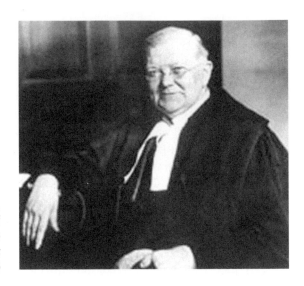

Hugh Kennedy of Newstead,
Clonskeagh road. First chief
justice of the Irish Free State
(*with permission: UCD archives
website*)

CHIEF JUSTICE HUGH KENNEDY AT NEWSTEAD, CLONSKEAGH

But before discussing that it is necessary to go back and discuss the other person who had taken up residence in Clonskeagh after the new state was founded and who, as we shall see, took a very different stance to that taken by the residents of nearby Roebuck house. He was Hugh Kennedy who, shortly before he took up residence in Newstead on the Clonskeagh road, had been appointed the first chief justice of the Irish Free State. Before being appointed to that position he had played an important role in both the Provisional Government and its immediate successor, the Government of the Free State, as law advisor in the former and attorney general in the latter.

Born in Dublin on 11 July 1879, he was educated privately and later at University College where he beat James Joyce in the election for Auditor of the Literary and Historical Society. He was the first UCD editor of the student magazine, *St Stephen's,* which that college had inherited from its predecessor Jesuit college; a magazine that was of very high standard, rarely equalled by subsequent student magazines. After study at the King's Inns, he was called to the bar in 1902 and became King's Counsel in 1920. He was a prominent member of the Gaelic League being on the *Ardchraobh* along with Patrick Pearse, Eoin MacNeill and Éamonn Ceannt. He was legal adviser to the Department of Local Government under the first Dáil. Shortly after the treaty was ratified by the Dáil in early 1921 he was appointed by the Provisional Government to a committee set up to frame a draft constitution for the new state when it would come into being. [8]

The task facing this committee was enormous as it attempted to bridge the gap between those who opposed the treaty and the demands of the British who wanted the terms of the treaty to be faithfully incorporated in the new constitution. Unable to agree on one draft, three separate drafts were presented to the Provisional Government but the British government rejected the chosen draft (the one prepared by the Kennedy group within the committee) as it had attempted to remove the crown from having any role in Irish affairs. Collins and Griffith were called to London by Lloyd George and given an ultimatum over the wording of the constitution; abide by the treaty or return to the position prior to its signing. Collins and Griffith returned to Ireland and left Hugh Kennedy to hammer out with lord chief justice Hewart ammendments that would be acceptable.[9]

It has been cogently argued that the compromise constitution which emerged was arrived at through a subtle understanding by Kennedy of the difference between the letter and the practice of dominion law, under which, according to the treaty, Ireland was to be governed, whereby the role of the crown would, in effect, be ficitonal; appointments, for example, would be made by the representative of the crown but only after their being nominated by the Dáil.[10] Kennedy had met strong opposition by the British in relation to the use of the name of the crown in matters such as the summoning of the Dáil or the appointment of judges and public officials.[11]

The Irish Free State Constitution Bill was passed by the Dáil on 6 December 1922; with that the Provisional Government ceased to exist and the Irish Free State came officially into existence exactly one year after the treaty had been

---

8   Henry Boylan, *A dictionary of Irish biography* (3rd ed, Dublin 1998) 205-6; Donal McCartney, *UCD, a national idea: the history of University College, Dublin* (Dublin 1999) 56-7; Nicholas Mansergh, *The Irish Free State: its government and politics* (London 1934) 44-5;

9   John A Murphy, *Ireland in the twentieth century* (Dublin 1975) 52; Tom Garvin, *1922: the birth of Irish democracy* (Dublin 1996)174-75; Michael Hopkinson, 'From treaty to civil war, 1921-2' in J R Hill (ed) *A new history of Ireland* VII 'Ireland, 1921-84' (Oxford 2003) 1-61: 20-21; Joseph M Curran, *The birth of the Irish Free State: 1921-1923* (Alabama 1980) 192-94, 201.

10   Thomas Towey, 'Hugh Kennedy and the constitutional development of the Irish Free State, 1922-1923' *Irish Jurist* 12 (1977) 355-70.

11   Thomas Jones, *Whitehall diary* (ed) Keith Middlemas (3vols. London 1969-71) iii 201-2.

signed.[12] Hugh Kennedy became its first attorney general although the office of the attorney general was not mentioned in the new constitution which he had done so much to bring about; its function, however, was i.e. that of legal adviser.[13]

The legal system at that time was in some confusion as the courts which had been set up by decree of the 1st Dáil, on 29 June 1920, had been suddenly closed down a few days after the outbreak of the civil war in June 1922; the government apparently feared that they would be used by those who opposed the Treaty. However, closure of courts proved not to be sufficient for that purpose since *habeas corpus* applications could still be heard; in fact, that is what happened. So the government decided instead to rescind the original Dáil decree by which the courts had been set up in the first case; this was done on 25 July 1922. Despite the appointment of two judges to tidy up affairs consequent on the decision, much frustration arose as a result of this rescission; it was also feared that the British courts would return. In early October the government set up a Committee on the Winding-up of the Dáil Courts; it reported to Kennedy within a week. Judicial commissioners were appointed by the Minister for Home Affairs; eventually, after much debate, the Winding-up Act was passed on 31 July 1923. Although Kennedy was only peripherally involved with the Winding-up commission he was very closely associated with the Courts of Justice Bill which was immediately introduced after the Winding-up Bill was passed. This followed on the Report of the Judiciary Committee; Kennedy had worked on this with lord Glenavy from October 1922 to April 1923, its purpose being to devise a new system of courts to replace those hitherto in operation. To help the passage of the Courts of Justice Bill through the Dáil and Seanad a special motion had to be passed to allow Kennedy to address the Seanad; it eventually got through into law in April 1924.[14]

By that time Kennedy had become a TD; he won a seat in South County Dublin for the newly launched Cumann na nGaedheal party at the elections of August 1923, the first to be held under the new regime. His tenure of the Dáil seat was short, however, for not long after the Courts of Justice Bill had been passed, he was appointed chief justice of the Free State on 5 June 1924.[15] In some

---

12 Murphy, *Ireland in the twentieth century*, 57.

13 Casey, *The Irish law officers*, 2.

14 Mary Kotsonouris, *The winding up of the Dáil Courts: 1922-1925* (Dublin 2004) 1, 17-26, 32-3, 37-41, 67-9, 76, 251; Eunan O'Halpin, 'Politics and the state', J R Hill (ed), *A new history of Ireland* VII Ireland, 1921-84 (Oxford 2003) 86-126: 109-110; Towey, 'Hugh Kennedy', 364.

15 Kenneth Ferguson, *King's Inns barristers: 1868-2004* (Dublin 2005) 219; Murphy, *Ireland in the twentieth century*, 59.

respects he could now be seen as being the equivalent of the lord chancellor in the *ancien regime,* a number of whom, as we have seen, had lived in the Clonskeagh-Roebuck area; in reality he was quite different given the major restructuring of the courts system which he had helped to bring about through the Courts of Justice Act. At his swearing in ceremony held in refurbished buildings in Dublin castle, speaking in Irish and English, Kennedy said 'This is surely a precious moment ... when, after a week of centuries, Irish courts, fashioned in freedom by an *Oireachtas* again assembled, are thrown open to administer justice according to laws made in Ireland by free Irish citizens for the well-being of our dearly beloved land and people. ... The judicial authority which we shall exercise ...is... derived under God from the people'. There was no reference to the crown or its representative in his address and the customary robes were not worn.[16]

The courts continued to transact business at Dublin castle for a period of seven years while the much-damaged Four Courts was restored. When the time approached for the return Kennedy sought to put preparations in train to have this done in a ceremonial manner. However, the Executive Council rejected his proposals; the country was not yet settled and it was thought that a formal opening ceremony might invite some opponent to wreck the building. In the event the Four Courts were re-opened on 12 October 1931 without any special formalities although Kennedy, at his first sitting, did make a point of thanking Mr Byrne, the principal architect of the Board of Works, for the quality of the restoration. One of the court rooms in the refurbished building is called after Kennedy.[17]

From the beginning, the Free State was determined to diminish the limitations imposed on it by its dominion status. This was the thinking behind its application to join many international bodies including the League of Nations. It was also there when attending Commonwealth conferences. Gradually the term 'British Commonwealth of Nations' replaced the older one 'British Empire'. Other members, especially Canada, had a stake in this process too. This would eventually lead to the enactment by the British Parliament of the Statute of Westminster in December 1931 which recognized that all members of the Commonwealth, including Britain itself, were equal; as well as that, dominion parliaments, including the Dáil, could repeal or amend any Westminster

---

16 Ferguson, *King's Inns barristers,* 104-06.
17 Gerard Hogan, 'Hugh Kennedy, the Childers Habeas Corpus application and the return to the Four Courts', Caroline Costello (ed), *The Four Courts: 200 years. Essays to commemorate the bicentenary of the Four Courts* (Dublin 1996) 177-219: 207-17.

legislation which affected them. In all of this Kennedy played a crucial role.[18]

The one office which had raised the ire of republicans most was that of governor-general as it was the visible representation of the crown in Ireland. It soon became an issue after de Valera came to power in 1932. A clash between James MacNeill, then governor-general, and the new government soon arose. Having been asked to resign he refused so de Valera requested the king to terminate his appointment. The king complied but before a replacement was appointed de Valera asked Kennedy to assume the office while still retaininig that of chief justice. Kennedy refused as he wished to retain the separation of the judiciary from the executive. De Valera tried to get the British government to accept a number of different possibilities including one which would combine his own office as president with that of the governor-general. All were refused. Eventually he adopted a suggestion made by Kennedy at the outset of the controversy; he recommended the appointment of a man of very modest standing. This man would hold the office without any quasi-royal trappings, living in an ordinary house in the suburbs of Dublin and carrying out only those duties which were specifically required of him for the functioning of government under the constitution, all of which were strictly on the advice of the Executive Council. Kennedy's advice was a further reflection of the sharpness of his mind when confronted with what appeared to be an intractable problem.[19]

Apart from the role he played in the political and judicial affairs of Ireland both before and immediately after the setting up of the new state Kennedy's other interests are reflected in his membership of the Royal Society of Antiquaries of Ireland of which he was a fellow and vice-president. He was also vice-president of the Statistical Society, a member of the Royal Irish Academy and a governor of the National Gallery.[20] He continued to live at Newstead on the Clonskeagh road until his sudden death in December 1936. His wife remained living there for only a short period thereafter.

SEÁN MACBRIDE AT ROEBUCK HOUSE: IRISH POLITICS

Up the road at Roebuck house meanwhile relations with the de Valera government had deteriorated after initial hopes were dashed. A new but short-

---

18 Murphy, *Ireland in the twentieth century,* 66; Lawlor, *Seán MacBride: that day's struggle,* 57.

19 Deirdre McMahon, 'The Chief Justice and the Governor General controversy in 1932', *Irish Jurist* 17 (1982) 145-67; Ward, *The Irish constitutional tradition: responsible government and modern Ireland,* 227-28.

20 Boylan, *A dictionary of Irish biography,*206.

lived political party, Cumann Poblachta na hÉireann, had been launched and
Maud Gonne represented it as a candidate in the June 1936 elections; neither she
nor any of its members were elected. At the same time de Valera clamped down
on the IRA. Once again there were political prisoners and hunger strikes were
back; Maud Gonne's protests began again. After a bombing campaign in
England had been approved by the IRA in 1938 Seán MacBride left the organisation and resumed his legal studies. Maud began to write her autobiography *A
servant of the queen*. The bombing campaign brought a response from the Irish
government; the Offences against the State Act, which allowed for internment
without trial, was enacted. Now once more, this time under a new government,
Roebuck house experienced the attention of the police; it was raided in May
1939. In the war, that soon afterwards broke out in Europe, the sympathy of the
MacBrides appears to have been, like so many Irish people at the time, aligned
with Germany and they entertained the German ambassador in Roebuck house
on a number of occasions. Coincidentally, the British representative in Ireland,
Sir John L Maffey, was living just a very short distance away at Farmhill – off the
Goatstown road. Around this time Maud Gonne's health started to deteriorate.
Her son Seán, on the other hand, saw his legal career start to blossom becoming
a Senior Counsel in 1943. In this capacity he attended the inquest of Seán
McCaughey a young IRA man who had died of hunger strike in prison on 11
May 1946. As a result of this and the publicity it brought to the plight of political
prisoners a major impetus was given to the founding of a new political party,
something which had been in gestation for a period of time beforehand.[21]

The first presidential elections under the 1937 constitution, held in 1945,
showed that there was substantial opposition to Fianna Fáil, then in power for
13 years and this was not just from their traditional opponents from the time of
the civil war. A combination of factors played their part in the growth of this
opposition not least of which was the economic situation but also dissaffection
among republicans with the performance of the government. Out of this grew
the desire to found a new political party. This party, Clann na Poblachta, was
inaugurated on 6 July 1946 and aimed to set new standards of public morality in
politics. Seán MacBride was chosen as leader. A new era was dawning on
Roebuck house. MacBride was now committed to achieving his aims through
political action; physical force as a means was now in his past. One of his close
associates in the party, Noel Hartnett, in fact moved into the gate lodge of
Roebuck house; it would later be called 'Redroof', a name it retains to this day.[22]

---

21 Ward, *Maud Gonne*, 168-83; Lawlor, *Seán MacBride*, 130-32.
22 Kevin Rafter, *The Clann: the story of Clann na Poblachta* (Cork 1996) 15, 21-25.

Substantial enthusiasm accompanied the early days of the new party and it grew rapidly. In 1947 it won two out of three by-elections, one of which was won by MacBride in Dublin county. Fearing that de Valera would call a general election and defeat the looming threat posed by the Clann before it had time to organize properly, MacBride challenged him in the Dáil to do so thinking that this would put him off. It did not work; an election was called.[23] MacBride campaigned tirelessly in what was to be a very bitter battle. His mother, Maud Gonne, now old and infirm was energised by it and left what she characteristically called her 'prison house' [Roebuck house] to cast her vote. Given its high expectations the Clann was disappointed with the number of TDs it got elected – 10; nevertheless the elections had left Fianna Fáil with 68 seats incapable of forming a government. The perennial issue of whether a small party shoud join a coalition in government now arose. There were of course a number of other small parties elected as well (there were six parties, counting Independents as one, apart from Fianna Fáil). In the event an inter-party government was formed after agreement was reached as to who would be Taoiseach. MacBride agreed to John A Costello whom he knew from the Law Library; his son, Declan who would later reside in Clonskeagh, was considered by MacBride to be progressive and an asset. The Clann got two ministerial posts in the new government; MacBride in External Affairs and Noël Browne in Health.[24]

Although this government is perhaps best remembered for the manner of its demise, the so-called 'mother and child scheme', there were many other events that characterised it; we are concerned here only with those associated with Seán MacBride. One of these was the rejection of the invitation to join NATO mainly because of the issue of partition. This rejection did not mean that they remained aloof from the countries of Western Europe; on the contrary, they co-operated with them in its economic reconstuction which was closely associated with Marshall Aid. A White Paper drawn up in January 1949 introduced a Long Term Recovery Programme – the first attempt at economic planning in Ireland – at the request of the Organisation for European Economic Co-operation. In July Ireland was represented at a Conference for European Economic Co-operation and she was the first country to agree to accept the jurisdiction of the Court of Human Rights. She was also a founder member of the Council of Europe out of which the EU would eventually emerge. In general, MacBride's time in External

---

23   Murphy, *Ireland in the twentieth century*, 118; Lawlor, *That day's struggle*, 138.
24   Ward, *Maud Gonne*, 189; Lawlor, *That day's struggle*, 138-39, 141, 145; J. Anthony Gaughan (ed), *Memoirs of Senator Joseph Connolly (1885-1961): a founder of modern Ireland* (Dublin 1996) 419.

Affairs saw its role in government become much more significant. However, the government did in time run into the sands with the 'mother and child scheme', the detailed working out of which is still controversial to this day. What is not controversial, however, was that it was a major blow to Clann na Poblachta; thereafter its decline was catastrophic.[25]

The break-up of the government also involved a political falling out between Seán MacBride and Noel Hartnett. John Horgan in his biography of Noël Browne puts this falling out rather colourfully when he writes "By the end of February [1951] the fallout from Noel Hartnett's resignation was still being felt, at least in Clonskeagh, where MacBride and Hartnett were writing to each other from opposite ends of the avenue of Roebuck house and, occasionally, meeting late at night to trade insults."[26]

After Hartnett had left Clann na Poblachta he, along with Noël Browne, organised the Independents TDs who supported de Valera back into power in 1951; in the same year he was elected to the Seanad. It is with the title Senator that his name appears as the occupant of the gate lodge to Roebuck house, Redroof, in 1952 and 1953. In the latter year he re-joined Fianna Fáil. In the election of 1954 the Clann only won 3 seats one of them being won by MacBride. Although offered a cabinet seat by the new Taoiseach, John A Costello, he was forbidden by his party from joining in the coalition; support was given from without. There were, however, tensions within the party. Late in 1956 Tom O'Higgins of Fine Gael visited MacBride at Roebuck house and asked him to propose a vote of confidence in the government which he did. However, within six weeks he was required to do the opposite by the executive of the Clann and the government fell. In the ensuing election Fianna Fail was returned to power; Clann na Poblachta won only one seat and MacBride lost his. He tried to regain his seat in the by-elections of 1958 and 1959 and the general elections of 1961 but was defeated on all occasions. The party stuggled on until 1965 when it finally dissolved itself. This phase of MacBride's political career was effectively over; the larger world stage beckoned. No longer would he have to endure taunts of people like Jack B Yeats who called him 'the gaunt knight, wistful yet severe, in the dilapidated La Mancha of Roebuck'.[27]

By that time his mother was dead. She had found old age and infirmity difficult to handle. She died in Roebuck house on 27 April 1953 after a painful

---

25   Rafter, *The Clann*, 104-06; Murphy, *Ireland in the twentieth century,* 123, 130-31,
26   John Horgan, *Noël Browne: passionate outsider* (Dublin 2000) 126.
27   Gaughan, *Memoirs,* 417 n; Jordan, *Seán MacBride,* 139, 145, 150-56; Murphy, *Ireland in the twentieth century,* 138.

final illness having received the last sacraments; she was 86 years old. Her funeral was large but without political tension; old comrades from Inghninidhe na hÉireann, Cumann na mBan and the IRA followed the hearse from the church of the Sacred Heart, Donnybrook to the republican plot in Glasnevin, stopping for a moment at the GPO. Her coffin had been carried by members of the Standing Committee of Clann na Poblachta from the church to the hearse. Even those who had not agreed with her activities conceded that she was a woman of courage and dignity and that she was sincere in following her cause.[28]

SEÁN MACBRIDE: WORLD POLITICS

With Seán MacBride's entry on to the world's stage Roebuck house would see a completely different type of visitor to those who had arrived in the 1930s. As already noted, as Minister of External Affairs, he was one of the founders of the Council of Europe and had signed the European Convention on Human Rights which included the European Court of Human Rights. It is probably more than a coincidence that he was also the first to take a case to this Convention and to have it heard before the Court in 1957; it was brought against the Irish state on behalf of Gerard Lawless who had been interned without trial. Although defeated it did set a precedent; an outside body could adjudicate on internal affairs within a state in certain circumstances. He succeeded in the same Court in the case of archbishop Makarios of Cyprus; his deportation to the Seychelles by the British government was deemed to be illegal and Makarios went on to become president of Cyprus. Both of these cases had something in common; an attempt to gain freedom for someone illegally detained in prison.

It is not surprising, given his lifetime experience, that when the English lawyer, Peter Benenson, wrote a letter to papers in England and France entitled 'An appeal for Amnesty 1961' urging six governments to release named prisoners one of the first to reply in support of his appeal was Seán MacBride. As a result and within a matter of weeks, Amnesty International was founded at a meeting in Luxembourg on 22/23 July 1961; MacBride was the first chairman of its Organising Committee. Quite soon afterwards he was sent to Prague to find out what had happened to archbishop Beran, the Primate of Czechoslovakia. He had been secretly imprisoned because of a conscientious objection he had towards sweaing allegiance to the communist government. The latter were surprised at MacBride's visit; after initial refusal to respond, the continued activity of Amnesty brought about the release of the archbishop. This was an early example

---

28   Ward, *Maud Gonne*, 191-93; Cardozo, *Maud Gonne*, 409-10.

of the influence Amnesty International was able to exercise on behalf of prisoners of conscience. It afterwards spread globally having branches in almost every country in the world and a huge membership. Its activities were at one with MacBride's earlier activities in Ireland where both he and his mother had worked over a long period on behalf of prisoners. During the early years of Amnesty's existence MacBride helped to develop its policy; he also insisted that the deed of trust for the Prisoners of Conscience fund be regularised. Other important areas also benefitted from his skill and attention at that time such as the internal structures of its Secretariat and the drafting of its constitution. He remained active on its International Executive Committee into his seventies leaving it only in 1974. The building which houses the Irish branch of the organisation bears his name today – Seán MacBride house.[29]

Around the time Amnesty was establishing itself, MacBride was appointed full-time Secretary General to the International Commission of Jurists (ICJ); this involved his taking up residence in Geneva. His wife and children remained at Roebuck house. The Commission of Jurists, a non-governmental organisation, with members from a diverse range of countries, attempted to promote respect for the rule of law; this fitted well with the work then being carried out by Amnesty. Although an institution with a western orientation MacBride nevertheless condemned America's war in Vietnam. His work with ICJ brought him into contact with many heads of government, leading opposition figures and a large variety of important institutions. When it became known that the ICJ was partly funded by the CIA MacBride protested vehemently and later resigned.

In 1973 he was appointed the first United Nations Commissioner for Namibia at the request of the African States of the United Nations; aware of his independence and skill as a diplomat, they held him in high regard. South Africa had refused to relinquish its mandate over Namibia which it had got from the League of Nations although it had expired. As a United Nations Commissioner, MacBride now had the task of getting South Africa out of Namibia; in its stead a UN council would administer the country. For his work there and, as President of the International Peace Bureau, MacBride won the Nobel Peace Prize in 1974. Three years later he was presented, in Dublin, with the Lenin Peace Prize, making him unique in his possession of both of these prizes. The latter was the highest award that the Soviet Union could bestow on a non-citizen and was

---

29 My thanks to Caitriona Lawlor, assistant to Seán MacBride and curator of his archive for providing me with this information which she had published in an article 'Seán MacBride and Amnesty International' in *Village Magazine*.

given in recognition of MacBride's 'selfless service to [the] noble ideals of peace and progress'. Perhaps even more uniquely he was awarded the American Medal for Justice in 1978 and was the first non-American citizen to whom such an award would be made. Many other awards such as honorary degrees were conferred on him by a variety of countries.

However, now 74 years, old he returned to live in Roebuck house. His wife, Catalina, had died there two years previously. After a requiem mass in the pro-cathedral she was buried in the republican plot in Glasnevin alongside Maud Gonne. Although she had been a political activist in her early years, her mature yeas were centred on Roebuck house looking after her family including Maud Gonne in her declining years. At Roebuck house MacBride received many distinguished visitors at this time including Bruce Kent of the Campaign for Nuclear Disarment in England, Paul O'Dwyer – an eminent Irish-American, bishop Desmond Tutu and other Anti-Apartheid as well as anti-colonial activists and Venerable Gyotsu Sato, a Buddist monk working with the International Peace Bureau; also visiting were many Russians, Namibians, UN staffers, Amnesty members, former IRA and Clann na Poblachta activists, politicians, academics and personal friends such as Una O'Higgins O'Malley, Proinsias MacAonghusa and Kevin White.

Although semi-retired, MacBride was still involved with a number of organizations such as Amnesty, the Campaign for Nuclear Disarmament, the Irish Council for Civil Liberties; he also supported Ireland's entry into the European Community. He even agreed to allow his name to be put forward as an agreed candidate for the presidency of Ireland; it did not happen as the political parties did not agree on the matter. The problems in Northern Ireland troubled him greatly. One particular aspect of this with which he became directly involved was an Irish-American movement set up to fight discrimination against Catholics – The Irish National Caucus; he became chairman of its Irish branch. In November 1984 his name was appended to a set of principles which it sought to have American companies, with subsidiaries in Northern Ireland, adhere to – the MacBride Principles. These were widely promoted in America; on this side of the Atlantic they were not welcomed by the British but also by others on the nationalist side including the Irish government in Dublin. After protests, some adjustments were made to them in 1986 with an input from a trade union representative from the North. In 1987 the British government announced that anti-discrimination laws would be introduced; they were enacted in the following year. But before their enactment, MacBride was dead. He died at Roebuck house on 15 January 1988 shortly before his 84th birthday. His funeral mass was held at the pro-cathedral where he regularly attended the Latin mass sung by the Palestrina choir; afterwards he was buried in Glasnevin beside his wife and his mother. With this, the active involvement of the residents of Roebuck house in Irish (and later international) politics which had begun when Mrs Despard and Maud Gonne bought the house in June 1922 and was continued by Sean MacBride, came to an end. It had spanned almost 66 years during which it was always centrally involved in a particular way with issues related to prisoners and, more generally, the human rights of all.[30]

---

30 Jordan, *MacBride,* 157-87; personal communication from Caitriona Lawlor concerning visitors to Roebuck house.

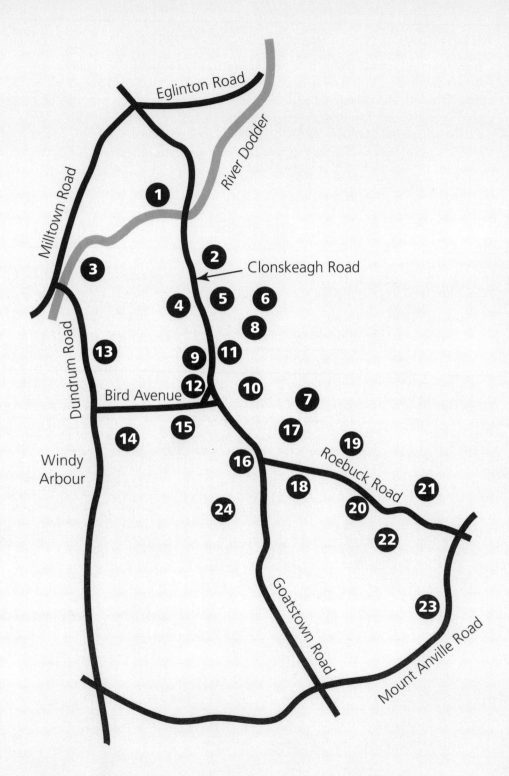

12

Clonskeagh emerges as a residential area in the late eighteenth century

I N 1659 THERE WERE ONLY 19 PEOPLE reported as living in Rabucke (Roebuck), 2 English, 17 Irish. Quite obviously the area comprising Roebuck, which would have included Clonskeagh, was at that time very much a rural area. This information only refers to those who lived on the south side of the river Dodder. There is no similar detail on the number living on the other side but it may be assumed that it was quite small also given the added factor that the area there, which may be considered part of Clonskeagh, was very much smaller than that for which we have the numbers (it was a little over 6 acres, while Roebuck was over 822 acres).[1]

Being close to Dublin would not in any way have, at that time, influenced the size of the population there. Up to the end of the 16th century Dublin was still, in effect, a garrison city which tried to govern a country which was only partly under its control. John Speed's map (1610) shows it to be enclosed by medieval walls with Trinity College located outside. A settled period began around 1660 after the end of the civil war and the restoration of the monarchy; expansion commenced and the walls disappeared. Halted for a while by the Jacobite wars later in the century it resumed when Protestantism was in the ascendancy after the Treaty of Limerick. The contrast between Speed's map and that of Brooking (1728) clearly shows that considerable development had by that time taken place. College green had by then been surrounded by buildings and the space between the college and Cork hill (i.e. Dame street) had buildings. Rocque's map of 1754 shows, inter alia, that the earl of Kildare had built himself a house in Molesworth Fields. By 1799 the map, included by Malton in his volume along with his plates, shows a city the boundary of which was seven

---

1   Pender, *A census of Ireland c1659*, 381; Ball & Hamilton, *Parish of Taney*, 2.

miles in circumference and with a population of 200,000; in Speed's day it was about one mile and a population of 20,000.[2] In 1800 it was easily the second largest city in the islands of Britain and Ireland.[3]

This expansion of the city in the 18th century took a considerable time before its effects were felt in Clonskeagh area. According to Samuel Lewis, writing in 1837, there had only been one house (i.e. substantial house) apart from Roebuck castle in the area 50 years previously i.e. in 1787.[4] That date, therefore, is an important marker. Only after it, can the houses which were about to be built in the area be dated. But the reference by Lewis contains within it an unstated notion that he finds it remarkable that in that 50 years so many houses, which he could see there in 1837, had been built. It is that which allowed the compiler of *Thom's Directory* of the 1840 to state that Clonskeagh was 'studded with gentlemen's seats and neat villas'. It is therefore within that period that the rise of Clonskeagh and Roebuck as a desirable place to live began to take hold.

The growth in the number of people with businesses in Dublin who now began to acquire houses in Clonskeagh and Roebuck can be seen in the effect it had on one particular item – transport. It is possible to detect this effect in the Dublin almanacs of the time. In these, notices appear regularly about the charges for transport to and from various areas within and around the city as set by the Carriage Office. Already in 1746, John Bush writing about a visit to Dublin stated that 'the rates of hackney-coaches and sedans, are established here [Dublin] as in London, for the different distances, or set-downs, as they are here called'.[5] These rates are given in various almanacs and directories for the city and surrounding countryside, although, of course, rates for sedans are confined to the city. One can observe in these, for example, the rates set by the Office for the years 1791, 1792 and 1793; these cover a variety of places near the city but no reference is made to either Clonskeagh or Roebuck. However, for the first time, in the year 1794 Clonskeagh (but not Roebuck) appears. In that year, the rate set is two shillings and two pence for a coach, one shilling and one penny for a noddy or a jaunting car (a noddy and a jaunting car were two quite separate types of vehicle). It seems highly unlikely that the Carriage Office is here operating pro-actively, that is,

---

2   Maxwell, *Dublin under the Georges*, 56-59.
3   Cullen, *Princes and pirates: the Dublin Chamber of Commerce*, 13.
4   Samuel Lewis, *A topographical dictionary of Ireland* (2vols, London 1837) ii 518-19.
5   J. B[ush], *Hibernia curiosa: a letter from a gentleman in Dublin to his friend at Dover in Kent, giving a general view of the manners, customs, dispositions, etc., of the inhabitants of Ireland, collected in a tour through Ireland in 1764* (2nd ed, London 1782) 23-4. The letter (and the book) ends with the author signing off as J. B., Lucas's Coffee-house, Dublin 1764 (ibid. 143).

setting the rate before the drivers of coaches, noddies or jaunting cars started to be hired by people wishing to be transported to Clonskeagh. It is much more likely that this service was being provided for some years beforehand which resulted in some complaints from disgruntled passengers who felt that they had been overcharged or had otherwise suffered from the whims of non-controlled drivers. These complaints are the most likely reason why the Carriage Office set the rate, probably in 1793, since it appeared for the first time in *The Gentleman's and Citizen's Almanack* compiled by John Watson Stewart for the year 1794.

If demand for the services of these hackneys had been growing in the years before 1794, then it is a good indication that the traffic of people, who could afford these considerable prices, between the city and Clonskeagh was on the increase; that, in turn would be a reflection of the number of such people both living and carrying out commercial enterprises in Clonskeagh and those visiting them for social or business reasons. The fact that in the early 1790s a critical mass of travellers, as it were, had been achieved would be sufficient to allow one to dub Clonskeagh a residential area in the neighbourhood of Dublin at that time even if lieutenant Archer, some ten years later, did not deem it to be a village.[6] Roebuck, incidentally, as a separate place to be given a rate by the Carriage Office for hackneys of the various types, did not appear in the almanacs until 1831 although it is possible that it may have appeared one or two years earlier since the sources for the years 1829 and 1830 are not readily available. Roebuck would have continued to be more residential, not having the industry that existed in Clonskeagh.

A further development in the provision of transport for people who wished to live outside the city but do their business within it was the proposal made in 1816 by Mr Robert Turbett that a public conveyance be established between Dublin, Dundrum and Enniskerry; the route taken would be via Clonskeagh. A committee of leading inhabitants was set up and plans submitted which envisaged one coach going to and from Enniskerry each day and another to and from Dundrum – the Enniskerry coach to be drawn by four horses with two spares while the Dundrum one by three horses without a spare. In the event, a scheme was established whereby two coaches, each carrying six people inside and twelve outside, travelled between Dublin and Enniskerry. One set out from each place in the morning and returned in the evening. The fare from Dundrum was 1s-3d inside and 10d outside. The starting point in Dublin was first Aungier street but later Molesworth street.[7]

In 1824 the coach leaving Molesworth street is called the Post coach in *Pigott & Co's Directory and Guide*; it left at 4pm every day except Sunday. In 1830

---

6   Archer, *Statistical survey of the county Dublin*, 102.
7   Ball & Hamilton, *Parish of Taney*, 201-203.

Watson's Almanack reports the timing of what it refers to as the Day Coach which leaves Enniskerry in the morning, arrives at 17 South Anne's street at 10 am and returns to Enniskerry at 4pm each day. It would appear that the demand for this public service continued to grow such that by 1848 *Thom's Directory* could report that 'Three omnibuses ply through Clonskeagh from and to Dundrum several times a day'. Although this makes no reference to the Enniskerry coach, it was still operating. During the next decade there is a subtle change in the wording of the report in *Thom's Directory*; in its 1858 edition it reports 'Three omnibuses ply to Clonskeagh from Dublin several times a day'. Clonskeagh, which previously had just been a stop on the way to other destinations, had in the middle of the 19th century become a destination in itself.

In keeping with the evidence to be gleaned from trends in transport demands which help establish a date for the emergence of 'modern' Clonskeagh and Roebuck, it is worth noting that until approximately the 1830s Dublin directories and almanacs confined themselves to the people living within the city. Around that time tentative efforts were begun to give information about the people living in areas close to and surrounding the city; these efforts improved as time went on. This would have reflected the growing number of people living just outside the immediate confines of the city and probably also to the growing needs of the ever-expanding postal services. Indeed, the Post Office itself did have a Dublin street directory published around this time.

In what follows, efforts are made to track the emergence of new houses in the Clonskeagh area from the late 18th century onwards. However, mainly because of the difficulty in finding the date on which the various houses were built, it is proposed that instead of taking a chronological approach to the subject a geographical one will be taken; that is, starting at the closest point to the city the houses are discussed as one proceeds outwards. Some exceptions to this will be highlighted at the appropriate place. Extensive use has been made of the directories but it has not been deemed necessary to footnote them all. To help pinpoint the location of the houses a special map is drawn to accompany this chapter; on it are found the numbers of each house which is assigned to it in the descriptions which are now given.

VERGEMOUNT HOUSE, LATER ISOLATION HOSPITAL, LATER STILL CLONSKEAGH HOSPITAL

Although it no longer exists, Vergemount house has left a legacy to the area in its name. Before its demolition, the house was located in the grounds of what is now Clonskeagh hospital (location no. 1 on map). It would appear that it was built as his country house by John Crosthwaite, a watchmaker of 27 Grafton

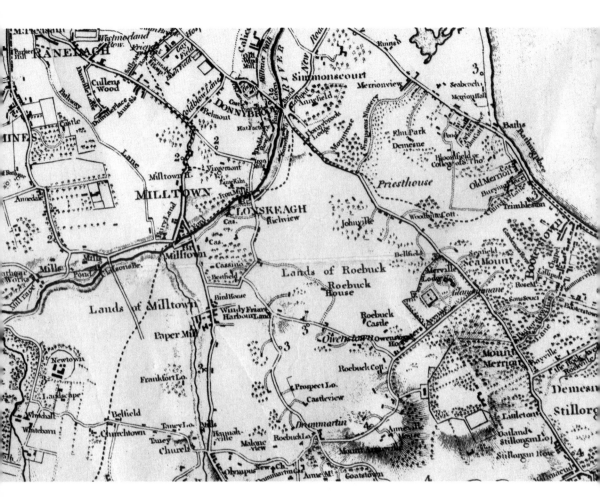

Taylor's map of the environs of Dublin (1816)

street in Dublin. The date of building has not been discovered but it seems to have been at some point in the late 1700s; there is no sign of it in Rocque's map of the area drawn around 1760 but it is clearly marked in Taylor's map of 1816.

Crosthwaite was born on 29 September 1745 and aged 15 he was apprenticed (1760) in Christ Church Yard. From about 1772 to 1775 he worked in Dame street and transferred his business to the Sign of Kings Arms, 27 Grafton street (formerly known as the Sign of Eagle & Watch). In 1795 he was joined formally by his son in the business as it then became known as J. Crosthwaite & Son, Watch and Clockmakers. It traded under this title until 1801 and then became known as J. Crosthwaite & Co. During this period a portrait of Mrs Crosthwaite of Grafton street was painted by William Cummings (in 1829 he was Treasurer and in 1830 he was President and Trustee of the Royal Hibernian Academy of Painting, Sculpture and Architecture, incorporated by Royal Charter on 5 August, 1823 (Watson's *Dublin Directory* for 1829, 1830)), a sure sign of the prosperity of his company at this period. From 1803 the company became known as Crosthwaite & Hodges and moved next door to number 26 in 1804 but apparently moved back to number 27 in 1810. He died on 30 January, 1829.[8]

It has been asserted that Crosthwaite called his country residence Vergemount house because 'he invented the verge watch'.[9] An investigation into the truth of this matter leads to the initial impression that it is unlikely since, what is known to watchmakers as the 'verge escapement' (an 'escapement' is what makes a watch or clock 'tick'[10]) has been known for over 500 years and was adapted to a pendulum in the seventeenth century, probably by the watchmaker Huygens, who was born in 1629. It is therefore untrue to say that John Crosthwaite 'invented' the verge watch; he is not listed among those who lodged horological patents in England at the time. However, the adaptation of the verge escapement to the pendulum by Huygens occurred perhaps less than a hundred years before Crosthwaite began his career in 1760 and the perfection of the adaptation, to improve the accuracy of timekeeping over the lifetime of the watch, was likely to have been still an ongoing process when he was working.

With that in mind, it is worth examining an extract from an entry given in an authoritative listing of the watchmakers and clockmakers of the world: "Crosthwaite – John. *Dublin.* 1760-1800. Experimented with pendulum supported by steel knife edges on diamond plates, and pub(lished) desc(ription) in 1788 and 1800." (1760-1800 are the dates of the earliest and latest known records.)[11] From this it appears most likely that he took a prominent part in the ongoing development of the process since he 'experimented with pendulum supported by steel knife edges on diamond plates' and, crucially, he published the results of his work as early as 1788 and again in 1800. Now this is not what one expects from an 'ordinary' or journeyman watchmaker, plying his trade. This is the work of a man actively interested in the science of watches, keen to make improvements in how they worked. Although it is not immediately apparent what his contribution was to improving the performance of the verge

---

8   William Gailland Stuart, *Watch and clockmakers in Ireland* (Dublin 2000) 26.

9   Hall, *The Bank of Ireland*, 484.

10   Stuart, *Watch and clockmakers in Ireland*, p. xvi.

11   G. H. Baillie, *Watchmakers and clockmakers of the world*, Volume 1 (London 1929, 3rd ed. repr. 1996) 71.

escapement, when it was adapted to a pendulum, by experimenting with the manner in which the pendulum was suspended, it would not be an exaggeration to say that he 'invented' at least some aspect of the verge watch.

In any case, these experiments carried out over such a long period indicate an ongoing involvement by John Crosthwaite with the problem of perfecting the operation of the verge watch and it is therefore reasonable to believe that he would include the word 'verge' in the name of his new country residence 'Vergemount house'. The fact that the name of this house and surrounding area was sometimes spelled 'Virgemount' need not take from this conclusion as pronunciation of words and their orthography can vary for a variety of reasons, not least the custom of a particular time. John Crosthwaite was not merely a watchmaker, albeit one of considerable substance; it would appear that he was also a business man of some standing since he was a director of The Grand Canal Company, the greatest infrastructural project of his day.[12]

John Crosthwaite died, as we have seen, in January 1829; whether at Vergemount or Grafton street has not been discovered. The last reference to him living at Vergemount is found in *Wilson's Dublin Directory* for 1818. The next definite information we have is that Rev John Clarke Crosthwaite was living there in 1832. He was born in 1801 in Dublin, possibly at Vergemount house; he was educated by the famous Mr White (or Whyte) of Grafton street and later at Trinity College. He was ordained a deacon in 1827 and a priest in 1830. In 1832, the year before he married Elizabeth Todd, he was living in Vergemount house. His father's first name was Charles; this rules out the possibility that he was a son of the man who had built Vergemount house, John Crosthwaite. It seems most likely, however, that he was his grandson as the evidence relating to John's sons places their birth at a considerably earlier date than 1801.

We have already noted that in 1795 John Crosthwaite had been joined by his son in his business in Grafton street, not, it should be added, as an apprentice but as a partner since the firm then took on the name of John Crosthwaite & Son; this suggests that the (unnamed) son was an adult in 1795. As well as that an older Rev John Crosthwaite, born in Dublin in 1783, would seem a more likely candidate to have been his son. He, incidentally, went on to become chaplain to the duchess of Kent, the mother of queen Victoria. In any case, we find Rev John Clarke Crosthwaite living at Vergemount house in 1832. In 1834 and in 1835 he is listed as having a boarding school there but no further details

---

12   A. L. Rawlings, *The science of clocks and watches*, British Horological Institute (Upton 1993) 106; Charles Aked, *Complete list of English horological patents up to 1853* (Ashford, Kent 1975); Hall, *The Bank of Ireland*, 484.

about this enterprise could be found. Between 1834 and 1844 he was a vicar choral at Christ Church cathedral; this may have stimulated his interest in editing the manuscript of the *Book of Obits and Martyrology* of that cathedral which he published in 1844. Most of the other works he published were concerned with ecclesiastical matters. In one of these, a collection of a series of articles that had already appeared in the *British magazine*, he was careful to point out that 'the greater proportion of these volumes had been printed before Mr Newman had declared himself a Roman Catholic, and while many of his friends were unwilling to believe that he had any intention of taking such a step'. During most of this period he lived at Vergemount house (1832- 1842) where it is most likely that his children, including Sir Charles Hawke Todd Crosthwaite, was born. Thereafter he served as rector of St Mary at Hill and St Andrew Hubbard, London until his death in 1874.[13]

After he had left Vergemount house in 1842 colonel Charles Gordon lived there for a few years before Dr Todd, FTCD, whom we have already met, took up residence in 1847. A brother-in-law of Crosthwaite he was joined by his mother, Mrs Eliza Todd in 1850; she remained on until 1856 when the last connection with the Crosthwaites was severed. It was then bought by J Donegan; his son Patrick who lived there, apart from a short interval, from 1860 to 1884 was, like the original owner, a watchmaker and jeweller with premises at 32 Dame street. Afterwards it was occupied first by Samuel Murray (1885-89), then by the Thompson family (1891-1900) before remaining vacant for three years. That was the end of its existence as a private dwelling house. It then became the site of an Isolation hospital under the control of the Conjoint Boards of Pembroke and Rathmines Urban Council and Clonskeagh hospital is still located in its grounds; the house itself has long since been demolished. (The history of the hospital is discussed in Chapter 16).

One final point about Vergemount house; the present entrance to Clonskeagh hospital was not always where the entrance to the house was located. Judging from Duncan's map of 1821 and the first Ordnance Survey map of 1837 it appears to have been where the entrance to Vergemount hall now is. However

---

13   Leslie & Wallace, *Clergy of Dublin and Glendalough*, 525-6; *The Post Office Annual Directory* for 1832; Stuart, *Watches and clockmakers in Ireland*, 26; Rev J C Crosthwaite, *Modern hagiology: an examination of the nature and tendency of some legendary and devotional works lately published under the sanction of the Rev J H Newman, the Rev Dr Pusey, and the Rev F Oakley* (2vols, London 1846) i, iv-v; *The Post Office Annual Directory* for 1833, 1838; *Pettigrew & Oulton Street Directory* for 1834, 1836, 1840; *Dublin Almanac and General Register of Ireland* for 1835, 1837, 1838, 1839, 1840, 184, 1842, 1843.

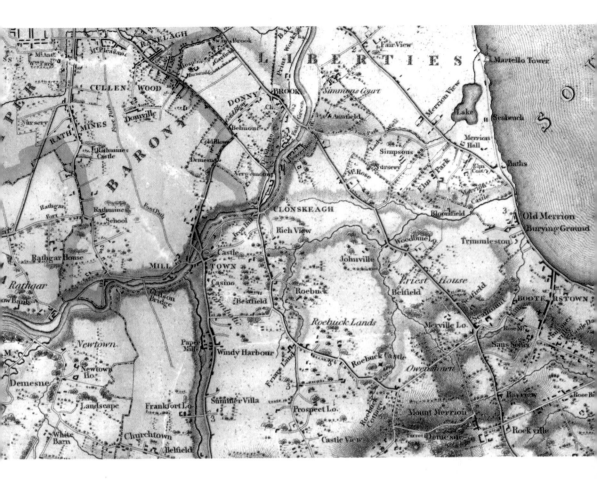

Duncan's map of the county of Dublin (1821)

it seems to have changed over the next number of years. To explain where it then was we first note the change in the shape of the road in front of the property that was made afterwards. At the present time there is a curving right-hand bend in a much widened road as it passes the grounds of Clonskeagh hospital but in previous years it was a sharp right-angled bend. The original road shape can be still seen immediately in front of Ashton's licensed house; the grounds of Vergemount house would have sloped down towards that road with the river a little farther on. A short distance after that right-angled bend the entrance was located. It was quite soon after the bend, not as far as Clonskeagh terrace which is on the opposite of the road. A gate lodge is marked at the point in the first Ordnance Survey map of the area. However, it can be more clearly seen in the map prepared for *Thom's Directory* by the Ordnance Survey in 1875.[14] In this, the driveway to the house is clearly discernible. From the entrance it goes parallel to the Clonskeagh road, almost as far as the end of the property before the bridge, then takes a sharp right hand turn and heads to the house which was situated to the very back of the grounds.

RICHVIEW HOUSE, LATER MASONIC SCHOOL, NOW SCHOOL OF ARCHITECTURE, DEPARTMENT OF REGIONAL AND URBAN PLANNING, AND DEPARTMENT OF ENVIRONMENTAL STUDIES UNIVERSITY COLLEGE, DUBLIN

Going southwards across Clonskeagh bridge one soon meets the entrance to Richview house (location no. 2 on map). It is on the left hand side immediately opposite where Whitethorn road meets Clonskeagh road; its piers with their spherical ornaments on top are still visible. This house was called 'Richview', a name that was later to be transferred to other entities such as Brown and Nolan's 'Richview Press' and the 'Richview Business Park'. The occupant in the late 1700s was James Potts, best known as the proprietor of one of Dublin's newspapers, *Saunder's News Letter*. Described as a bookbinder, bookseller, printer, publisher and lottery office keeper, he was born c. 1733 and his working career spanned the years 1747-1796. His first known work is dated 1759 and he was in business on his own from 1761 after serving his apprenticeship to George Faulkner; his place of work and office was the Swift's Head, 74 Dame street. In April of the same year he married Elizabeth Irwin in St Werburgh's church. By 1766 he was a master printer employing 4 journeymen and 5 apprentices. Two years later he began selling lottery tickets at his office and in 1780 he joined in with a group of three other men to buy 500 lottery tickets costing upwards of £7,000. In 1783 he was admitted as a free member of the Guild of St Luke the Evangelist with which a number of Dublin booksellers were associated. He stood for election to the Common Council of the Corporation in 1786.

He published the *Dublin Courier* from 1760 to 1766; in 1771 he started the *Hibernian Magazine*. From 1755 he printed *Saunders News Letter and Daily Advertiser*; along with John Giffard, he purchased this publication in 1772. He also joined others in publishing Shakespeare's *Midsummer Night's Dream* (1764), his *Works* (1766) and *Timon of Athens* (1772) and Smollet's *Humphrey Clinker* (1771). As well as that he tendered for the bookbinding of Parliamentary Journals

---

14   This may be seen in the Gilbert Collection, Dublin City Library and Archive, Pearse street, Dublin 2.

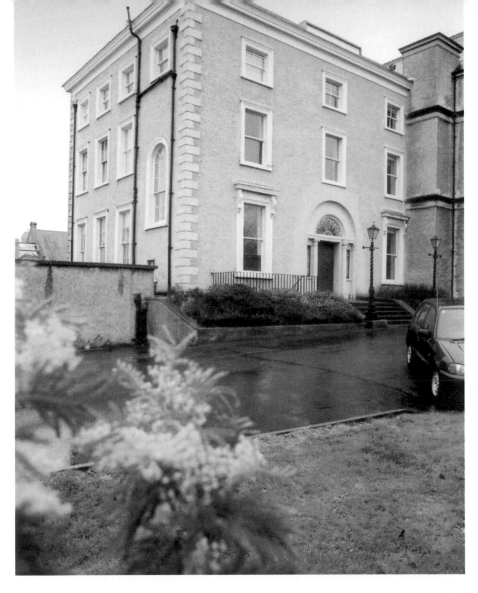

Richview house today: part of the School of Architecture, UCD
(*Photographer: Matt Walsh*)

in 1785. In 1783 he was among the original subscribers of capital (£2,000) to the newly founded Bank of Ireland; by 1786 he was reported in Exshaw's *Magazine* as being in possession of £3,000 worth of Bank Stock. In 1792 he entered a partnership with an anonymous person in a calico and cotton business, his investment in the business amounting to £3,000.[15] Politically *Saunder's News*

---

15 Ball, *History of county Dublin*, ii 80; Munter, *Dictionary of the print trade in Ireland*, 212-13; Pollard, *A dictionary of members of the Dublin book trade*, 463-64; Hall, *The Bank of Ireland: 1783-1946*, 509.

Letter was pretty innocuous; it relied in the main on advertisements. For the rest it depended upon news from abroad which it published without editing. This led the historian R. R. Madden to remark that 'it could not have been more destitute of Irish news if it had been published in Iceland'.[16]

However, this did not prevent its owner from becoming embroiled in a much publicized row over an item it contained in 1794. By this time the man with whom Potts had originally bought the paper, John Giffard, had gone his own way and had become the proprietor of the *Dublin Journal*. This publication was fanatically in favour of the government and, to quote Madden again, its owner Giffard was 'a privileged bully and state protected ruffian of the press'.[17] Perhaps because the *Saunder's News Letter* published much foreign news unedited and since the French Revolution occurred in 1789, there was a lot about it in that paper; or perhaps it was personal animosity since their co-ownership had broken up but Giffard, in the *Dublin Journal* during 1794, accused Potts of propagating Jacobinism (i.e. a form of radicalism that arose in Paris during the Revolution). Potts was furious since the accusation appeared to suggest that he was under the control of the United Irishmen. He replied in his own paper by writing a satirical piece about Giffard in which he referred to him by his nickname 'The Dog in Office'. This led to a much reported confrontation between the two protagonists.

This happened just outside the church at Taney in Dundrum. Although James Potts had his business premises at 62 Dame street and, presumably, his city home at that address too, he was, nevertheless, a churchwarden at the old Taney church; he was also one of the two governors of the first known school associated with it. The connection with this church would have come about through his country residence at Richview in Clonskeagh. On Sunday, October 19th 1794, while Potts was performing his duty as churchwarden after service in the church the sexton brought a message to him to the effect that Mr Giffard wanted to see him. When Potts went to Giffard, the latter suggested that they go to an adjoining field as the church door was too public a place. When there, Giffard pulled the previous day's *Saunder's News Letter* from his pocket and challenged Potts to a duel. While moving towards Giffard's house, where preparations for the duel were to be made, Giffard exclaimed 'A parcel of rascally printers. And you (addressing Potts) the greatest rascal of them all'. When Potts demurred Giffard struck him on the mouth. Then knocking Potts to the ground Giffard and his son Hardinge horsewhipped him.

---

16 B. Inglis, *The freedom of the press in Ireland: 1784 –1841* (London 1954) 84. The citation from the work of R. R. Madden: ibid 21.

17 Madden, *History of Irish periodical literature*, ii 104, 117.

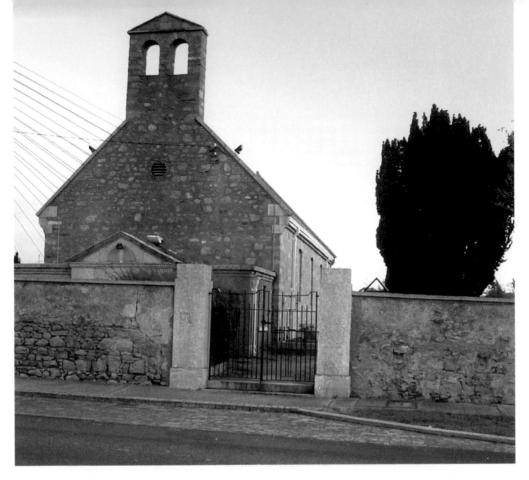

Old Taney church

At the trial to which the incident gave rise, Hardinge was acquitted but the jury found Giffard guilty of assault and of provoking Potts to a duel. Giffard was sentenced to five months in prison for the assault; however, he served only one month, the rest was commuted by the lord lieutenant, 'the humane earl Camden'. Giffard was, after all, a fanatical government supporter. Potts never recovered from the beating. He died, aged 63, in April 1796 at Richview according to a report in the *Dublin Evening Post* – a tragic end for its early occupant who was described as an 'upright, inoffensive, unassuming and courteous trader'. He was buried at St Werburgh's church.

He was succeeded by his nephew, James Potts who continued the business at 74 Dame street. However, *Saunder's News Letter* became the property of John Potts of Athlone who was joined by James' widow, Elizabeth. Together they continued to print *Saunder's News Letter* 'on Tory and genuine Protestant principles' up to 1800; despite this it is believed to have been the most important periodical for its reporting of the rebellion of 1798. It is not clear whether

Richview remained in the Potts' family after his death. They, however, continued to hold *Saunders News Letter*, in *Wilson's Dublin Directory* for 1825, 1828 and 1829 John D Potts, Proprietor of *Saunders News-letter* is listed with an address at 74 Dame street. There is no reference made to any attachment that he may have had to Richview in these entries.

However, in the following year, 1830, *Wilson's Dublin Directory* contains a list of barristers which includes the entry: John Duffy, Richview, Clonskeagh; it further tells us that he had been called to the bar during the Easter term in 1827. Duffy remained in residence at Richview until 1834.[18] The name of the person or persons who resided at Richview between James Potts' death in 1796 and the reference to John Duffy being in residence there in 1830, therefore, remains undiscovered. However, it is possible that John Duffy's father was already there in 1806. In Walker's *Hibernian Magazine* it is reported that in July of the same year John Duffy, Roebuck, Co Dublin married Catherine Nolan, also of Roebuck.[19] Given the similarity of name, the Roebuck address, the date of the wedding and the fact that he was of sufficient importance to have his wedding reported in the *Magazine*, there is a possibility that this John Duffy was the father of the man whom we have already identified as living at Richview in the early 1830s. It could, however, have been in fact the same John Duffy rather than his father although, if this were the case, it would seem a little strange that he was called to the Bar twenty one years after his marriage in 1806. Whichever was the case, it is a possibility that the Duffy family succeeded the Potts at Richview at some date around the turn of the eighteenth and nineteenth centuries. However, one must be cautious with such a conclusion as, according to a report in the *Freeman's Journal* dated 2 November 1843, John Duffy, merchant (i.e. not the barrister) of Roebuck, was a member of the Special Jury Panel of the county of Dublin for that year. He could have been the man whose marriage in 1806 was, as noted above, reported in Walker's *Hibernian Magazine*. If he was and if he was the father of the John Duffy, barrister, who we know lived at Richview until 1834, then he must have lived at a different house in Roebuck; our sources are simply not sufficient to come to any definite conclusion.

---

18   Inglis, *Freedom of the press in Ireland*, 59, 84; Madden, *History of Irish periodical literature*, ii 104, 117, 126, 132; Munter, *Dictionary of the print trade in Ireland*, 213; Pollard, *Dictionary of members of the Dublin book trade*, 463-64; *Wilson's Dublin Directory* for 1830, 1831; *The Post Office Annual Directory and Calendar* for years 1832 & 1833; *Pettigrew & Oulton Street Directory* for 1834 & 1836; Ball & Hamilton, *The parish of Taney*, 138, 188.

19   Henry Farrar, *Irish marriages: being an index to the marriages in Walker's Hibernian Magazine 1771 to 1812* (London 1890) 448.

After John Duffy ceased to reside at Richview in 1834 Michael Powell, who had a city address at 3 Merrion street East, moved in and remained there until at least 1844.[20] His name is of special interest since it has been stated, without the sources on which it is based being given, that Richview was 'built about 1790 for the Powell family'.[21] If that is the case, then James Potts who we know lived there at least as early as 1794 (the year he was churchwarden at Taney church) would have been a very early lessee. For the next few years after Michael Powell's departure, 1845 to 1847 inclusive, the sources are silent. However, in 1848, Richview was occupied by the Venerable John Torrens D. D., archdeacon of Dublin, who also had an address at Narraghmore Glebe, Ballitore. The Rev Torrens was born in 1768 in co. Derry and was educated at Trinity College, Dublin where he received his BA in 1789, his MA in 1811 and his BD and DD in 1824. After serving as curate and rector in various parts of the country he was appointed archdeacon of Dublin and rector of St Peter's, Aungier street in 1811, offices he held until his death on 9 June, 1851 at Narraghmore rectory. He was the last archdeacon of Dublin in whose Corps (i.e. possession) Taney had been since 1274 (this is discussed in the chapter which deals with the ecclesiastical history of the area). One of his daughters, Elizabeth Grace, married Rev William Chichester on 8 April 1858. In 1868, Rev Chichester was made 1st baron O'Neill of Shane's Castle.[22]

The following is a summary of subsequent residents of Richview with dates as found in *Thom's Directory*: 1858 -59 Captain Stirling Stewart; 1860/1 no entry; 1862-64 George McDowell FTCD; 1865-68 Herbert Manders, esq.; 1869 General Archibald Little, CB.; 1870-71 Herbert Manders, esq.; 1872-73 Thomas H Pitt, Captain, RN; 1874-83 Mrs Herbert Manders; 1884 Vacant; 1885 Charles Barden Hely esq. (Charles Barden Hely, Son & Co, Wholesale and Export Stationers, 17 Dame street); 1886 *Masonic Boys' Orphan School*.

Much of Richview's subsequent history can be found below in Chapter 15 where the Masonic Boys' Orphan school is dealt with. After this school ceased to function, University College, Dublin (UCD) bought, in 1980, the house and its grounds (17.4 acres at the time) at a cost of £2.1 million which was provided by the government in return for the college's agreement to vacate the part of the buildings in Merrion street which it had occupied. This is now the Department

---

20   Ibid. for 1835, 1836; *Dublin Almanac and General Register of Ireland* for 1837, 1838, 1839; *Pettigrew & Oulton Street Directory* for 1840; *Dublin Almanac* for 1841, 1842, 1843, 1844.

21   McCartney, *UCD, a national idea*, 397.

22   *Thom's Directory* 1848; Leslie & Wallace, *Clergy of Dublin and Glendalough*, 1116-7; Ball & Hamilton, *The parish of Taney*, 3, 229.

of the Taoiseach but for years was known as the College of Science. The buildings at Richview were adapted to UCD's needs by Professor Cathal O'Neill. They are now used to house the college's School of Architecture, Department of Regional and Urban Planning and Department of Environmental Studies. UCD subsequently sold 6.5 acres of Richview grounds to the Department of Posts and Telegraphs. The proceeds of this sale were used to purchase Rosemount in 1981, at the time the property of the distaff side of the Corballis family (to be discussed later).[23] The name of Richview lives on still in other properties which are located close to the original house such as those in Richview Office Park.

CLONSKEAGH CASTLE

The entrance to Clonskeagh castle, no longer in existence, was located at what is now the end of Whitethorn road where it meets Clonskeagh road; it was directly opposite to the entrance to Richview house. Located at a considerable distance from the castle itself the entrance, described by D'Alton in 1838 as 'cumbrous [and] castellated',[24] was at the beginning of a long curving driveway up to the castle (location no. 3 on map). Comparing maps from the early 19th century with those of today it appears that Whitethorn road follows the contours of this driveway until it meets what is now a roundabout in front of the castle. This is most clearly seen in the first printed Ordnance Map of the area where also the two entrances, one to Richview house, the other to Clonskeagh castle, can be seen directly facing one another across Clonskeagh road. There was a gate lodge beside the entrance to the castle and it continued to exist until relatively recently; it was then occupied by a family called O'Neill.

Considerable detail relating to the building, in the late 18th century, of this castle by Henry Jackson, the United Irishman and radical, has already been discussed in Chapter 5. The castle was reputed to have cost him £20,000 to build.[25] Although it has not been possible to find any evidence to back it up there remains a tradition in the area that the present castle was built on the site of a medieval castle. Something that might add some substance to this claim is the statement made by Lewis in his *Topographical Dictionary* published in 1837. In this he wrote 'On digging in front of the mansion, a few years since (i.e. a few years before 1837), a layer of muscle shells, about three feet thick, and imbedded in clay, was found about eight feet below the surface.' Rather surprisingly, however, when the first Ordnance Survey was carried out in the area around the

---

23 McCartney, *UCD, a national idea*, 397.
24 D'Alton, *History of the county of Dublin*, 808.
25 Ball & Hamilton, *Parish of Taney*, 146.

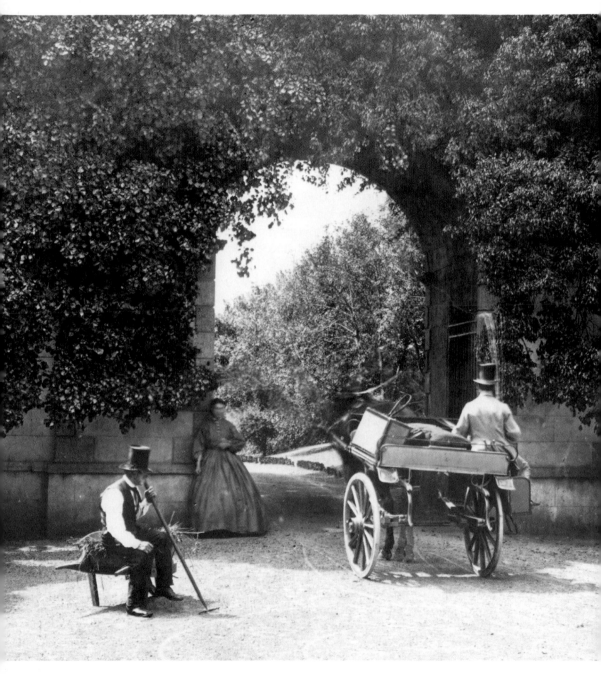

Entrance to Clonskeagh castle, located where Whitethorn road now meets Clonskeagh road (*Courtesy of the National Library of Ireland*)

same time as Lewis was writing the only thing the surveyors had to say was that they had found in the castle two brass cannon which had been recovered from an Armada vessel lost off Kerry.[26] These seem to be more like antiques or trophies rather than anything to do with a medieval castle.

It is possible that the tradition got this castle mixed up with Milltown castle; certainly that was the name which D'Alton, whose views on the architecture of the entrance we have just quoted, called it. Furthermore, there is a curious item in Taylor's map of the environs of Dublin, drawn in 1816, where he has two castles marked in close proximity to one another. One of them, at the end of the long curving driveway from Clonskeagh road is clearly Clonskeagh castle. The other, located a little behind that one is simply marked 'cas'. However, this is the only map out of four drawn between 1760 and 1840 which makes any reference to a second castle in the area. It seems most likely that what it is referring to is Milltown lodge which the first Ordnance Survey shows to be in much the same position as that which Taylor calls a castle. Until there is more evidence available, whether it be archaeological or documentary, with the present state of knowledge it is impossible to say whether the present castle was or was not built on the site of a now extinct medieval castle.

After Henry Jackson's arrest and departure for America following the 1798 rising it appears that the castle was bought by George Thompson, second son of David Thompson of Oatlands, county Meath by his wife Anne Acheson. George was born on 16 August 1769. David Thompson of Oatlands was 5th son of William Thompson of Clonfin, county Longford who married Miss Metge of Athlumney castle, county Meath. He was a grandson of captain William Thompson of Yorkshire, one of three brothers who accompanied king William III to Ireland in 1688. The king gave captain Thompson land that had been confiscated and he settled and married in county Longford.

At the time George Thompson bought Clonskeagh castle he was working in the Treasury in Dublin castle. He was, on a number of occasions, churchwarden of his parish church in Taney – in 1804, 1814, 1817 and 1818. During one of those periods he was, as we have seen in Chapter 7, part of a protest against the window tax during which he disagreed with the then curate of the parish, Rev Ryan. It was all the more remarkable that he was involved in such a protest given his position in the Treasury at the time. His first wife's name was Eleanor and with her had 6 children, 3 sons and 3 daughters. He had two further marriages, the first of these to Catherine daughter of general Robert Alexander of Derry and the second to Jeanett, 4th daughter of William Butler of Drame, county

---

26   Herity, *Ordnance Survey Letters*, 74.

Kilkenny by hon. Caroline Massy, 6th daughter of Hugh, 1st lord Massy. With his third wife he had a son, Massy Wade, who was baptised in Taney church but died leaving no progeny.

George's eldest son by his first wife, David, became a barrister, being called to the bar during Michaelmas term in 1824, and later a magistrate attending Petty Sessions every alternate Monday at Dundrum. Later still be became a Justice of the Peace for county Dublin. He lived all his life at Clonskeagh castle and died without any progeny in 1875. His father George, who had lived with him at the castle, died in May 1860, aged around 91 years. Perhaps because of his father's increasing age, the directories which had listed both of them as living at the castle with George's name first, this situation was reversed in 1853. Thereafter David was listed first and listed on his own after 1860 until his death in 1875. For the next two years, Mrs Thompson, probably George's 3rd wife, is the only occupant recorded as living there. After that, we find Thomas Higginbotham Thompson in residence. He was the second son of George and brother of David. He was a Justice of the Peace for both counties Galway and Dublin. He married Martha daughter of Thomas Wallace KC of Belfield, Stillorgan road, in Taney church on 6 February 1836. Together they had nine children, 5 sons and 4 daughters. All the daughters married and lived elsewhere; they probably never lived at Clonskeagh since their father did not take up residence there until 1878, forty two years after his marriage.

When he did his first two sons were already dead; George, baptised in Taney church died in 1865 and Thomas Wallace died in 1864. So too had his 4th son, Hamlet Wade, of the King's Own Borderers Regiment who died in 1866. However, his other two sons did live there with him in 1879. The first of these was Robert Wade Thompson, BA, TCD, a barrister (c. 1873) and Justice of the Peace for county Dublin (c. 1885). From around 1888 he became a captain of the Dublin Artillery Militia. He married, at Taney church on 10 March 1876, Edith Isabella, daughter of Rev William Jameson by his wife Eliza, daughter of Arthur Guinness of Beaumont, county Dublin. They had nine children, the first of whom Thomas Wade (Ball & Hamilton call him Thomas William but this seems to be a mistake) we will meet a little later. The second son who came to live at Clonskeagh castle in 1879 was Arthur William who became a major in the Dublin Artillery Militia c. 1885.

From 1887 neither he nor his father Thomas Higginbotham are listed at the castle; the reason for this is not clear. At that date the sole occupant is given as Robert Wade; he would be listed with his title of captain from 1889 onwards. An interlude in his occupancy occurred in 1912-13 when a brigadier-general T Capper with a military address at the Lower [Dublin] castle yard is the sole occupant listed. However, from 1914 captain Thomas Wade Thompson, the eldest son of Robert Wade lived there. In 1916 the letters DL (i.e. deputy lieutenant of the county) are added to his name and from 1920 to 1931, after which year he disappears from the directory, he carries the title 'lieut. colonel'. During his last few years there, from 1927 to 1931 the future occupant of the castle, H M Whitton, is listed as living with him at the castle. A barrister, he would continue to be listed there until 1951 and Mrs Whitton, presumably his wife, until 1954. After that, Dr M McMahon is recorded as the occupant until 1963 and, significantly, it was listed as just another house on Whitethorn road during his occupancy. Also of note is the fact that when its rateable valuation is first given in 1895 it is a relatively modest one – £174. It would remain at that value until 1922 when, during the occupancy of lieut. col. Thomas Wade Thompson, it was reduced to £76 and remained at that level. Finally, from 1965 onwards for a number of years it is recorded as being 'let in flats'.[27] One of the lasting memories of the long association of the Thompsons with Clonskeagh castle was a construction down near the river Dodder below the castle called Thompson's Tower in the first Ordnance Survey map of the area; it was still surviving within living memory.

SPRINGFIELD, LATER ST BRIDGET'S (BRIGID'S)

A little further up the Clonskeagh road the entrance to St Bridget's was located on the same side as the entrance to Clonskeagh castle; it was just short of where Clonskeagh motors now is. After the entrance, as can be seen in the early maps, especially Taylor's (1816) and the somewhat later first Ordnance Survey one, the driveway took a long angled approach to the house (location no. 4 on map). After initially going straight in from what is now Clonskeagh road it then took a fairly sharp bend to the left before reaching the house. As will be discussed in a later chapter on ecclesiastical history, St Bridget's well was located at a point to the left of that bend; it is clearly marked there on the map made as part of the Pembroke Estate survey in 1866.[28] All of these maps show a considerable amount of buildings on the site with a large garden at the rear of the house; however it is impossible to tell from them whether these buildings represented the main dwelling house alone or that house together with out offices; the latter seems more probable.

The first name of the house that we know of, Springfield, could possibly

---

27 Ball & Hamilton, *Parish of Taney,* 144-46, 185; *Thom's directories.*
28 Pembroke Estate Papers: Private sources at the National Archives of Ireland (NAI) 97/46/4/31; Taylor's map of the environs of Dublin; Ordnance Survey Map of 1837, NAI OS/ 105 E 295 P. I.

reflect the presence on its lands of the holy well dedicated to St Bridget. This had been the centre of pilgrimage for very many years, a fact that would have been well known to the person who chose the name. Later we will note that it was changed to one that more closely reflected the presence of the well.

It has not been possible to discover who the original owner or builder of the house was. It is possible to speculate that it might have been Alexander Jaffray, who we know lived in the area in the late 18th century but we do not know where; however, it is no more than pure speculation to suggest that this was his country seat. As to the first person known to have lived there it was Matthew Franks, eldest son of Thomas Franks (1729-87) of Ballymagooly, county Cork, by Catherine, daughter of Rev John Day and sister of the hon. Mr Day. He is said to have bought Springfield in 1806 but we do not know from whom. Later his brother Sir John Franks, who was away from Ireland for some time, lived there; in the meantime others resided there after Matthew.

In 1834 it was occupied by Michael Powell; (he would subsequently move across the road to live at Richview)[29] and in 1835-36 by John G Schoales, KC.[30] Sir John was listed there in 1837 although Boase says that he was already in residence in 1835.[31] He continued to retain the name Springfield for the next five to seven years. However, in 1843 the property is listed under the name St Bridget's, almost certainly because of the presence of the well; this name was retained until the demolition of the house over a hundred years later.[32]

Franks was born, second son of Thomas Franks in Loher Cannon, near Tralee, county Kerry, in 1769. He was educated at Trinity College, Dublin where he graduated with a BA in 1788, an MA in 1791 and an LL.B also in 1791. He was called to the Irish bar in 1792 and went on the Munster circuit. He became a King's Counsel on 25 November 1822. Later he would become one of the judges of the Supreme Court of India in Calcutta in 1825 and was presented to the king on his appointment; at that stage he received his knighthood at Carlton house on 20 April 1825. He resigned from his judgeship in 1834 and returned to Ireland in 1835 taking up residence in Springfield, Clonskeagh around the same time. After his return home he acted as a bencher of the King's Inns in Dublin until 1840. He married for the first time Catherine, daughter of Thomas Franks of Carrig, county

29   *Pettigrew & Oulton Street Directory* for 1834; *Dublin Almanac & General Register of Ireland* for 1836 and subsequent years..

30   Ibid. for 1835; *Pettigrew &Oulton Street Directory* for 1836.

31   *Dublin Almanac* for 1837; Lewis, *Topographical dictionary of Ireland,* ii 519; Boase, *Modern English Biography,* i 1099-1100.

32   The first reference to the title 'St Brigid's' (subsequently 'St Bridget's') is in the *Dublin Almanac* for 1843.

Cork. They had five children, 2 sons and 3 daughters. He married, secondly, Jane daughter of John Marshall and, thirdly, Sarah Wollaston. There does not appear to have been any issue from the latter two marriages. He died at St Bridget's, Clonskeagh on 10 or 11 January, 1852 and is buried in Taney graveyard.[33]

An indication of the size of the property he held at St Bridget's can be seen by the rateable valuation assigned to it in 1848 – £157.[34] After his death, Lady Franks, remained in the house until 1857; she then moved elsewhere since we know that she, his last wife, died on 22 February 1874 and like her husband is buried in Taney graveyard. In 1858 St Bridget's had a new resident; major-general Sir Richard Dacres, KCB, RHA commanding Royal Artillery in Ireland. He in turn was shortly thereafter replaced by colonel John William Ormsby, also commanding Royal Artillery. By 1870, John Reilly, esq., Deputy Keeper of the Rolls, had taken over. Earlier he had been Clerk of Records and Writs in Chancery. He was born 16 November 1817, the eldest son of James Miles Reilly and married the hon. Augustus Sugden daughter of Edward, 1st lord St Leonard. They had three children. He was called to the bar in 1842 and was churchwarden in Taney church on three occasions, 1869, 1872 and 1873. He died 1 July 1875.

However, it would appear that the property was merely rented to these people during this period since, in 1878, we find that John Franks, esq., DL had re-established the family's connection with St Bridget's. He was the eldest son of Sir John by his first wife. He continued to be listed there until 1881; in the following year we find H. W. Franks, esq., and Mrs John Franks living there, presumably the latter being the wife of the aforementioned John Franks. In the 1883 entry H W Franks has the title 'lieut. col.' attributed to him. From 1883 to 1921, Thomas Cuthbert Franks, esq. is in residence. He was the son of John Franks and the grandnephew of Matthew Franks who had bought the property in 1806. Thomas Cuthbert was a solicitor and one time President of the Incorporated Law Society of Ireland. He was also a Justice of the Peace for county Dublin. During his time living there the property, like many others in the area, was revalued in 1895 and reduced to £105. Thomas Cuthbert was the last of the Franks to live in the house; it had been in their family for around 115 years.[35] According to the directories the following then took residence there: 1922-23: Miss Sarah Magill, 1924-36: H C Poulter, St Brigid's and 3 College-green (during

---

33 Boase, *Modern English Biography*, i 1099-1100; Ball & Hamilton, *Parish of Taney*, 171-72.

34 *Thom's Directory* for 1848.

35 Ibid. throughout the rest of the century and up to 1921; Ball & Hamilton, *Parish of Taney*, 171.

his time the spelling of the house name changed to St Brigid's); 1937-42: W T Anthony (rateable valuation reduced to £99-5s in 1932 most likely because of land being sold for house building on the Clonskeagh road); 1943-47 John Kearney, St Brigid's (£90-5s) (rateable valuation had again decreased); 1948-56: T R A Turgeon, Canadian Ambassador; 1957-58 Alfred Rive, Canadian Ambassador. The Ambassador apparently had left by 1959/60 as the entry in the 1960 directory is blank. The next appearance in the directory (1963/3) has John O'Farrell as occupier but crucially the rateable valuation had dropped substantially to £32-5s. And what is more, in the same directory Embassy lawn, a new development of houses, made its first appearance. The land on which it was built was part of the property associated with St Bridget's; that would account for the drop in valuation. The entry in the directory for 1965 is placed on the other side of Clonskeagh Motors from that on which the original entrance to St Bridget's had been. Its record for that year is 'St Bridget's – Leinster Homes – Flats 1 to 19'. In 1974 Leinster Homes Ltd., and P V Doyle Holdings Ltd is listed followed by the names of people in St Brigid's Flats (nos 3 and 8 to 20). St Brigid's Flats continued to be listed for a number of years although it is not clear whether these were part of the original house or newly built flats. This situation lasted into the new century – in the year 2000, the listing was 'vacant premises – St Brigid's – 3-20' with no name of occupants, if they still existed, given. By 2005 this had been reduced to 'vacant premises, 3-20-', that is, the reference to St Brigid's had been omitted. Thus the last remaining link, no matter how tenuous, with an ancient site which, we will argue in the chapter on ecclesiastical history, carried the name of St Bridget for more than a thousand years had finally disappeared. None of the new buildings on the grounds of the old house, as far as can be ascertained, adopted the name; it had gone without trace.

ROSEVILLE, ROSE VILLA, ROSEVILLE, LATER ST ANNE'S *A QUA* ANNSBROOK

A short distance further along the road from the original entrance to St Bridget's, but on the other side, one comes to a place where once a house called Roseville stood (location no. 5 on map). This house no longer exists. On its grounds, a number of houses have been built and have an address 'Annsbrook'. Tracing this house from its origins presents some difficulties as houses which incorporate the element 'Rose' in their name were relatively common and can lead to some confusion; e.g. in this case it is called Roseville, later Rosevilla before reverting to Roseville; it was also called Rosevale on occasion. One thing is clear, however, there was no house there when the Ordnance Survey map of the area was drawn up in 1837. In 1866, on the other hand, when a map was produced during a survey for the Pembroke Estate a house there was clearly marked 'Rosevilla'. We are safe, therefore in putting the origins of the house between these two dates. In fact we can even get a clearer date from the directories of the time. In these we find that David Alexander lived at Roseville (as he called it; we will see shortly a slight change in the spelling to the second variation of the name) from 1855 to 1858. The reason that we may be confident of this is that when Roseville appears two years later in the 1859 directory, with a new occupant, it is placed among those directory entrants which are grouped together under the heading of 'Clonskeagh (Roebuck, part of)'. This confirms that we are not referring to the house called Rose vale, which was located further out in Roebuck; it appears near the house entitled Harlech in the Ordnance Survey map of 1837. Also the house with its revised name, 'Rose Villa' is clearly marked on the map in the Pembroke Estate Papers (*National Archives*: 97/46/4/31) surveyed in 1866 and on the map prepared by the Ordnance Survey for *Thom's Directory* in 1888 and is located exactly where Annsbrook is today. The house would appear therefore to have been built for Mr Alexander although his short stay there might suggest that some speculative builder was behind it and Mr Alexander merely rented it. His successor there, John Moss MD, is also listed for a few years only but is followed by Mrs Moss who remained until 1870. She, incidentally, seems to have changed the name of the house to 'Rose Villa' in 1865. This is how it appears in the directory for that year and it is how it appears, as we have seen, on the Pembroke Estate survey map of 1866. After Mrs Moss, Samuel Murray lived there from 1871 to 1884 and then Michael Brophy, grocer and purveyor, Clonskeagh took up residence in 1885. While there the description of his business changed slightly to 'grocer, tea, wine and spirit merchant, Clonskeagh'. He remained until 1891 and was succeeded by a man in a similar business, Mr D O'Connell, described as 'grocer &c'; he resided there until 1895. In that year there was a general revaluation of houses in the area, most commonly resulting in a reduction in valuation; his house had a rateable valuation assigned to it of £37 in that year. During the period of residency of the next occupant, Samuel Wilmot, Government Stockbroker, there was some confusion over the name appearing first as before, Rose Villa, then, Rosevale before reverting to its original name Roseville in 1897. It would retain that name throughout his stay in the house until 1929. During his stay the rateable valuation rose slightly during the First World War to £38-10s.

He was succeeded by Lady Oswaldena Redmond. She renamed it once again but this time there is no 'Rose' element in the name; she called it 'St Anne's'. The change in the name during Lady Oswaldena's tenure is easily detected by comparison of the entries for the years 1929 and 1930; Samuel Wilmot, Roseville, rateable valuation of £38-10s in the former is replaced by Lady Oswaldena Redmond, St Anne's, with similar valuation in the latter. She remained in the house until her death in 1941; it was subsequently bought by Dr C J McSweeney who remained there until 1953. Dermot J Clarke lived there afterwards and he was still there well into the 1970s. Eventually, it was demolished and a new scheme of houses was built on the site. This housing development retained an element of the name St Anne's which Lady Oswaldena had given it; the new name chosen was Annsbrook.

Of all these people who had lived there from the outset it has been possible to find out more detail about Lady Redmond than about any of the rest of them. She was the daughter of James Nelson, JP, Liverpool, a man with a very interesting career.[36] He had begun his life as a butcher in county Meath, perhaps the most important of the cattle-raising counties in Ireland. As well as a butcher he was also a cattle breeder. In both of these capacities he began to send large numbers of cattle to Liverpool where he later set up a butchery business under the title of James Nelson and Sons. As business flourished, he began to open shops all around England. Soon he discovered that he was unable to get a sufficient supply of cattle from Ireland, so he turned to South America. Resulting from this, his son Hugh, a brother of Oswaldena, went out to the Argentine in 1888 where he founded the Las Palmas meat factory at Zarata, near the mouth of the Parana river. This factory was run by a company which he founded, Nelsons River Plate Meat Company; it sent meat back to England to the Nelson butchery business. The next step was the acquisition of steamers to ensure that sufficient ships were available to transport the growing amount of meat being sent to England.

In 1889, James Nelson and Sons bought the first such steamer, newly built with a specially designed refrigerating plant. Primitive in design, it was a pioneer in its field. Oswaldena's brothers Hugh and William managed a company set up to operate it; with new ships added this was the beginning of what would become known as the Nelson Line (Liverpool) Ltd which carried other cargo and passengers as well. James Nelson, Oswaldena's father, died in 1899 but by that time the company had a firm grip on the South American trade.[37] The company

---

36   Sir Charles A Cameron, *History of the Royal College of Surgeons in Ireland* (2nd ed, Dublin 1916) 808.

37   Material on the origins of the Nelson shipping line was first published in the October 1966 issue of *Sea Breezes* magazine. Derived from this with the permission of the editor and with extra material added by FJW and T Robins an article entitled 'Nelson Line's 42 years' was posted on the Merchant Navy Officers' website: [http://www.merchantnavyofficers.com/nelson.html]. Acknowledgement is made in the article to T A Bushnell "Royal Mail 1839-1939" and to the Central Record of the World Ship Society for certain historical details.

continued to prosper and by 1911 it had a fleet with a refrigerated capacity of nearly six million cubic feet. It was now a major competitor for the Royal Mail Steam Packet Company. As a result of overtures made from the latter in 1913, William Nelson, now Sir William, retired and the Royal Mail Steam Packet Company bought the whole of the Ordinary Shares of all the Nelson companies. These, however, continued to operate and with their ability to import large quantities of meat were of great help to Britain during the 1914-18 war. They did, of course, suffer many losses during that time; later all Nelson vessels were transferred to the Royal Mail Lines Ltd thus ending a forty-two year existence.[38]

At a time when the Nelson business was soaring ahead in England, Oswaldena Nelson married, in 1898, Joseph Michael Redmond whose medical career in Dublin was then in the ascendant. The son of Denis Redmond of Belmont lodge, Sandford, Dublin and his wife Bridget E, daughter of Patrick Gorman of Dublin, he received his early education at St Francis Xavier College, Dublin. Later he studied at the Catholic University and the Carmichael Schools; also in Jervis street, Baggot street, the Meath and the Mater, in the latter he was a Resident. Further studies were carried out in London at the Hospital for Diseases of the Throat and Chest. In 1876 he received the Diploma of the Royal College of Surgeons, in 1878 the Licence of the College of Physicians, in 1881 Membership and in 1884 Fellowship. He was elected President of the College of Physicians in 1906, a post he held for two years.

Earlier, in 1877, he was appointed Demonstrator at the Catholic University School in Cecilia street. Six years later he became a Lecturer on the Practice of Medicine and Pathology in the Ledwich School. The following year he became Pathologist to the Coombe Hospital and Guinness Dispensary. In 1879 he was appointed Assistant Physician and two years later, Physician to the Mater hospital in Dublin. In time he became consulting physician to various hospitals such as Cork street, the Coombe, the National (Maternity) Holles street, St Michael's, Kingstown (now Dún Laoghaire), the Cottage, Drogheda. He was also President of the State Medicine Section of the Academy of Medicine. As well as all this he made a number of contributions to journals such as *Transactions of the Royal Academy of Medicine*.

In 1911 during a visit to Dublin of king George V he was knighted and in 1915 he was awarded, *honoris causa*, the degree of MD by the National University of Ireland.[39] It has not been discovered where he and Oswaldena lived immediately

---

38 Appendix V 'A short history of the Nelson line: 1890-1932' in T A Bushnell, *"Royal Mail": a centenary history of the Royal Mail Line, 1839-1939* (London 1939) 265-68.

39 Cameron, *History of the Royal College of Surgeons*, 807-08.

after their marriage but it is known that Joseph Michael Redmond bought Gortmore in Dundrum; today that house now much extended for institutional purposes is called Gort Mhuire. It was while living there that he received his knighthood. It is believed that he never used his new title but his wife did use hers. After his death, Lady Oswaldena moved to Clonskeagh.[40]

The latest date of Lady Redmond's occupancy of St Anne's, which appears in the directories, is 1942 but we know from another source that she had in fact died the previous year. This source is a catalogue prepared for the public auction of 'the late Lady Redmond's well-known collection of antique furniture' which was held on Monday 9 June 1941 and lasted for three days. The catalogue, interestingly, informs those who would attend how to get to her house where the auction was to take place. It states 'St Anne's is situate on the main Clonskeagh road practically opposite Clonskeagh castle [then located at the entrance to what is now Whitethorn road]. It is only 10 minutes easy walk from the terminus of the Clonskeagh bus route No. 11 [then at what are still called the Terminus buildings at Vergemount]'. That the No. 11 bus only went as far as Vergemount as late as 1941 gives a very good indication of how little of Clonskeagh had been developed as a suburb by that year although, as we will see later, that development was well under way at that stage. Included in the sale, the catalogue tells us, were Chippendale, Sheraton, French and other furniture; Broadwood Boudoir grand piano, spinet, valuable oil paintings, prints, Waterford glass; China including Dresden, Copeland, Worcester, Minton, Capo di Monte, Bohemian and Venetian glass; Turkey, Dún Emer and Donegal carpets; silver and Sheffield plate etc etc. Bedroom furniture including crucifixes, shrine and lamp, religious pictures. Atco motor mower – 620 lots in all. At the end of the 3 day auction there would be then sold 'the contents of two maids' bedrooms, back stairs, sculleries and kitchen – including Moffat Electric Refrigerator'.[41]

---

40   This information is contained in 'The history of Gort Muire: 1944-1994' by Peter O'Dwyer, O.Carm. abridged for the Irish Carmelites' website [http://www.carmelites.ie/Ireland/Gort%20Muire/gmhistory.htm] Evidence adduced in this that Lady Oswaldena died in 1924 is countered by other evidence that she was still alive in 1928. It was presumed that she had died thereafter but this cannot be the case as we know that she moved to Clonskeagh most likely in 1929 since she appears as a resident there in the 1930 directory.

41   Allen & Townsend, *Catalogue of the late Lady Redmond's well-known collection of antique furniture and fine art property at St Anne's, Clonskeagh road, Clonskeagh to be sold by Public Auction on Monday June 9th 1941 and following 3 days at 12 Noon prompt.*

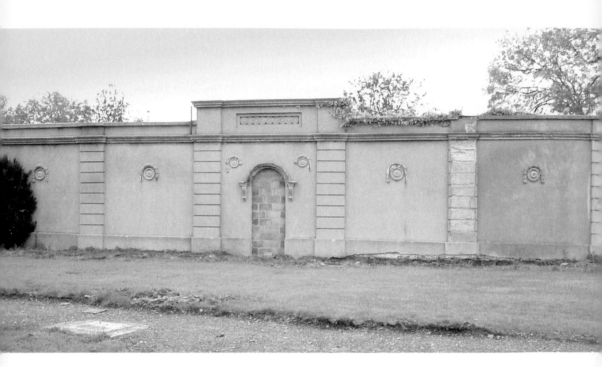

Only remains of Newstead (later Philips Electrical (Ireland) Ltd), Clonskeagh road: camouflaging the outhouses

NEWSTEAD, LATER PHILIPS FACTORY, NOW PART OF UNIVERSITY COLLEGE, DUBLIN

The next house on the same side of Clonskeagh road was originally called Newstead; at a later date the business premises of Philips Electrical (Ireland) would be located there (location no. 6 on map). Newstead first appears in the directories in 1849. It does not feature on the Ordnance Survey map of 1837 (*National Archives*: O/S 105 E 295) but does appear on the Pembroke Estate map which was the result of a survey carried out in 1866 (*National Archives*: Pembroke Estate Papers 97/46/4/31). This suggests that it was built in the interim between these two dates and that fits well with its first entry in the directories in 1849. The occupant then is given as P Scott, solicitor. According to the Griffith Valuation records his full name was Patrick Scott. In 1855, John Scott, who was also a solicitor, is listed as being in residence there. He was succeeded in 1858 by William Cruice, barrister with Henry W Cruice listed there at the same time. The latter worked in the Chief Secretary's Office in Dublin castle. In the following year we learn that William, whose surname is now given as Cruise though it appears as Cruice again in the 1862 listings, worked in the Fines and Recoveries office, Dublin castle, later called Fines and Penalties office. In 1862 Patrick Scott appears as well as William Cruice under the Newstead heading; his city office was at 73 Dame street. This suggests that the Scott family retained ownership of the house a point that is supported by the fact that from 1906 to 1913 Scott names return again as residents of Newstead. In the meantime the property was probably rented.

The following names are given in the directories from 1863 to 1905: Colonel R A Fitzmayer, CB (1863-64); Robert Ross Todd esq. (1865-67); Charles Tuthill, barrister (1868-88) – the death of his son, Arthur Hendley Tuthill, aged 27 years was reported in the *Cork Examiner* on 4 September 1878; Mrs Tuthill (1889-90); J J Stopford (1891-92); Edward J Greene, Queen's (later 'King's') Bench Div., (1893- 1905). In 1906 major Scott is in residence there but in the following year William E Scott, DL, JP moved in and remained there until 1913. For the last two years of his residency another name is listed alongside him as living at Newstead, that of Edmund Loftus Phillips who also had an address given as 'St James's gate brewery', apparently his business address. But curiously, his name precedes that of William E Scott in the listings for these two years and he would subsequently be listed from 1914 to 1923 as the sole occupant of Newstead; he is listed in 1924 separately from another listing which gives B W Whyte as the occupant. Despite the similarity of the names, it has not been possible to connect Edmund L Phillips to the subsequent business use of the premises that was to be made by Philips Electrical (Ireland) from 1955 onwards. In the meantime, after lying vacant for a while in 1925 Aodh Ua Cinneidigh (The hon Hugh Kennedy), chief justice of Saorstát Éireann, took up residence there in 1926 and remained until his death; the last listing of his name is in 1937. After him came John Hanlon; he lived there from 1938 to 1954 and in the following year a radical change was made when it ceased to be a private residence. In that year Philips Electrical (Ireland) Ltd. arrived and set up their business there.

There is a certain curiosity attached to the name chosen for this house, Newstead. It is the same name as that of the ancestral home of the famous poet Lord Byron. He had died in 1824 not long before we first meet the house in the directories and his memory would have still been quite fresh; indeed his fame grew even more after his death. As well as that there is a further, although tenuous, connection with the name of Byron's ancestral home. Both were on occasion referred to as Newstead abbey or simply Newstead. In the case of the Clonskeagh house, it first appears under the simple name Newstead; that remained until 1859 when William Cruise changed it to Newstead house. However, that only lasted for approximately three years and was changed back to Newstead when Patrick Scott returned in 1862. It continued under that name until Charles Tuthill took up residence in 1868 and changed the name to Newstead abbey the name it would retain until shortly before the return of the Scotts when it was, once again, changed back to Newstead, the name which it continued to hold. Although the evidence is slight, it is not unreasonable to suggest that the house was indeed called after Byron's ancestral home. That house is in Nottinghamshire in England where it is a popular place for visitors to this day.[42]

Newstead in Clonskeagh was the home to some people who are of particular interest. One, Hugh Kennedy, has been dealt with in Chapter 11. Another will be discussed here – Dorothy Stopford Price. She was born there on 9 September 1890, the third child of Jemmett Stopford who, as we have already noted, most likely rented the house for a short period in the early 1890s. Prior to that he had lived for a number of years at Roebuck lodge further out along what is now the Goatstown road. Jemmett Stopford was an accountant who worked for the Irish Land Commission and was the brother of the well-known historian Mrs Alice Stopford Green. Given the latter's strong and well articulated views, her staunch support for Irish independence (she was subsequently elected as an independent in the first three elections to the Seanad, 1922, 1925 and 1928) and her increasing awareness of the role to be played by women, it seems most likely that she had a substantial influence in the early formation of young Dorothy. Of course Dorothy's mother, Constance Kennedy, daughter of Dr Evory Kennedy, a Master of the Rotunda hospital was also likely to have been an important influence, given the career that Dorothy was to pursue.

She attended St Paul's Girls' school in London where the family had moved after the sudden death of her father; at that time Dorothy was only twelve years old. While in London she worked with the Charity Organization Society for a number of years before returning to Dublin where she studied medicine. After qualification she worked for some time in a district dispensary in county Cork but soon returned to Dublin where she set up a private practice. Along with some others she established St Ultan's hospital for infants in Charlemont street. In 1925 she married Liam Price, a district justice. She attended a post-graduate course in Vienna in 1931 and there came in touch with a man who had established a proper system for treating children with tuberculosis. Soon this became for her the compelling focus of her work; she realised then how little was known in Ireland about the diagnosis of childhood tuberculosis although this

---

42 Newstead Abbey, Nottinghamshire [http://www.nottinghamcity.gov.uk/newstead/house/default.asp]; *Thom's Directory*: various dates.

knowledge was well established on the continent. Lack of knowledge of German, she believed, was the reason that text-books on the subject were unknown in Ireland; she therefore learned German and pursued further post-graduate work in Bavaria. On return to Ireland she lectured on the modern methods of testing for tuberculosis and later wrote a book *Tuberculosis in Childhood* which was published in 1942.

She was appointed paediatrician in Baggot street hospital in 1932 and received an MD for her thesis 'The diagnosis of primary TB in children'. Once again she travelled abroad, this time to Sweden and Denmark and invited men closely associated with the rapidly advancing knowledge of tuberculosis at the time to come and give lectures in Ireland. Perhaps even more importantly, she had begun to do research on BCG vaccination. Soon she, along with Dr Patricia Alston, was vaccinating children at St Ultan's hospital. This was pioneering work and it led in time to the BCG scheme set up by Dublin Corporation in 1948.

However, her efforts in setting up an Anti-Tuberculosis League did not meet the same acceptance; medical treatment was still caught up in the miasma of opposing religious standpoints at that time. Although very disappointed and even hurt she was not embittered; she kept going. She threw all her efforts into the BCG campaign and did all in her power to get a BCG unit in St Ultan's hospital.

Her standing on the subject of Tuberculosis was such at this time that she was appointed physician to Newcastle sanatorium and Sunshine home, Stillorgan. When Dr Noël Browne became Minister of Health he appointed her as chairman of his new Consultative Council on Tuberculosis. One particular recommendation which emerged from this was the setting up of the National BCG Committee to which Dr Browne gave full autonomy. She was chairman of this committee and it held its inaugural meeting at St Ultan's on 4 July, 1949; it marked a major milestone in her work up to that time. She entered into its work with energy and enthusiasm; her own home was used in the wide range of activities it got involved in. It was a mark of her practical patriotism; in her youth she had supported Ireland's bid for freedom, in her maturity, she worked hard to make that freedom live up to its name. However, soon after the committee was set up she suffered the first stroke that was to affect her ability to work at the level she would have wished. Despite it, however, she continued to contribute although unable to return to the BCG Committee; she did, however, keep on writing. Another stroke occurred on 28 January 1954; this time it proved to be fatal and she died two days later. However, true to her indefatigable nature an article she had written appeared in the *Journal of the Irish Medical Association* in the same issue as that which contained her obituary. In that, her obituarist wrote: 'Given the circumstances of her time and place on earth she fulfilled herself more completely, and used her talents to greater effect than any physician I have known'.[43]

As noted earlier, Newstead was taken over by Philips Electrical (Ireland) Ltd in 1955 thus ending the residential character of the house. New buildings emerged in its place as, presumably, the old house was not suited to the new purposes for which it was bought. The house was, therefore, demolished and no traces of it are apparent today. There is, however, one trace of the original property still extant. That is the ornamental work on the rear walls of the outhouses which are to the left of the place where the old house once stood. The impression given as it is viewed from the house would have been that of an important building with access to it through a centrally placed door. When one went through and was out of sight of the house, the true nature of the building, however, became apparent. The purpose of the ornamentation, therefore, was to camouflage the view of these outhouses as seen from the house.

Philips Electrical is no longer at Newstead but their new premises at Fonthill, in the Liffey valley, still retains that name. University College, Dublin now own the Clonskeagh property and are currently developing it.

ROEBUCK HOUSE

Although the next house along the Clonskeagh road is Winstay/Wynnstay, the house in which Gypsum Industries Ltd until recent times was based, for a particular reason it is necessary to pause first before discussing it. The reason for this is that it is most likely that it was once called Roebuck or Roebuck house and there is considerable confusion in the sources about the use of the name 'Roebuck house'. For example, during the 1830s there are three apparently different houses which carry this name; from 1835 to 1838 J D Farrer occupied one such house while Roderick Connor was listed as being in residence during the same time (i.e from 1837 to 1838) in another. However, it is possible to positively identify a third one carrying this name during and after the same period; other later examples can also be identified but with a lesser degree of certainty. Before the chronology of occupancy (together with rateable valuation, where available) of these is attempted, the third one, referred to above, is considered first.

---

43   H E Counihan, 'In Memoriam: Dr Dorothy Stopford Price' in *Journal of the Irish Medical Association* 34 (1954) 84, 72; J B Lyons, *Brief lives of Irish doctors* (Dublin 1978) 161 -62.

ROEBUCK HOUSE, LATER GROVE HOUSE AND LATER STILL ROEBUCK GROVE

This house, which no longer exists having been demolished in 1980, was located in what is now UCD grounds at a little distance in from the Clonskeagh entrance over to the right, near where the UCD crèche is now located (location no. 7 on map). It was approached originally by a carriage driveway which began on Clonskeagh road just behind and to the left of the well-known house called 'The Cottage'. That carriage driveway eventually emerged on to Roebuck road opposite Harlech grove; there is a pedestrian gateway now at the point where it emerged. An exceptionally clear image of this driveway is recorded on Taylor's map (1816). As the house no longer exists and given that it appears to have been the original Roebuck house it is perhaps worth recording the description given to it around 1879 when it was unoccupied and available for sale: 'Comprises the Mansion House ... standing in a Demesne of about 18a. 2r. 33p., statute measure, which is handsomely timbered, with Gate Lodge at entrance. It is approached by a carriage drive, and contains entrance hall, diningroom, library, breakfast room and pantry on same flat, large drawingroom, and 3 bedrooms on first floor, and 4 attic rooms, conservatory off landing, and w. c.; basement storey, extensive out-offices enclosed, large walled-in garden. The house, with some outlay, could be made a most comfortable residence. The situation is most desirable being in a select and fashionable neighbourhood, and within fifteen minutes' drive of the city; also being indemnified against rent it forms a good investment, or a nice residential property. Immediate possession can be had by purchaser'.[44] The first known resident of this Roebuck house is John Power, the whiskey magnate. The house is one of the few on Taylor's map (1816) which are named. John Power was described in the *Freeman's Journal* on 24 July, 1841 as 'an eminent distiller in Dublin who is a DL for the city. His son James Power, co Wexford, a Repealer, sat for the county since 1837. Lived at Edermine house, Wexford. [Member of the] Reform Club, London'.[45] James may have been born but was certainly raised in Roebuck house before moving to Edermine house when elected MP for Wexford. The date of his election given in the *Freeman's Journal* is somewhat at variance with that given in the House of Commons records; there it is stated that he was returned on 27 January 1835.[46] John Power is described in Boase as follows: 'Sir John Power,

44   Archives of the Carmelite monastery, Roebuck road.
45   Guide to Irish Commoners, written especially for the *Freeman's Journal* and published on 24 July, 1841.
46   RETURN to Two Orders of the Honourable The House of Commons, dated 4 May 1876 and 9 March 1877: *Ordered by* The House of Commons, *to be printed* 1 *March* 1878. p. 331.

Baronet, born 1771; a distiller in Dublin; alderman of Dublin; created baronet 18 October 1841; a supporter of Daniel O'Connell by his purse and influence; laid foundation stone of O'Connell's monument in Glasnevin cemetery 1854. Died Roebuck house, co Dublin 25 June 1855; buried in cathedral, Marlborough street, Dublin'.[47] His vault under the pro-cathedral has a plaque over it with the following words etched on it: 'Sepulchral chamber dedicated to the family of Sir John Power Bar[t] Roebuck House C[o] Dublin Anno Domini 1834'. Given that he was not created baronet until 1841 it may be assumed that the plaque was erected at a date later than that but that the vault was there since 1834. After the death of Sir John Power, the house was bought by Abraham Brewster. Shortly thereafter the name of the house was changed first for a short period to Grove house then to the more long-lasting Roebuck grove. There are two definite sources of evidence for the change of name from Roebuck house to Roebuck grove:

i.)   Ball & Hamilton wrote as follows: 'Sir John Power (1814-55) who was one of O'Connell's most influential supporters resided at Roebuck house (now called Roebuck grove) for over 40 years. He was a DL and JP of Dublin and was created baronet 18 October 1841. He died 26 June 1855. The house was then bought by Rt Hon Abraham Brewster; he resided there between 1855 and 1874. He was leader of the Irish bar and became lord chancellor of Ireland in March 1867. He held that position until the resignation of the government in December 1868.'[48]

ii.)   The Carmelite archives show that the property adjoined Mount Dillon into which the Carmelite sisters moved in August 1877. In the Deeds, which they acquired around that time, reference is made to the adjoining property as follows 'The Mansion house, out-offices, garden, and part of the demesne lands, formerly called Roebuck house, now called Roebuck grove, situate in the Townland of Roebuck, and county of Dublin'. The size of the property is given as 11 acres 2 roods 9 perch (Irish) or 18 acres 2 roods 33 perch (British). The property was unoccupied at the time and was for sale. These Deeds were probably drawn up during 1879, as the entry for that year in the *Thom's Directory* indicates that it was vacant.[49]

The reason for the name change is likely to be the confusion caused by the many different houses using the name 'Roebuck house', although it should be

---

47   Boase, *Modern English biography*, ii 1613.
48   Ball & Hamilton, *The parish of Taney*, 179.
49   Archives of the Carmelite monastery, Roebuck road, Dublin.

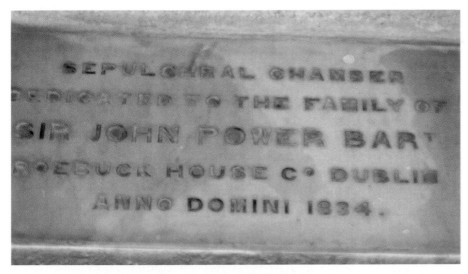

Inscription over burial vault under the pro-cathedral, Dublin, of Sir John Power, baronet, Roebuck house (later Roebuck grove, now part of UCD campus)

pointed out that there was one other property (and possibly two) in the vicinity which was also called 'Roebuck grove'.

From 1835 to 1836 Alexander Brewster, barrister, resided at Castleview, Roebuck and from 1837 to 1840 Abraham Brewster, barrister, was in residence there (that house would have its name changed later to 'Charlton'). It is not certain, but most likely, that he is the same Abraham Brewster who came to live at Roebuck house, later called Roebuck grove, in 1855. Incidentally, the entries in the directories alone do not allow us to state that he lived at Roebuck grove during 1856 to 1859; they merely give 'Roebuck' as his address. Ball & Hamilton, however, allow us to clarify that he did move into the house where John Power had recently died. The use of the address 'Roebuck' on its own was relatively common and may not have any other significance other than that a particular person lived in the townland of that name. On the other hand, 'Roebuck' is clearly the name given to John Power's Roebuck house on the Duncan map of 1821 and it is separate from the general name which is written as 'Roebuck lands'.

It is not clear if Abraham Brewster changed the name of the house immediately or some years later. The directories give 'Grove house' first as the new name (1860-63) and 'Roebuck grove' from 1864 onwards. The following information about him is taken from Boase and from Ball's *Judges in Ireland*. The detail in it is, in general, to be preferred to that given in the directories cited above. 'Abraham Brewster, the eldest son of William Bagenal Brewster of Ballinulta, co.

Wicklow and Mary, daughter of Thomas Bates, was born at Ballinulta in April 1796. He was educated at Kilkenny college and at Trinity College where he gained his BA in 1817 and his MA in 1847. He was called to the Irish bar during Michaelmas term in 1819; he married Maryanne, daughter of Robert Gray of Upton house, in co. Carlow, the same year and went on the Leinster circuit. He became a King's Counsellor on 13 July 1835, a legal advisor to the lord lieutenant of Ireland on 10 October 1841, a bencher of the King's Inns Dublin in 1846, solicitor general for Ireland from 2 February 1846 to 16 July 1846, retiring on the fall of the ministry; proceeded master of arts 1847; became attorney general from 10 January 1853 to 10 February 1855 in lord Aberdeen's ministry retiring on its fall; Privy Counsellor Ireland January 1853; lost his wife in 1862; lord justice of Court of Appeal in Ireland July 1866 and lord chancellor of Ireland from March 1867 to 17 December 1868, retiring on fall of the ministry; resided in Dublin in Merrion square and near Dublin at Roebuck house. He died at his city residence in Merrion square, Dublin on 26 July 1874 and was buried at Tullow in co Carlow; left issue.'[50] From this, we can see that Abraham Brewster lived in Clonskeagh during his later years when he was at the height of his career. It can also be seen that he lost his wife quite soon after taking up residence there.

It has not been possible to discover anything in particular about the next occupant of Roebuck grove, David Coffey, apart from the fact that he was the taxing master in Chancery and that the office he held was of relevantly recent origin. The appointment of a taxing master in 1845 added a new department to Chancery, one of the most ancient of the six superior courts in Ireland at the time, although by the time of Coffey's appointment these six courts had been remodelled by the Supreme Court Judicature Act of 1877. The appointment was made by the lord chancellor.[51]

However, we do know something about his successor in the house, Sir Christopher F Nixon, a man who had an illustrious career both in the practice of medicine and in education. He was born in Dublin in 1849; his father was a railway agent and died before Christopher was born. Educated at Terenure college, he became a licentiate of the Royal College of Physicians of Ireland at the early age of nineteen; later, in 1879, he gained an MB from Trinity College in 1879. Before that he had been appointed assistant physician to the Mater hospital in 1868 and physician in 1872. Some years later he became secretary to its Medical Board.

In 1877, at the young age of 28 he was given the chair of the Institutes of

---

50   Boase, *Modern English biography,* i, 393-94; F Elrington Ball, *The judges in Ireland, 1221- 1921* (2vols, London 1926) ii 365-66.

51   R B McDowell, *The Irish administration:1801-1914* (London 1964) 104, 131.

Medicine (physiology) at the Catholic University School of Medicine in Cecilia street, founded around 22 years earlier by John Henry (later, cardinal) Newman. The 1860s and 1870s saw numerous efforts made to get government endowment for the Catholic University but all failed for a variety of reasons. However, the impasse was broken, in the short term, with the introduction of the University Education (Ireland) Bill (1879) by the Disraeli government; this led to the incorporation by charter of the Royal University, a non-teaching, degree-awarding institution located in Earlsfort terrace, in 1880. It was endowed by the government and a number of its senators were drawn from the Catholic University thus gaining government funds indirectly for the latter. Three of these came from Cecilia street and among them was Christopher Nixon, despite the fact that he was very critical of this new departure in university education. Unlike the other part of the Catholic University, the School of Medicine had gained recognition for its graduates by the appropriate licensing bodies.

After the deaths in 1881 of Thomas Hayden and Robert Cryan, both of whom had been appointed by Newman when the school was founded, Christopher Nixon was appointed to the, now combined, chair of anatomy and physiology. After the death of another appointee of Newman, RSD Lyons, in late 1886 Nixon was appointed to succeed him in the chair of Medicine. Two years after he had got this promotion he took up residence at Roebuck grove in Clonskeagh. He would remain there, while still professor of medicine, until his death in 1914. Of course by that time, Cecilia street had become the UCD faculty of Medicine as a result of the Irish Universities Bill (1908) which saw the end of the long running battle between the Catholic church and the government on the university question. Christopher Nixon had thus worked, not just in the Catholic University School of Medicine and University College, Dublin but also in what may now be seen to have been the interim Royal University of Ireland. He had also contributed to the efforts made to bring about the transition which saw the emergence of that Bill in 1908. For example, he gave a detailed submission to a Royal (the Robertson) Commission in 1901-02; in this he said that the Catholics wanted a university that stood in the same relationship to them as the University of Dublin stood to Episcopalian Protestants. That, of course, is not what was eventually achieved but it gives a flavour of the struggle that was going on prior to the University Bill of 1908.

During the early years of the twentieth century students were becoming more interested in national affairs; this was especially evident in the debates of the Literary and Historical Society (popularly known as the L & H) which had originated in Newman's time but was restored during Fr Delany's presidency of University College in St Stephen's green (1883-1907). Perhaps the most dramatic interventions by students occurred at conferring ceremonies held in the Royal

University's great hall where many national minded students objected to *God save the king* being played on the organ. Given that a number of senators of that university were also on the staff of the Catholic University tension was bound to arise between them and some students. Things came to a head at the conferring ceremony of 27 October 1905 when the organist's seat was commandeered and approaches to the organ blocked; instead of the anthem being played as usual some students sang *God save Ireland*. Much fuss was made of this incident. A special meeting of the senate was called for 7 November to deal with it; Sir Christopher, the first to arrive for the meeting, was booed 'but not very loudly', while variations in greeting awaited the others. Decision was deferred at the meeting and afterwards others outside the university got involved. Because of the uproar, the inaugural meeting of the L & H for that year was delayed from 8 to 22 November at Fr Delany's request. Some guest speakers to the topic 'Higher education and national life' decided not to turn up, including Dr Mahaffy of Trinity College, but others did; Sir Christopher Nixon spoke and in his speech praised Fr Delany highly but he was continually interrupted by loud calls from the back of the hall. Fr Delany was highly embarrassed by the behaviour of the students and made an impassioned speech in which he deplored those interrupters whom he referred to as 'blackguards'. As if to compensate Nixon for the indignity he had suffered he said that he had been for twenty years a colleague of his in educational work and 'during that time a stauncher colleague I could not have in the defence of Catholic interests. He has been at all times ready to do all that lay in his power, at great professional sacrifices, to advance university education in Ireland, and above all to advance and promote in every way the interest of the establishment of which he is dean of the faculty' – a sentiment which was greeted by applause. Later the students whom Delany had called 'blackguards' wrote, in a letter published in Arthur Griffith's *United Irishmen,* that they intended no personal insult to Sir Christopher but were protesting at what they saw as the anomaly of 'one who accepted honours and emoluments from the government' while protesting 'against the government's policy and parsimony'. Nixon had received his baronetcy c. 1896.[52]

There is another aspect to Sir Christopher that is of interest; he played a major part in having a veterinary college established in Ireland at the turn of the twentieth century. In previous years, Irish veterinary students had to travel abroad for their education to places like Scotland. As Professor of Medicine in

---

52 F O C Meenan, *Cecilia street: the Catholic University School of Medicine 1855-1931* (Dublin 1987) 7-13, 40, 42, 46-50, 62-4; McCartney, *UCD, a national idea,* 16-17, 22-7; Thomas J Morrissey, *Towards a National University, William Delany SJ (1835-1924): an era of initiative in Irish education* (Dublin 1983) 244-55.

1894 he brought together a group of physicians to progress a plan to provide such education at home. Eventually he managed to get £15,000 from the government; this together with funds privately raised allowed work to go ahead in building a veterinary college. It got its charter in 1900 and Sir Christopher became its first president. He laid the foundation stone of the new college at Ballsbridge on 21 May 1901. In doing that he used a silver trowel which was held later by his family as an heirloom. It was some coincidence then that the same silver trowel would be used a century later when the foundation stone of a new veterinary college was being laid in the year 2000. The trowel was provided for the occasion to University College, Dublin by descendants of Sir Christopher and they attended the ceremony. But the coincidence goes even further; Roebuck grove, the home in which Sir Christopher lived in from 1889 until his death in 1914 was subsequently bought by University College, Dublin in 1961 some years prior to its transfer from its city premises at Earlsfort terrace to the new Belfield campus. The new veterinary college was founded, therefore, in a campus that now incorporated the land on which Sir Christopher's home had stood and in which he had lived at the time when he laid the foundation stone of its predecessor.[53]

An interesting insight into the lifestyle of the Nixons may be gleaned from a note which they inserted in one of the social journals of 1904 and which Meehan cites: Sir Christopher and Lady Nixon 'do not intend to move into their Dublin house, 2 Merrion square, this winter, although Sir Christopher attends daily on professional business there'.[54] From this it may be assumed that in previous years they left their house, Roebuck grove, in Clonskeagh during the winter and, given that the announcement was made in a social journal, they must have conducted a fairly substantial social round of activity at their house there. Social activities based within a house would be easier to carry out in the city rather than out in what was then the countryside, Clonskeagh. Why they should have ceased to do so in 1904 is not clear.

After Sir Christopher's death his wife, Lady Mary Agnes, remained on at Roebuck grove until 1920. The connection of the family to the area, however, was to a certain extent re-established in 1930 when their daughter Josephine Francesca married Charles Aloysius Barnewall, 18th baron Trimleston. He, of course, was no longer living at Roebuck castle; the Trimleston connection with it had been severed some time during the incumbency of Nicholas, the 14th baron, around the year 1800. Charles Aloysius died in 1937 and she in 1945.[55]

After the Nixons, Walter Riddell Martin took up residence at Roebuck grove

---

53   UCD website: www.ucd.ie/vetmed/html/news/peg
54   Meehan, *Cecilia street*, 70.
55   Gibbs, *Complete peerage*, xii/2 §45.

and stayed until 1953. The next, and last, private resident was captain Alaster Stewart who is still listed there in 1963. However, by that time the property had been bought by UCD; in 1961 it had paid £66,000 for the house and 35 acres of ground. It would appear from this that land had been added to that which had earlier surrounded the house in 1877; then, as we saw above, they consisted of a little over 18 acres. Roebuck grove is now an integral part of the UCD campus.[56]

ROEBUCK HOUSE, LATER WINSTAY/WYNNSTAY

We now come back to Winstay/Wynnstay on the Clonskeagh road (location no. 8 on map). John Ennis and James Forrest occupied a house called 'Roebuck house' at dates from 1847 to 1849 and 1851 to 1867 respectively – there is no entry for 1850. Because of the continuity of dates it is assumed that the house in question is the same house. Two other houses had an identical title during at least some of the same period but they can be excluded (i.e. those occupied by John Power (see previous item) and Henry Deane Edwards (see the following item)) since they were in possession of their own similarly-titled houses both before and after the house we are now discussing had changed its owner; in other words, when James Forrest took up residence in Roebuck house it could not have been in either of the other two houses as they were known to be in the continuous possession of these other people at that time.

In 1847 John Ennis is first given the specific address of Roebuck house in the directory for that year; in the same entry his city address is given as 9 Merrion square east. A few years earlier, according to a report in the *Freeman's Journal* of 2 November 1843, which lists the members of a Special Jury panel for the county of Dublin, John Ennis of Roebuck and High street, merchant was on that panel. It would appear from this that he had changed his city address in the meantime. In Chapter 8, we have seen that Andrew Ennis, described as being 'of the very first mercantile rank' of 21 Harcourt street & Roebuck, a baker in North Great George's street and father of John Ennis was, in 1829, among the treasurers elected to supervise the collection of a Testimonial to Daniel O'Connell. His address, given simply as 'Roebuck' rather than 'Roebuck house' will be discussed shortly but first the change in name to Winstay will be considered.

This change is assumed on the basis of the fact that, in the year following Forrest's last date of occupancy, i.e. 1867, a new entry is found, called Winstay, in the section of the directory in which Forrest's 'Roebuck house' had been in the previous year. In support of this assumption is the fact that in the first Ordnance Survey maps of the area (1837) a substantial property, called simply

---

56   McCartney, *UCD, a national idea,* 397.

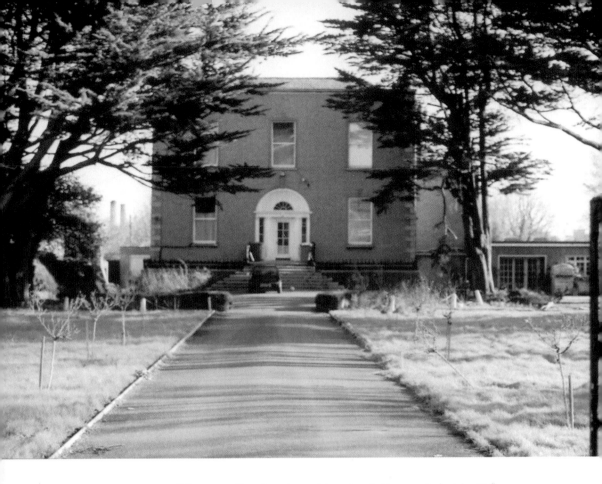

Wynnstay, Clonskeagh road (previously Gypsum Industries Ltd)
(*Photographer: Matt Walsh*)

'Roebuck', is seen to occupy the place where it is known Winstay was later located. It is also called by that name in the Pembroke Estate Papers (*National Archives*: 97/46/4/31) surveyed in 1866. The substantial difference in the rateable valuation of the property, from £206 in 1847-49 when John Ennis was in residence to £88 in 1895 can be accounted for by the hiving off of a very considerable part of the land, perhaps to allow for the building of Newstead which bounds it and which does not appear on the Ordnance Survey Map of 1837 but does appear on the Pembroke Estate map of 1866. Similarly, Rose villa/Roseville (later St Anne's, now Annsbrook) is not in the Ordnance Map 1837 but is in the Pembroke Estate map 1866 and is first listed in the directories in 1855. It too could have been built on lands that were originally part of the property in which John Ennis lived. However, it could also be accounted for by a drop in rateable valuations generally during this period. Note, in particular, the example of Roebuck house/Roebuck grove discussed above; its valuation was assessed at £230 in 1847 and at £117 in 1895.

Just as his father's address was given simply as 'Roebuck' in 1829, from the first time the directories include Clonskeagh in 1836 John Ennis appears under that heading but without getting the full title 'Roebuck house'. He continues to appear in this way until the 1847, when the directories were giving more detail. He is then reported as living in 'Roebuck house' and the rateable valuation given to it indicates that it was a quite substantial property. Thus John Ennis and his father before him were living in a property called simply 'Roebuck' that later, during John's occupancy, came to be known as 'Roebuck house'. This was in the approximate area where Wynnstay is today located. An indication of the date when the first house was built in this area can be got from a comparison between Taylor's map of 1816 and Duncan's of 1821. In the former there is no indication of a house to be found in the area while in the latter there is a clear sign, not alone of a house but also of a driveway going towards it. The house was therefore built between 1816 and 1821. Since we know that Andrew Ennis lived there in 1829 it seems quite likely that he was the original owner of the house. No name is given to it by Duncan in his map but in the first Ordnance Survey map of 1837 it is clearly marked and called simply 'Roebuck'. In a later map made by the Ordnance Survey for *Thom's Directory* in 1888 it is still called 'Roebuck'; in this map both Newstead house and Rose Villa are seen to be already in existence with the land around 'Roebuck' much reduced and somewhat similar in its extent to that of Wynnstay today except that it then had a curving driveway coming from Clonskeagh road at the point where Wynnsward drive today intersects with that road. There was a gate lodge at the entrance.

Andrew Ennis was, as already noted, a top ranking merchant in Dublin with a city address at 21 Harcourt street. His core business was the bakery trade located at North Great George's street. However, he had other interests which included being a director of the Hibernian Joint Stock Banking Company, Marlborough street; his fellow director lived very close to him in Clonskeagh – Richard Corballis of Rosemount. During his life he bought a large tract of land in county Westmeath. Politically he was, as we have seen, a strong supporter of Daniel O'Connell. Although the dates of his birth and death have not been found, it seems certain that he was buried in the crypt of the pro-Cathedral since one of the vaults there bears the inscription 'Family Vault of ANDREW ENNIS Esq'.

His son, John, was perhaps even more successful. He too, like his father, was principally a merchant. He was born in Dublin on 15 August 1800 and educated at Stoneyhurst college, in England. At the age of 36 he became a director of the Bank of Ireland for the first time. He would become a director again on a number of occasions and governor between 1856 and 1858. A leading figure in Irish commercial life, he was at one time chairman of the Midland and Great Western Railway. He became sheriff of Westmeath in 1837 and, while living in

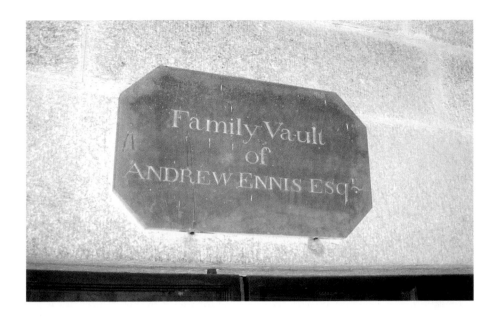

Burial vault under the pro-cathedral, Dublin, of Andrew Ennis, of Roebuck house
(later Wynnstay), Clonskeagh road

Clonskeagh, a sheriff of county Dublin in 1849. Later in April 1856 he contested Athlone in the elections of that year and became MP for the same constituency from April 1857 to July 1865. On 27 July of the following year he was created a baronet. He was a commissioner of charitable bequests- the importance of which has been discussed in an earlier chapter – a position he held until his death at no. 9 Merrion square east on 8 August 1878. He had held that city address while he lived in Clonskeagh; he also had an address at Berkeley square, London and a country house at Ballinahown Court, Westmeath where he owned around 9000 acres of land. On his death, the *Freeman's Journal* described him in an obituary as 'an earnest Catholic and a moderate Liberal, who held aloof from later popular movements'. His son, Sir John James Ennis, 2nd baronet, was sheriff of Westmeath in 1866 and MP for Athlone from 1868 to 1874 and from 1880 until his death in 1884.[57]

---

57 Boase, *Modern English biography,* i 993; Hall, *Bank of Ireland,* 486-87. There is a difference between these two sources as to who the father of John Ennis was. The view expressed in the latter source has been accepted as it seems to fit more accurately with the other evidence we have about both father and son, in particular the fact that both of them – Andrew and John – lived in Roebuck at certain times.

The house-name, Winstay, appears for the first time in the directories in 1868. The first occupant is given as captain John Wynne, Royal [Horse] Artillery. Is the name given to the house in any way related to his name? There is no definitive proof but it seems to be quite possible. That spelling of the name remained while captain Wynne was living there but soon afterwards it was changed to Wynnstay. It may be that subsequent occupants of the property corrected the directory entry to what may have been the proper spelling of the name from the outset. It was, incidentally, also spelled Wynnestay in an entry in the *Dictionary of National Biography* relating to captain Wynne's son, to be discussed later; sources used for this would have come originally from the Wynne family records. Also note that Wynne is retained in the name of roads e.g. Wynnsward drive/park which are on either side of Wynnstay.

Another possibility for the origin of the house name is an estate in Denbighshire, Wales called Wynnstay. Its Estate Records are now lodged with the National Library of Wales. This estate came into the possession of Sir John Wynn († 1719) through his marriage to the heiress of Eyton Evans of Watstay, its original name; he changed the name to Wynnstay. On his death, the estate passed to his kinsman, Watkin Williams (1692-1749), who added the name Wynn to his own; this was the name by which he came to be called later. It was he who was the real founder of what became the great Welsh house of Wynnstay; he built a new mansion on the estate to replace the old one. His grandson, Sir Watkin Williams Wynn (1772-1840), raised a cavalry regiment, 'The Ancient British Fencibles', in 1794; it subsequently took part in the defeat of the participants of the 1798 rising in Ireland. It was during his son's occupancy that the old mansion of Wynnstay in Wales was almost completely destroyed by fire in 1858; it took six years, from 1859 to 1865, for the house to be restored. Just three years later, captain John Wynne took possession of a house in Clonskeagh, hitherto apparently called 'Roebuck house', and called it Wynnstay. There is no record of any close family relationship between captain Wynne and the Wynns of Wynnstay in Wales but the fire and restoration of Wynnstay would have been widely reported around the time that he was moving into his new residence in Clonskeagh; it may have influenced him in his choice of name for that residence.

At that time he was already married to Anne, daughter of admiral Sir Samuel Warren, KCB GCH. A son of theirs was destined to become quite famous for his military exploits that would, in the end, cost him his life. He was Warren Richard Colvin Wynne, born in Collon house, county Louth on 9 April 1843. His early military career saw him serve in Gibraltar before returning to England in 1871. Quite clearly he was in close touch with his family in Clonskeagh at this time since he married a local lady in 1872, Eleanor, third daughter of J P Turbett, of nearby Owenstown.

He was promoted captain in 1875; three years later he set out for Africa where he was engaged in the Zulu war. Being a captain of the Royal Engineers he was initially responsible for building some forts. However, when military reverses indicated that a retreat from existing positions was considered necessary by superior commanders, Wynne sought permission to hold his position. This he did with considerable ingenuity thus reversing some of the earlier military setbacks. Wynne, however, was soon struck down with fever thought to have been brought on by the exertions involved in stabilising the situation. He died on his 36th birthday, 9 April 1879, and was buried in a hillside cemetery overlooking one of the forts which he had laid out and built, Fort Tenedos. He was posthumously promoted major on 5 March 1880, the appointment being made a week prior to his death. His name has been commemorated by his military corps in Rochester cathedral. That of his wife Eleanor Turbett is remembered in a tablet erected in St Thomas's on Fosters avenue, the chapel of ease attached to Taney church, built around the time of Eleanor's death. It reads 'To the praise of God and the hallowed memory of Eleanor, wife of Warren Wynne, Lieutenant, Royal Engineers, and seventh daughter of James Turbett, Esq., and Sophie, his wife, of Owenstown, Co Dublin who, at the age of 24 ... fell asleep on the Lord's Day 14 December 1873'.[58]

Occupants of the house (under its contemporary name) and rateable valuation, where available, as found in the directories and other sources, are as follows: *Roebuck*: (Andrew Ennis given an address of Roebuck in 1829); *Roebuck*: John Ennis (1835-46); *Roebuck house*: John Ennis, DL, 9 Merrion–square, east (*£206*) (1847-49); no directory entry (1850); James Forrest, silk mercer, 98, 100 & 101 Grafton street (1851-67); *Winstay*: Captain John Wynne, Royal Artillery (1868-84); Captain W H C Grattan (1885); Michael Nugent (1886-87); *Wynnstay*: John Forster, John M Forster (1888-94); do. (*£88*) (1895-97); John Forster, (*£88*) (1898); do. & Charles William E E Forster (1899-1900); Mrs Forster (*£88*), Charles William E E Forster (1901-02); Mrs Forster (*£88*) (1903-19); do. (*£67-10*) (1920-33); John O'Hagan Ward (*£67-10s*) (1934-36); do. (*£64*) (1937-46); D E McCarthy (*£64*) (1947-54); D E McCarthy (1955-58); Dermot McCarthy (1960);

---

58 Sidney Lee (ed), *Dictionary of National Biography* (London 1909) vol. xxi, 1174, 1179; Website of the Archives-Network-Wales [http://www.archives network-wales.info/(and links)]; Boase, *Modern English biography*, iii 1543; British military website – South Africa 1878-79 [http://glosters.tripod.com/south.htm]; personal communication from John Young, who has been in contact with the Wynne family; his book on the Zulu war: John Young, *They fell like stones: battles and casualties of the Zulu war, 1879* (London 1991); Ball & Hamilton, *Parish of Taney*, 198.

do. (*£42-12s*) (1962/3); Gypsum Industries Ltd., Building Materials and Systems (1965-2006); vacant (2007).

A separate listing for a house called Winnstay, in the same section of the directories as that of Wynnstay, appears between 1892 and 1906; it was occupied by H Goodisson but was vacant in 1906. It ceases to be listed after that and no rateable valuation is given to help assess its size. It is possible that it was a house or a lodge in the grounds of Wynnstay. As we will see in the next chapter, the grounds around Wynnstay were reduced in size in the middle of the twentieth century as new houses were built on both sides of it. By way of compensation, as it were, 'Wynn' was adopted as an element in the address assigned to these roads. Eventually, the house was taken over by a company called Gypsum Industries Ltd which located its offices there. However, in the early years of the twenty first century the house became vacant awaiting some further use. Unlike other houses in the area, that had been changed from residential to other uses and were subsequently demolished, Wynnstay is likely to avoid that fate as it has been dubbed a listed building by the appropriate Local Authority.

ROEBUCK HOUSE (MOUNT ANVILLE)

The following is the only information relating to this house as found in the directories: John Edwards (?1830-31 and 1841-42?); Henry Edwards (?1843-45?); Henry Edwards (1846); Henry Edwards (*£89*) (1847-48); Henry Deane Edwards (1849-56).

The Edwards family are the only known people to have lived in this house while it bore the name 'Roebuck house'. It was a relatively modest sized house given that its rateable valuation was £89 in 1847. Only one item has been discovered about a member of this family. That is found in a report in the *Anglo-Celt* newspaper, dated 13 April 1849. There it is stated that Henry Deane Edwards, esq., of Roebuck was appointed captain of the Cavan Militia. After his departure from the house in 1856 there is no clear succession of occupants of a house bearing the name 'Roebuck house' in Mount Anville. It is possible that Samuel Anderson took possession of the house along with Matthew Anderson since they first appear with the address of 'Roebuck house' in 1857. However, it seems likely that they did not remain there and, as a result, the name of the house in Mount Anville may not have been retained; it is likely to have been changed to some other, as yet undiscovered, name. Because of this, the exact location of the house in Mount Anville has not been located.

ROEBUCK HOUSE (CLONSKEAGH)

The Andersons continue to be listed with the address 'Roebuck house' until 1860. However, there is a problem pinpointing the exact location of this house due to some confusion in the way the directories are organised during these years. In 1857 and 1858 all houses in the Roebuck area are listed under Dundrum but from 1859 they are split in two; some are then listed under Clonskeagh, the rest under Dundrum. The Andersons in 'Roebuck house' appear under both headings in the entries for both 1859 and 1860 and cease to be listed thereafter.

Then in the following year (1861) there are two entries giving different people (captain Miller and Mrs Fulton) with an address at 'Roebuck house' and both are clearly entered under the heading of Clonskeagh. It is not possible to determine whether these are two separate houses; that seems unlikely as there is only one house bearing that name and suitably located in the Pembroke Estate Papers (*National Archives*: 97/46/4/31) surveyed in 1866 (location no. 9 on map). We do, however, have definite evidence that this house was owned by Mrs Fulton at that time. But before discussing that it must be pointed out that there was a house already located there in 1837 according to the first Ordnance Survey map. On that map it is named simply 'Roebuck' thus compounding the problems of identification which has already been discussed in relation to the early occupancy of the house that ultimately became Wynnstay. From its earliest existence, most likely some time before 1837, until Mrs Fulton took up residence, there is no definite information available as to who the owners or occupants were. The first definite information we have comes from a list of Documents of Title of Roebuck house drawn up by a later owner, Seán MacBride. This begins with a Landed Estate Court Conveyance to Mrs Anne Fulton in 1863;[59] this Court, incidentally, had only been established five years earlier absorbing in the process the Encumbered Estates Court.[60] This Conveyance eliminates captain Miller from ownership of the house (and, indeed, the associated land) as the dates of his entries in the directories overlap those of Mrs Fulton. It is possible, of course, that he could have lived there during the period he is listed in some capacity other than ownership.

The clearest evidence of ownership we have, therefore, begins with Mrs Fulton but for completeness the other names found in the directories and discussed above will be included in brackets in the following list of occupants of Roebuck house, Clonskeagh: {Samuel Anderson (1857); Matthew Anderson,

---

59   My thanks to Caitriona Lawlor for giving me sight of this document.
60   McDowell, *The Irish Administration: 1801-1914*, 110.

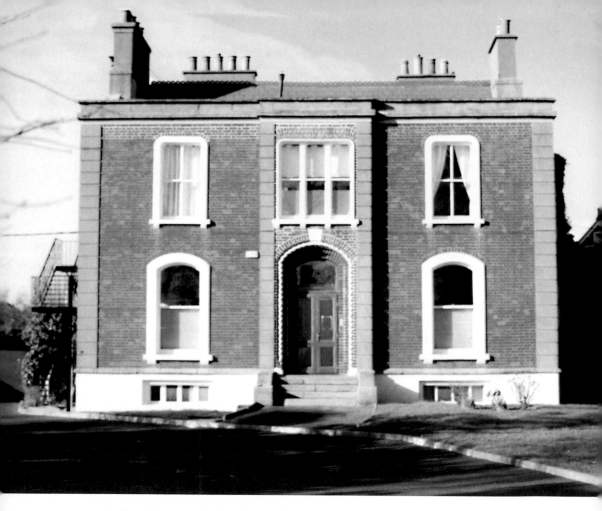

Roebuck house, one-time home of Madame Maud Gonne MacBride
(*Photographer: Matt Walsh*)

Samuel Anderson and 2 Inn's Quay (1858-60); Captain Henry Miller, R N (1861-73)}

    Mrs Fulton (1861-64); Joseph Fulton, LRCSI, Mrs Fulton (1865-70); Mrs Fulton (1871-75); Francis M Crozier (1876-78); vacant (1879); Henry J Gill, AM TCD (1880); do. MP (1881-89); do. but no longer MP(1890-1903); Mrs Gill, Michael J Gill, BA, R A Gill (1904); Mrs Gill (1905); vacant (1906); C Dunkan Blake (1907-08); Brig-Gen. Stratford Cecil Vernon Wingfield (1909-12); Col. H C de la M Hill, East Kent Regiment (1913); do. (*£85*) (1914-17); vacant (1918-19); Arthur Payne, engineer, and 43 Dawson street (*£85*) (1920-21); Mrs Despard (*£85*) (1922-33); Madam Maud Gonne MacBride (*£85*) (1934-53); Seán McBride, SC TD (*£85*) (1954); do. (*£35*)* (1955-63); do. (*£62*) (1965-1988). *Note: the valuation of £35 given is probably a printer's error for £85.

    The above list is drawn from the directories; greater clarity between owners and tenants or leaseholders can be gleaned from the Documents of Title that has already been mentioned. Although in residence from 1861 it was not until 19 December 1863 that the Landed Estates Court Conveyance to Mrs Fulton came through. Three months later on 23 March 1864 she got a Fee Farm Grant from Sir James Power. He, as already discussed, was the son of Sir John Power who, until his death in 1855, had lived in what was then called Roebuck house but later Roebuck grove. James would have inherited his father's property interests in the locality including the house, which it seems was held on a Reversionary Lease originally from Nicholas, lord baron of Trimbleston[61] and was sold after Sir John's death. But it would appear that Sir John had interest in property outside his own house, the nature of which is unclear; this, or at least part of it, was now being passed on to Mrs Fulton.

The month before this transaction took place Mrs Fulton leased three fields to James Dillon Meldon, then the occupant of Casino on Bird avenue. These were most likely to have been behind Roebuck house and thus in close proximity to Casino. This lease, incidentally, would suggest that although Meldon was a solicitor he must also have dabbled in some form of farming; he had been living at Casino since 1843. He is no longer listed there in 1882 and the fields then, according to a Memorandum of Agreement endorsed on the Lease document, were leased on 13 June 1883 to James Turbett of Oak lawn, now Farranboley house; he too was a solicitor with offices at 3 Bachelor's Walk. There is no subsequent reference to this lease.

Mrs Fulton made a will on 19 June 1869 which, shortly after her death, was admitted to probate on 15 June 1875. Her property, including Roebuck house, passed to her daughter Elizabeth Fulton. It appears that she never took up residence there and four years later, on 5 June 1879, she leased the house for 40 years to Henry Joseph Gill; that this did not include the surrounding land is suggested by the leasing of the three fields, already discussed, to James Turbett in 1883. The forty years lease on the house would have lasted until 1919. However, as can be seen from the list of occupants compiled from the directories various members of the Gill family were in residence only until 1905. The other

---

61   The basis on which this statement can be made is as follows. From documents in the Archives of the Carmelite monastery there is evidence that this is the manner in which Mount Dillon was held. A Certified Copy of the Reversionary Lease, dated October 1799, is listed among the Schedule of Documents held at the monastery. Another Document in the same archives shows the monastery to be Lot No. 1 of two lots, the second of which is the Roebuck house which Sir John Power had owned. It also states that Lot No 1 holds primary liability for payment of the entire headrent payable on both Lots.

people who lived there between that date and 1919, including the two military gentlemen, would have been tenants of the person who ultimately inherited Henry Joseph Gill's lease.

While the house was still on lease Elizabeth Fulton died and the property passed to her nephew, Henry Fulton, according to her will, admitted to probate on 23 April 1903. On the expiration of the lease in 1919 this nephew, now colonel Henry Fulton, leased the house to Arthur Payne. This soon ran into trouble as Payne became bankrupt. On 13 May 1921 there was a Court order for the sale of his interest in the lease. The house now was put up for sale and was sold on 8 June 1922 according to the document 'Conveyance Colonel Henry Fulton to Mrs Charlotte Despard and Maud Gonne MacBride'. Although this Conveyance and one to be discussed shortly makes it clear that the house was sold to both ladies only Mrs Despard appears in the directories until the time she sold her share to Maud Gonne MacBride suggesting, perhaps, that she had the greater share in ownership. On the 10 January 1934 Mrs Despard sold her share to Maud Gonne MacBride according to the Document 'Release and Conveyance Charlotte Despard to Maud Gonne MacBride'. The house remained in the MacBride family until finally sold. It is now divided into apartments.

Nothing of consequence has been found about Mrs Fulton. The Joseph Fulton, LRCSI who is said to be living in Roebuck house with her from 1865-70 was most likely her son and was presumably a surgeon. It seems almost certain that she had a daughter, Anne, living with her at the same time although not recorded in the directory. She is recorded as owning 294 acres of land in county Donegal in 1876 and her address is given as Roebuck house, Milltown, co. Dublin. It is indicative of the confusion often met in regard to where the boundary between Clonskeagh and Roebuck lay that in this particular record Roebuck house is actually stated to be in Milltown[62]

The forty year lease taken on the house by Henry Joseph Gill commenced, as already noted, on 5 June 1879. It may be a coincidence but early in the following year, on 13 April 1880, Gill was returned as MP for Westmeath county. His address given in the House of Commons records was most likely his business address in Dublin – 90 Middle Abbey street.[63] Did he lease the house in anticipation of his being elected? That must remain an open question but he did continue as MP until late in that decade. A chronology of the life of the poet

---

62   www.ulsterancestry.com

63   RETURN to an Address of the Honourable The House of Commons, dated 13 March 1890: *Ordered by* The House of Commons *to be printed,* 8 *April* 1891, p. xxvii.

William Butler Yeats (1865-1939) indicates that he visited the Misses Gill at Roebuck house on Wednesday 2 March, 1887 when he 22 years old. It is an interesting coincidence that in the same house a number of years later the woman he courted so ardently (from 1889), but unsuccessfully, came to live and eventually (1953) die there, Maud Gonne. She married John MacBride in 1903. It is worthy of note that some military gentlemen of officer rank lived there from 1909 to 1917 during the 1916 rising and the 1st world war. However, nothing of any substance has been found out about their military activities.

Arthur Payne, the engineer with offices at 43 Dawson street, who lived at the house from 1919 to 1921 was a tenant of Henry Fulton; he received a lease from him on 4 March 1919. However, it would appear that in 1921 Payne became a bankrupt and an Order of Court was issued on 13 May in the same year which ordered the sale of Payne's interest in the house. The house was once again fully in Fulton's possession and on 8 June of the following year a Conveyance was made out from col. Henry Fulton in favour of Mrs Charlotte Despard and Maud Gonne MacBride.[64] A new era had dawned in the house; this has been discussed in some detail towards the end of the chapter which deals with the affairs, political and others, of the twentieth century.

ROSEMOUNT

The next house is one of the exceptions referred to at the outset of this chapter; it was skipped over because of complications attending the discussion of Roebuck house. We now return to it (location no. 10 on map). It no longer exists but was once located in what is now UCD grounds at a little distance in from the Clonskeagh entrance over to the right as one progresses towards the college. It was approached originally by the same carriageway which served Roebuck house/grove a little further on. The entrance to Rosemount was on the right hand side of the carriageway not too far along it from the Clonskeagh entrance; it now has a formidable galvanised gate blocking it off with notices attached: 'No admittance except on business' and 'Rosemount Horticultural Field Station'. Inside, looking through the gate, one sees a well kept ground but there is no sign of Rosemount house from the gate. The reason is that it was demolished in 1985 after it came into the possession of UCD.

In this house the Corballis family lived from the time it was first purchased

---

64   'Documents of Title to Roebuck house'; an undated list of documents related to title of Roebuck house, drawn up by one-time owner of the house, Mr Seán MacBride.

from a speculative builder by Richard Corballis in 1793 until it was sold to UCD in 1981. This is almost 200 years and is by far the longest period of occupation of a house in Clonskeagh by the same family (apart from the lords Trimleston of Roebuck castle) that it has been possible to find even though the name Corballis did not survive for the whole of that time. This is because succession changed to the female line on one occasion and with that the name changed to Woulfe-Flanagan. In 1851 a daughter of John Richard Corballis, Mary Deborah, married Stephen Woulfe Flanagan, the second son of Terence Flanagan of Knockhall, co Roscommon and Mary Johanna, daughter of Stephen Woulfe, sister of chief baron Stephen Woulfe. Mary Deborah (or simply 'plain Mary' as she referred to the name when discussing what a new granddaughter might be called) and Stephen lived in Fitzwilliam place and in co. Roscommon. In a codicil to his will, added in 1864, John R Corballis expressed the hope that 'by his [Stephen's] care and advice he will keep my son Richard out of trouble and litigation'. Stephen at this time was a Queen's Counsel and would later become a judge of the Landed Estates Court, an Irish privy councillor, a justice of the Chancery Division and finally an English privy councillor. In fact he and his son John were both invited to attend the service at Westminster Abbey on June 21st 1887 to celebrate the golden jubilee of queen Victoria.

Richard, by comparison, did not seem to be a high achiever – at least in the conventional sense; his father's request to his son-in-law in the codicil referred to above suggests that this was already apparent to him in 1864 when Richard was 33 years old. Nevertheless he did manage to become a Justice of the Peace around 1885 and was apparently well able to manage his inherited wealth. That was something other younger members of his extended family seemed not to be able to do. He told his niece, a nun who on one occasion sent a 'begging letter' on behalf of her convent, 'that junior members of the family were not worthy of their progenitors and it was a great worry for him to be constantly called on for help'. Said to be something of a recluse he never married. Rosemount had been left by John Richard to his 'beloved wife' Jane in his will which was proved on 9 April 1879. After her death, it was passed on to Richard in 1884; he continued to live there until his death in 1931 after which it passed on to Stephen Woulfe-Flanagan, his nephew and son of his sister Mary Deborah and her husband, Stephen Woulfe-Flanagan. Hence the change in name but the continuation of the Corballis family connection with Rosemount. It had stayed in the family from the time that it was built until it was finally sold, along with its 13_ acres of land, to UCD in 1981.

The political, church and other public activities of both Richard (1769- 1847) and his son John Richard (1796-1879) have already been extensively discussed in an earlier chapter. Not mentioned, however, was Richard's involvement in a committee set up after a meeting held in Taney church in 1812 to establish a dispensary in Dundrum to promote 'the comfort of the poor'. Neither was mention made of John Richard's involvement in famine relief work carried out in the same place. Apart from that, there were a number of other activities which attracted his interest. He served on the committee of the Union Club from 1837 to 1840. However, the fact that he did not continue membership of the committee for any substantial length of time after the club had been taken over (and its name changed to the Stephen's Green Club in 1840) by the more radical repealers led by Daniel O'Connell would suggest that his views on the Union were moderate.

He was also a trustee for the project that saw the erection of a monument to John Philpot Curran in Glasnevin and was one of the two trustees of the Netterville Charities; these had been founded under the will of lord viscount Netterville. They were regulated by a decree of the Court of Chancery and provided maintenance and clothing for widows and orphans. They also provided education and medical services. Early in his career, in 1830, along with archbishop Murray and Daniel O'Connell he was on the committee of the Association for the Suppression of Street-begging, an association under the patronage of the lord lieutenant; this was a voluntary charitable organisation, established in 1818, which gave food and employment to paupers as an alternative to begging. Given his close connection with archbishop Murray and the Catholic church in general it is not surprising that he donated a scene depicting the Nativity in stain glass that is located in the apse of the Catholic church in Donnybrook, his parish church newly consecrated in 1866; inscribed at the bottom are the words 'Pray for Richard R Corballis and his deceased relatives'. His wife was also involved in charity work associated with the Catholic church. She was one of the Governesses of the House of Refuge, Stanhope street, founded in 1811. This institution was under the Sisters of Charity 'for the benefit of young women of good character in distress'.

Finally, given the illustrious career pursued by John R Corballis an interesting insight may be got into how he received help at an early stage in it from a man whose nephew would, in time, marry his daughter; that man was chief baron Stephen Woulfe. This may be seen in a memorandum drawn up by John R Corballis himself at some unknown date. Headed "Right Hon. Stephen Woulfe, L(or)d Chief Baron" it goes on to say 'We were school fellows for a short time at the Lay College of Maynooth, then the first class school for Roman Catholics. ... Stephen Woulfe always shewed a great regard for me – when Attorney General the place of Crown Counsel on the Home circuit becoming vacant, he was pressed to appoint others – His answer was, no, I shall appoint no one but Corballis – He has been damn badly treated – & accordingly he appointed me the junior Counsel, from which I rose to the senior in time. I was with him shortly before his death to ask him at Blake's desire to attend Mrs Blake's funeral – But his state of health would not permit his attendance – he died soon after'. Blake, it is reasonable to assume, was Anthony Blake, the very influential friend of Corballis whom we have discussed on a number of occasions.

It is not clear what was meant by the statement that Corballis was 'damn badly treated'; he had at that stage already served on the commission set up by the House of Commons to inquire into the state of municipal corporations in Ireland. In any case, the private views of attorney general Woulfe, as noted in the memorandum, are nowhere to be seen when the *Connaught Journal* commented on the appointment in 1840: 'Mr Corballis, who has been appointed by the Attorney General to conduct the crown prosecution on the Home circuit, (noticed in last publication) is a Roman Catholic, but a gentleman of high legal and literary attainments and unobjectionable in other respects. He never mingled in agitation or sought for pre-eminence at the bar, on account of religion, or politics'.[65]

The Corballis family have a sepulchral vault in the crypt of the pro-cathedral in Marlborough street where many of the family are buried. The plaque over it, when first inscribed, read 'Family Vault of Richard Corballis Esqr'. This would suggest that, at the very least, Richard Corballis was buried there; not surprising since, as we noted elsewhere, Dr Murray, archbishop of Dublin, stayed at Rosemount for some days around the time of Richard's death in 1847. One final word about the vault; the original inscription which is on the plaque above it has been subsequently slightly altered. The name CORBALLIS was changed, for some undiscovered reason, to CORBALAS by superimposing the letter A over the letters LI which had originally been on it.

It is, perhaps, appropriate at this juncture to point out that the directories make reference to another house in the general area which was called Rosemount. The entries for them are as follows: Lewis Edward Leipsett, M.D., Rosemount (1837-39); James Dillon Meldon, esq., attorney (1840-42); Edward Hornsby, esq (1843-46); do. (1847 (*£69*)); vacant (1848); William Gillespie, esq., Rosemount cottage (1849); Wm Barrett, esq (1850); lacuna 1851-53; John

---

65 Various Dublin directories; Danny Parkinson, 'The Corballis-Corbally Families of Co. Dublin', *Dublin Historical Record*, 45/2 (1992) 91-100: 97-9; McCartney, *UCD, a national idea*, 397-9; Cornelius F Smith, 'In the beginning: 1837 – 1875' in Cornelius F Smith & Bernard Share, *Whigs on the Green* (Dublin 1990) 36-59: 38, 185; Ball, *The judges in Ireland, 1221-1921*, ii 372; Irish National Archives: Private Sources 1189/2/7; 1189/16/4 &10; 1189/17/9; *Connaught Journal*, Thursday February 27, 1840.

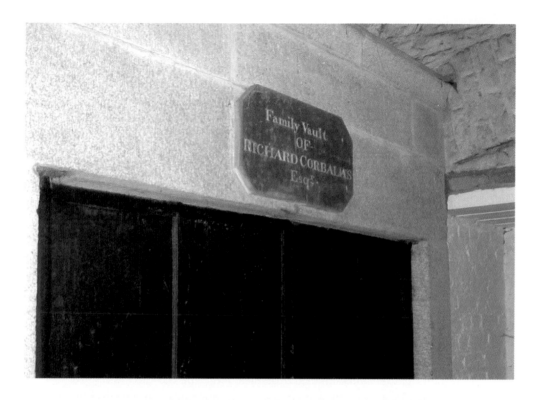

Burial vault under the pro-cathedral, Dublin, of Richard Corballis, Rosemount, Clonskeagh

Parkinson, Rosemount (1854); Mr Kavanagh (1856); William Kavanagh and 12 Dame street (1857-59); C Kavanagh, esq., and 12 Dame street (1860). This is the last entry and it is assumed that the name of house must have changed thereafter. This second Rosemount is clearly seen on the first Ordnance Survey map of 1837 in the same place as Trimleston lodge is seen to be on the Pembroke Estate Survey map of 1866 thus suggesting that the house name had been changed to Trimleston lodge. Furthermore, although there is a slight overlap in entries between 1858 and 1860, when this Rosemount disappears from the directories it is replaced by Trimbleston (later Trimleston) lodge. That they refer to the same house but under different names seems to be confirmed by the fact that they had similar rateable valuations; £69 for Rosemount and £65 for Trimleston lodge in 1915, the first year that the directories give a valuation for the house under this name. The location where this house existed has recently had a large number of apartment blocks built on it which retain the name Trimleston.

ROEBUCK LODGE, LATER THE COTTAGE

After Rosemount the next house to be considered is that which originally was called Roebuck lodge but later changed to The Cottage. Its location is well-known as it is prominently visible on the Clonskeagh road just beyond Wynnsward drive as one travels outwards from the city (location no. 11 on map). The ownership of the house at one time by John Richard Corballis, its occupation by his sister Miss Maria Corballis between 1849 and 1877 and the change by her of the name of the house from Roebuck lodge to The Cottage has already been discussed. So too has the death in it of the prominent Irish parliamentarian Isaac Butt. It only remains here to chart the names of the other occupants from the earliest date for which we have that information up until modern times.

In some of the early maps of the area (Taylor's of 1816 and Duncan's of 1821) there is a building indicated at the spot where we now know The Cottage to be located but there is no name given. Similarly in the first hand-drawn Ordnance Survey map of 1837 there is no name given; however, in the first of its printed versions (1843) the building carries the name Roebuck lodge. However, in the same map there is another Roebuck lodge that is located much further out in Roebuck and, what is more, that house is marked by name on Taylor's map of 1816. There is something of a dilemma in trying to decipher who the early occupants of the house named Roebuck lodge in the directories were. John Elliott Hyndman is given that address from 1833 to 1845 and during those years three other people are given the same address: General Haynes (1839), Rev Richard Barton (1840-43) and Rev Edward Day (1844-46).

There are two different ways of tackling the problem. On the one hand, observing the first year in which two different people are given the same address i.e. 1839, it would appear that the compiler followed a certain route when listing each entry. It appears that he began at the city end and progressed outwards taking a left turn at the junction of what is now Roebuck road and Goatstown road and proceeded along that road then turned right up Mount Anville road until he turned right down the Goatstown road finally ending at the junction where he had earlier turned right. Along this route he named a number of the houses and their occupants. If he remained true to this and did not, for some unknown reason, interject some house name and occupant at a point other than the logic of the route followed, then it must follow that the early occupant of the Roebuck lodge which later became The Cottage would have been Alderman John Elliott Hyndman. On the other hand, we are told by Lewis in his 1837 *Topographical Dictionary* that among the 'handsome villas, situated in tastefully disposed grounds' is 'Roebuck lodge, the residence of J E Hyndman, Esq., formerly the manor-house and about fifty years since the only house in the district with the exception of the castle'. The Cottage does not fit this description and since the evidence based on the description by Lewis is more direct than that which is deduced from the manner in which the directory of 1839 was compiled the former is to be preferred. That being the case, then the three gentlemen whose names are given above seem to have been the residents of what later became The Cottage between 1839 and 1846.

After them came Joseph Conroy, a civil engineer who remained there until Miss Maria Corballis took up residence in 1849. As already noted, she changed the name to The Cottage in 1861 or 1862 (information from directories comes, by definition, at an unspecified time after the event but not greater than a year later unless the compiler erred). Around this time we also discover that the rateable valuation of the house was £46; this confirms the view that the property was not substantial enough to meet the description given by Lewis to Hyndman's house. After her death and the house lying vacant for some time, Thomas Colquhoun moved in. A solicitor, he was married to Elizabeth, the daughter of Isaac Butt. It is through this connection that it came about that the latter died at the house. However, Thomas and Elizabeth did not remain long at The Cottage; within a short time of her father's death they moved to an address in Leeson street. The Cottage was then occupied by The Misses Colquhoun whose name would suggest that they were someway related to Elizabeth's husband Thomas. In 1885 the house was again vacant after these ladies moved on but soon a Mr Edward Holland took up residence and while there managed to have his status raised somewhat in view of the fact that after a few years he graduated from being plain Mr Edward Holland to being Edward Holland, Esq.; what he did or achieved to acquire such status has not been discovered.

After being occupied for a number of years in the 1890s by a Mrs Bailey the house got, for the second time, an engineer as a resident, Maurice Pitman. He was an electrical engineer which for the period was at the advanced edge of technology and he had his offices at 17 Cope street. He remained at The Cottage from 1898 until 1943 and seems to have retired around 1932 judging by the fact that the entry in the directory for that year no longer referred to his having an office. After a number of years in the middle 1940s when Terence De Vere White lived there, Stanley Huet moved in around 1950. By this time, the rateable valuation of the house had dropped from the £46 at which it had stood since at least 1860 to £25-10s. The reason for this seems to be clear; some of its ground was taken over for the building of houses in a new development, Wynnsward drive which was listed for the first time in the directories in 1949. Stanley Huet was still listed as residing in The Cottage in the mid-1970s, when the valuation had increased to £40-15s. In 1990 Ursula Huet was given as the occupant while in the year 2000 it was Brendan O'Sullivan.

OAK LAWN (OAKLAWN, ON OCCASION OAK PARK) LATER FARRANBOLEY AND LATER STILL FARRANBOLEY HOUSE

After The Cottage we move across the road and a few doors beyond the intersection of Embassy lawn with Clonskeagh road we come to Farranboley house (location no. 12 on map); this house was called Oak lawn in the earliest records we have. Now entered directly from Clonskeagh road, it was originally approached by a driveway from Bird avenue; indeed as late as the 1960s Farranboley house is listed in the directory under Bird avenue and alongside this entry is one for a Gate lodge which was probably originally associated with the start of this driveway. The entry and driveway can be seen on Duncan's map of 1821 but not on Taylor's of 1816. On the first printed Ordnance Survey map the gate lodge is specifically marked in the same location. This is opposite the entry to Bloomville/Gledswood house, to be discussed later, and would therefore suggest that it was located where later the entry was to the College of Surgeons' Sports Ground, now a housing estate called The Maples.

Not much is known about the origins of this house. However there is one important item that allows us to suggest that it was the home of Alderman John Exshaw in the late 1700s and early 1800s; Exshaw was twice lord mayor of Dublin around that time. When discussing the land held by Robert Emmet's father at Casino in a previous chapter it was noted that, in the Registry of the deeds of his main holding, the land attached to Casino was bounded 'on the eastern side by ground in the possession of Alderman John Exshaw'.[66] If, as we have seen, the entrance to the house, which the earliest records we have call Oak lawn, was some distance up along Bird avenue, then it seems reasonable to assume that the land around this entrance and driveway would have been associated with Oak lawn. That being the case, it could very easily have bounded the land associated with Casino since there is no record of any house being in between the two. In support of this is the address given to Exshaw in *Wilson's Dublin Directory* from 1816 onwards: '103 Grafton street and Windy Harbour'. This latter address may have been seen at the time to have taken in Bird avenue since it is in the townland of Farranboley. It is worth noting that in both Taylor's map of 1816 and Duncan's of 1821 the land to the rear of Oak lawn is called 'Bestfield'; nothing further, however, has been discovered in relation to that name. It should, however, be pointed out that this evidence regarding Oak lawn being Exshaw's house is fairly slight and one has to bear in mind the possibility that the land to the east of the Casino property was that associated with Roebuck house since there is a record of the owner of Casino, James Dillon Meldon,

---

66   Kerr, *Emmet's Casino*, 6.

renting three fields from Mrs Anne Fulton of Roebuck house in 1864. However, the same fields were rented in 1883 by the then occupant of Oak lawn, James Turbett. The land was, therefore, likely to have been adjacent to both of these properties.[67]

As Exshaw and his political involvement at the time – he was strongly against the United Irishmen of the 1790s – have been discussed in some detail in Chapter 7, it is not considered necessary to repeat it here. After him, we have to wait until the directories of the 1830s to find Francis Codd in residence there. From 1834 to 1842 he is merely given the address of Bird avenue; only from 1843 onwards is Oak lawn given specifically as his address, although rather curiously in an other part of the directories for the early 1840s his address is given as 'Oak park, Bird avenue', most likely a mistake for Oak lawn. As in the case of other subsequent residents it is possible, by a process of elimination, to infer that he was living at Oak lawn from 1834 and most likely at an earlier date. The process of elimination is accurately used since at that time and throughout all of the rest of the nineteenth century there were only four houses recorded in the directories in Bird avenue; a missing house-name is, therefore, easily found. Codd family members remained at Oak lawn until 1850 and during their residency the rateable valuation of the property is given as £118. In the 1830s a Francis Codd had a city address at 23 Harcourt street but another entry in 1833 has a Francis Codd, merchant, with an address at 52 Townsend street. Whether they both refer to the same person is not clear nor is it clear that one or both is the man who lived at Oak lawn in the same year. In 1847 the entry in the directory gives the name Francis A Codd; on first sight, this appears to be just extra detail. However, in 1850, the Chamber of Commerce is listed as having as secretary Francis Codd and he is also included among the members of its committee along with Francis A Codd. They are therefore two distinct people, probably father and son. Francis Codd had been in charge of the Corporation for Preserving and Improving the Port of Dublin in 1836. He was elected a director of the Corn Exchange Building Company in Burgh quay on 29 September 1849 while Francis A Codd was on the committee of the Commercial Building Company of Dublin in 1850; the latter was also a member of the Ouzel Galley Society where his address, perhaps of his business, is given as 168 Townsend street.

Around 1851, after the Codds moved out, George Kinahan, junior, took up residence at Oak lawn. He was soon joined by Daniel Kinahan who was most likely his father as his name took precedence in the listing in the directory. The

---

67   Document of Title to Roebuck house, drawn up by a subsequent owner of Roebuck house, Seán MacBride.

Kinahans were a well established family in the area with their main residence at Roebuck park. There is a problem in trying to decipher which branch of the family the people in Oak lawn belonged to since both names George and Daniel were common in the family. The first Daniel, of interest here, was born in 1756 in Churchtown and married in 1791. He had, among others, two sons George and Daniel born in 1791 and 1797 respectively. The son Daniel lived at Belfield which is located on what is now the Goatstown road. His brother Robert Henry was lord mayor of Dublin in 1853. Daniel married in 1825, had 15 children and died in 1859. It seems most probable that it was his son, called George but using the qualification 'junior' since his uncle George of Roebuck park was still alive, who moved into Oak lawn around 1851 followed by his father Daniel some years later. Daniel had been a churchwarden in Taney church during the years 1834, 1836 and 1840.[68]

After a short interlude during which Shapland Sweeny was in residence in 1855/56, James Turbett, junior, took up residence at Oak lawn around 1856. Like the Kinahans who had lived there shortly before him, James belonged to a well established family in the area, their main residence being Owenstown house just beyond Roebuck road. We have already met his grandfather Robert earlier in this chapter; he was the man who in 1816 devised a scheme to run a coaching service between Dublin, Dundrum and Enniskerry resulting in the establishment of two coaches operating between Enniskerry and Dublin. James himself much later in the century and while he lived at Oak lawn ran a coach between Dublin and Bray. He was the second son of James Exham Purefoy Turbett of Owenstown who had married in 1823. James, junior, would therefore have been born probably in the mid to late 1820s. He married Harriet, daughter of John Powys, esq., of West Wood Manor, Staffs. We have already met his youngest sister Eleanor who married lieutenant Warren Richard Colvin Wynne, RE of Wynnstay, Clonskeagh road which is but a short walk from Oak lawn. James was a churchwarden at Taney church in 1855. He shared his father's city office at 3 Bachelor's Walk and continued to use it after his father's death in 1868. In the years after this his entry in the directories dropped the qualification 'junior' and he remained at Oak lawn until 1886. [69]

After James Turbett came Maurice Brooks, esq., JP, DL whose city office was in Sackville place. He remained at Oak lawn until 1905 and his wife remained a short while longer, presumably after the death of her husband. With her was E Clive Brooks, perhaps her son. The arrival after them of Michael Cartan O'Meara saw the first name change of the house. He called it Farranboley, presumably after

---

68   Ball & Hamilton, *Parish of Taney,* 120-24.
69   Ibid 146-48, 201-03.

the name of the townland in which it is located; that name remained up until quite recent times. O'Meara was a solicitor, a commissioner of oaths and a Justice of the Peace for county Tipperary. While at Farranboley he apparently kept in contact with Tipperary since the entries in the directories always give his address there – Bouladuff, Tipperary. In Dublin, his office was at 44 Kildare street. He remained at Farranboley until 1918 and was replaced by Thomas Condren Flinn, chartered accountant who had his office at 31 Dame street. During his stay, between 1918 and 1929 the house was, for the first time, listed in the directories under the heading of 'Roebuck, part of; Clonskeagh' instead of 'Bird avenue' under which it had always previously appeared. After him the house was occupied for relatively short periods by different people being, also, on occasion listed as vacant: Joseph Dowling (1930-33); vacant (1934); J A Burke (1935-39); vacant (1940); Miss M Gartland (1941-53). During the next short occupancy the house got another name change; it became Farranboley house in 1954 when William Brennan-Whitmore was in residence. Thereafter the name remained with J Holland there from 1955 to around 1959, Mary Holland from 1960 to around 1962, Robert W G Burton c1965, Miss Margaret Gartland at the latter part of the 1960s before being taken over by the Marist Brothers in the 1970s. The name remains to this day. Occasionally spelled Farrenboley, the correct spelling, according to the Ordnance Survey, is Farranboley.

CASINO, LATER MOUNT ST MARY'S HOUSE OF STUDIES

As we have noted when discussing Oak lawn, later Farranboley house, the lands that were once associated with it were to the east of those associated with Casino (location no. 13 on map). Casino, now the property of the Marist Fathers with an entrance from the Dundrum road, originally had its main entrance from Bird avenue; the Dundrum entrance was then a side or back entrance. Throughout the 19th century it is always listed under Bird avenue in the directories. It lost its main entrance when it donated land for the new church on Bird avenue; around the same time the gate lodge associated with it was demolished. A good description of both the entrance gates and the avenue up to Casino was published in the 1920/21 annual produced in the first year in which the Marists took up residence at Casino; it was republished by Fr Kerr in his work on Emmet and Casino. The following is an excerpt: 'The main entrance, with its massive gates and stag-crowned piers is by Bird avenue ... On entering the impressive portals, the visitor is confronted with a magnificent and extensive property ... Advancing up the winding avenue, a pretty view is shortly gained of the stately mansion ... .'[70]

---

70   Kerr, *Emmet's Casino*, 11-12.

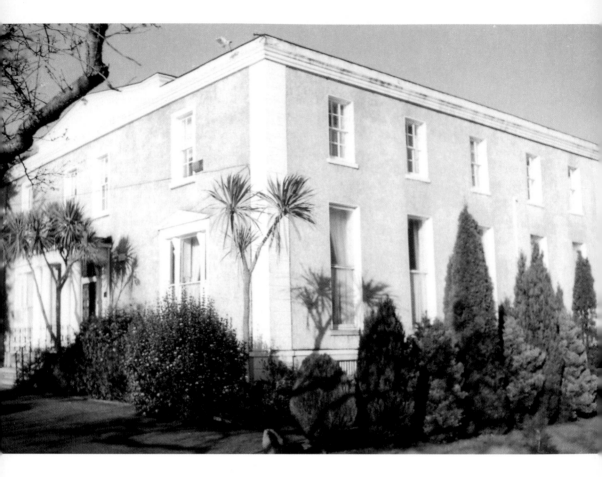

Emmet's Casino, now House of Studies, Marist Fathers (*Photographer: Matt Walsh*)

The historical connection of Casino with Robert Emmet has been discussed in Chapter 6 (above) as well as the writings of Fr Kerr on the subsequent owners. Because of that only the bare details of what has emerged from an examination of the directory entries will be given here. They are as follows:

George Stapleton (1834-41); James Dillon Meldon, solicitor (1843-47); do. (1848 *(£216)*); do. (1849-61); do., James F Meldon, solicitor, John J Meldon, solicitor (1862-64); Charles Meldon, barrister, and 3 Fitzwilliam street lower, James Dillon Meldon, solicitor, James F Meldon, solicitor, John J Meldon, solicitor (1865-67); Charles Meldon, barrister, and 3 Fitzwilliam street lower, James Dillon Meldon, solicitor, James F Meldon, solicitor (1868); A G Meldon, barrister, Charles Meldon, barrister, James Dillon Meldon, solicitor, James F

Meldon, solicitor (1869-71); Michael Errington (1872-74); no entry (1875); J D Meldon (1876-80); J D Meldon, James F Meldon (1881); Henry L Harty and 14 Fitzwilliam place, Allsopp F Harty, LRCSI, LM, Lionel L Harty (1882); Henry L Harty, coroner co. Dublin (JP from 1888), Allsopp F Harty, esq., LRCSI, LM, Lionel L Harty (1883-94); do. (1895*(£114)*); Henry L Harty, esq., JP, coroner co. Dublin, *(£114)*, Allsopp F Harty, esq., LRCSI, LM (1896-02); Sir Henry L Harty, bart., JP, coroner co. Dublin, *(£114),* Allsopp F Harty, esq., LRCSI, LM (1903-04); Sir Henry L Harty, bart., JP, coroner co. Dublin, Casino (1905*(£114)*-06); Sir Henry L Harty, bart., JP, Casino (1907*(£114)*-13); Casino – vacant (1914*(£114)*); J C Meyers (1915*(£114)* -20); Mount St Mary's House of Studies (1921-to date).

IVY LODGE > FARM BOLDING COTTAGE > FARM BOLIE > FARNBOLEY > FARNABEL > ARDNABEL > ARDNOBEL > ARDNABEL > ARD-NA-BEL > ROEBUCK MANOR > THE MANOR

As has already been stated, throughout the 19th century there were only four properties consistently listed under Bird avenue. After Oak lawn and Casino the next one of these to be dealt with (location no. 14 on map) carried a variety of names throughout the century, many of which appear to be variations of the same name as can be seen in the title over this piece. When Robert Billing is listed under Bird avenue from 1834 to 1842 there is no house name associated with him. However, Samuel Lewis in his *Topographical Dictionary* gives his house name as Ivy lodge. This must therefore have been his house in Bird avenue at least while Lewis was doing his research. In 1843, for the first time, the name of Billing's house is given; it is Farm Bolding cottage. It is most likely the same house renamed since, as we have already noted, there were only four houses listed from 1834 onwards. Its first recorded name is likely, therefore, to have been Ivy lodge and was changed to Farm Bolding cottage at some unknown date between 1837 and 1843. That name, however, may be a corruption of the name Farranboley cottage which appears in the appropriate location in the first printed edition of the Ordnance Survey map (1843); it was, on that map, approached by a curving driveway from Bird avenue at a point near the centre of the avenue although Duncan's map of 1821 shows the driveway coming from the Windy Arbour end of the avenue. In any case, Farm Bolding cottage is the name of Robert Billing's house given for the years 1843 to 1848.

Billing was a solicitor belonging to the King's, Chancery and Exchequer courts and had his office at 4 Palace street; he was also described as being an 'agent'. He was the son of Thomas Billing, esq., and married for the first time in 1794 Elinor, daughter of John Meyler, esq., with whom he had 4 children. In

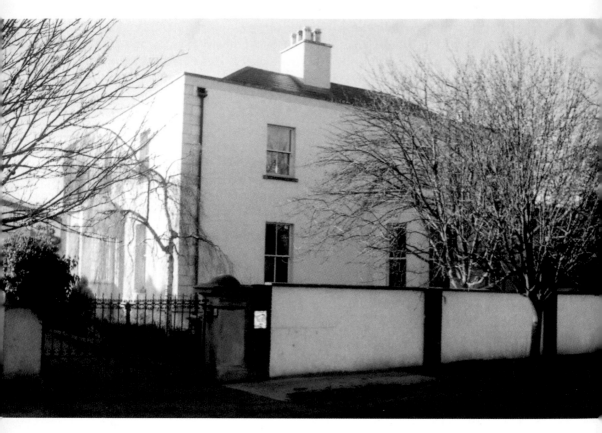

The Manor, previously inter-alia, Ardnabel: accessed through Beechwood drive, Bird avenue (*Photographer: Matt Walsh*)

1805 he married for the second time Martha, daughter of John Busby, esq. In 1821 he was a churchwarden at Taney church. It is likely, therefore, that he was living in the area, perhaps in the same house for a considerable length of time before the information we get from the directories which only begins in 1834.

In the directory for 1844 we find Robert Billing of Farm Bolding cottage described as being a barrister. This, it would appear, was Robert Billing's son and we know that he was called to the bar only a few years earlier during Michaelmas term of 1838. Robert Billing, solicitor, continues to be listed in directories among attorneys up to 1844 and then is de-listed. However, according to Ball & Hamilton he died on 18 April 1840.[71] If this is correct, then his son must have taken over the house shortly thereafter. It had a rateable valuation of £82 around

---

71   Ball & Hamilton, *Parish of Taney,* 99.

that time. While he was living there the house name underwent another change. From 1849 it is listed as Farm Bolie; perhaps that is the way Farranboley was pronounced locally at the time. In this regard, it is worth noting that in Duncan's map of 1821 the general area in which the house is located is marked Farmbolie. Further transformations in the name occurred later during his stay there; in 1870 it became Farnboley, in 1873 Farnabel and in 1876 Ardnabel. When Miss Harriette Billing, probably Robert's daughter, took over the house in 1885 she retained the name Ardnabel. During her time there the rateable valuation dropped to £63. She remained in residence until 1899.

In 1900 it is listed as being vacant but in the following year William S Archdall moved in and stayed until 1909; it was vacant again in 1910. However, when T J Waters took up residence in 1911 the name changed again, this time to Ardnobel. This, however, may have been an error on the part of the printer of the directory since, in the following year, it changed back to Ardnabel. Later in 1915 and 1916 it was vacant until Justin MacCarthy took up residence in 1917. A solicitor and commissioner of oaths with an office at 19 Merrion street, upper he did not stay long there. He, nevertheless, left his imprint on the house since the name underwent another change, although minor, during his occupancy; it was now called Ard-na-bel. His successor in the house retained this name. He was James Berry Kenny, LRCP & SI and he lived there from 1919 until 1935 after which Mrs Anna Kenny, probably his wife, remained on until 1948. During her stay, the rateable valuation fell from £63 to £60-10s. She was succeeded by John J White (c.1949); he changed the name to Roebuck manor. This new name bears no relationship to the previous one, Ard-na-bel. One can be sure, however, that it refers to the same property for three reasons. First they both have the same valuation (£60-10s) and, second, Mrs Anna Kenny, Ard-na-bel, disappears from the listing of Bird avenue properties in 1949, having been there for many years, and is replaced by John J White, Roebuck manor, its first time to appear in the same listing. Finally, the road leading up to Roebuck manor was called Ardnabel road when it (the road) was first listed in 1952; that was four years after the house name Ardnabel had been dropped and the new name adopted. This road would itself be soon renamed Beechmount drive. The name seems to have changed again to simply The Manor; that is how it appears while John J White was still in occupation in 1974.

BLOOMVILLE (BLOOM-VILLA), LATER GLEDSWOOD, LATER STILL GLEDSWOOD HOUSE

We now come to the fourth and final property which was regularly listed under Bird avenue throughout the 19th and well into the 20th centuries (location no.

15 on map). When it was built has not been discovered but the first record available of a resident there is for the year 1815. In *Wilson's Dublin Directory* of that year, the list of Nobility and Gentry contains the entry 'A C Macartney, esq., 47 Stephen's Green, east and Bloomville, Roebuck'. That entry continues for a number of succeeding years. However, by 1832 we find in the *Post Office Annual Directory* that Hutchins Thomas Williams, esq., 38 Dame street is listed as living in Bloomville, Roebuck; he was also said to be a churchwarden in Taney church. He continues to be listed in other directories until 1836 although they spell the house name as Bloom-villa. This version of the name was also used by Lewis in his *Topographical dictionary* when he gives the occupant as col. Thackeray. However, the name is spelled Bloomville in the first Ordnance Survey map of the same year, 1837; it shows the entrance to the house as being on Bird avenue and opposite to that to Oak lawn which, as already suggested, was located at the entry to the housing estate The Maples.

That year also saw the return of a Macartney; from 1837 to 1842 Clotworthy Macartney is listed there. We get more detail on him and the house in subsequent entries; from 1843 onwards he is described as a solicitor with offices at 38 Gloucester street, upper and in 1847 the rateable valuation of the property is given at £248 indicating that it was of substantial proportions. Elsewhere in the directories we find that he was clerk of the crown for county Down and that he was also in a partnership practice in the same office under the style 'Joseph and Clotworthy Macartney, solicitors'. He continues to be listed at Bloomville until 1854.

Then in 1855 the name of the occupant changed; T Robertson, Bloomville appears that year. The next year lists James Robertson there but with the house name changed to Gledswood; he remained there until 1859 to be succeeded the following year by John J Robertson. As for the change in the house name, it was probably derived from that of the village of Gledswood, Melrose, Roxburghshire, Scotland. If that is the case, then it seems most likely that the Robertsons originally came from that village; Robertson is a relatively common name in Scotland. When John J took up residence he was approximately 50 years old. That can be deduced from the notice of his death which appeared in the *Cork Examiner* on 22 February 1882 which gave his name, address and age: 'John James Robertson, Gledswood, Clonskeagh, Dublin aged 72 years'. Mrs Robertson, presumably his wife, is listed from the following year as being the occupant of the house and continues to be recorded there until 1899. During her occupancy, the rateable valuation was substantially reduced to £93. The reason for this is not clear but it appears that a number of properties in the area had their valuations reduced in that year. Following the departure of Mrs Robertson the house was taken over by Miss Alice Robertson and she was to remain living

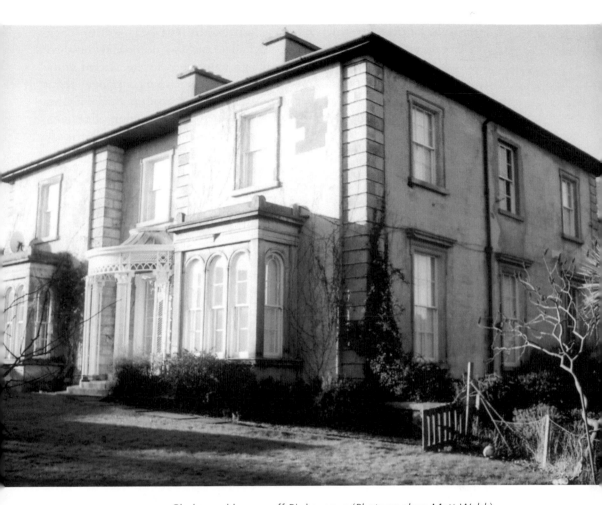

Gledswood house, off Bird avenue (*Photographer: Matt Walsh*)

there until 1944. Towards the end of her tenure another change in valuation occurred; instead of the original £93 the property was then rated £93, £17. This may be to include a separate house that was in some way part of the overall property and it may already have been rated separately but not recorded in the directories.

After the last listing of Miss Robertson in 1944, the property was vacant for some time being occupied by lieut. col. Wm Robinson, DSO from 1946 to 1952. It then was divided into three separate dwellings. In 1953 the entry is as follows: Gledswood – Kearon, Leslie, solr. (£40); White, E (£35); Polden, H R (£35). It is worth noting that the sum of the rates on the three houses (£40+£35+£35 =

£110) is the same as that which had previously existed (£93 + £17 = £110). There would subsequently be a number of changes in the occupancy of these individual units and from around 1955 the group of houses were entered in the directories under the title Gledswood house. The name change brought about by the Robertsons was to have lasting consequences in the area in that a number of new roads, which emerged with the expansion of the population of the area, adopted the word Gledswood in the address given to them. They had been built on land that previously had been part of the Gledswood property.

FRIARSLAND (FRIAR LAND, FRIARS LAND), LATER FRIARSLAND HALL, LATER GLENARD UNIVERSITY RESIDENCE

Taking a right turn into Roebuck road after leaving Bird avenue, one encounters Friarsland. The house which originally carried this name, now called Glenard University Residence, is located on the right hand side of the road just before the junction of Goatstown road and Roebuck road (location no. 16 on map). The original name was, quite obviously, based upon the name of the townland in which it is located although the latter is spelled in a slightly different manner – Friarland. This townland is quite small and is squeezed in between the much larger ones of Roebuck and Farranboley. Its name could very easily lead one to the suspicion that it was once the property of some House of Friars, perhaps one located in Dublin. However, it is necessary to be very careful about that as the etymologies of such words are not always as simple as they seem. In any case, a search of the extents (i.e. possessions, including lands) of monastic houses, including friaries, which were dissolved at the time of the Reformation does not indicate that any of them had property in the Clonskeagh or Roebuck area.[72].

It is not clear when the house was built; it appears in Taylor's map of 1816 but not very clearly. However, there is definite evidence of a substantial building there in Duncan's map of 1821 while the house is named on the first Ordnance Survey map of 1837. The land associated with the house bordered that of Bloomville, later Gledswood. As to the early residents, the first evidence in relation to this comes from the *Pettigrew and Oulton Street Directory* for the year 1836. In this we find Charles Copland there; he may have been living there for some time prior to that but unfortunately we do not have the evidence. After he left, the house was occupied by The Misses Johnson for two years, 1843-44, following which it appears to have lain vacant for two further years. It was at this time that a person of particular interest, Henry William Curran, moved in. We will return to him but first we give the subsequent occupants. They are: Colonel

---

72   Newport B White (ed), *Extents of Irish monastic possessions 1540-1541* (Dublin 1943).

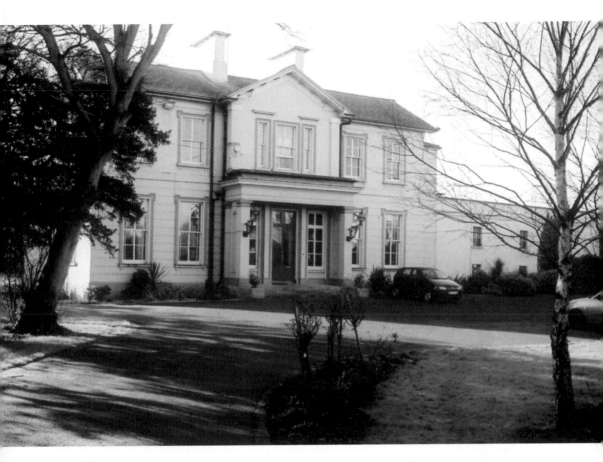

Friarsland, Roebuck road: now Glenard University Residence (*Photographer: Matt Walsh*)

Augustus Debutts or De Butts (1859-64); John R Somers, JP (1865-77); vacant (1878); Hugh M Macken (1879-86); Richard Davoren (1887-1914); vacant (1915-16); Reginald Stafford Phillips, sometime JP, for most of the period of his occupancy the house was called Friarsland hall (1917-28); Thomas Smalley (1929-39); Mrs Dorothy Smalley (1940-42); W J Clarkson (1943-51); Mrs Clarkson (1952- c. 1961); Friarsland hall – Glenard University Residence from c.1962; later the Friarsland hall was dropped and it was called, as it is today, Glenard University Residence.

A peculiarity about the entries for Friarsland throughout the 19th century is that they never, unlike the majority of other entries, include the rateable valuation of the property. This is unfortunate as it does not allow an assessment to be made of its comparative size during that period. The first indication of this

197

we get is for the year 1910 when it stood at £132; this suggests that it was a property of substantial size. It increased slightly to £140 during the time Mrs Clarkson lived there. An interesting item is shown on the Pembroke Estate Survey map of 1866 (*National Archives*: 97/46/4/31); it has a gasometer in close proximity to the house suggesting that it was lit by gaslight. J Edmundson & Co, Capel street, advertised such private gasworks in *Thom's Directory* (1867).

At the time Henry William Curran took up residence in Friarsland (1847) he was a Commissioner of Insolvent Court. This position was then of relatively recent origin. The court had been inaugurated in 1821 for the relief of insolvent debtors and was composed of two commissioners. These had to be barristers with ten years experience and were appointed by the lord lieutenant. Another court with a somewhat similar purpose and structure was set up in 1836 when a commissioner in bankruptcy was appointed by the lord lieutenant with another appointed the following year. However, in 1857 the two courts were coalesced into one, the court of bankruptcy and insolvency, which had two judges; these were crown appointees and held the tenure and approximate status of a judge of one of the superior courts. Before this coalescing took place, it would appear that Curran had ceased to hold his commission as he is no longer listed with that title in the directories from 1855; indeed his retirement may have facilitated that coalescing. It seems that he returned to practice as a barrister since his office address in Fitzwilliam square is given from that date onwards. He thus held his commission in a time of evolution of thinking on the matter of insolvency and bankruptcy when the legal distinction between these two conditions still held; indeed, a glance at the *Freeman's Journal* during his time as commissioner shows his court to be quite busy although reading the detail could not be described as exciting. However, his salary of just below £3,500 per annum – a not inconsiderable sum in those days – would have compensated for any tedium the job may have entailed.[73]

He was called to the bar in 1816 and became a bencher of the King's Inns in 1848. It is not, however, his legal career or his role as Commissioner of Insolvent Court that makes him of particular interest; instead, it was his familial connection with events of great historical significance that brings him to our attention. He was the son of John Philpot Curran and brother of Sarah Curran, Robert Emmet's lover; the latter being of special interest in the context of Clonskeagh in that Friarsland is but a short distance away from Casino in Bird avenue, Emmet's home at the time of his abortive rising, although it should, of course, be pointed out that Sarah never lived at Friarsland.

---

73   McDowell, *The Irish administration: 1801-1914*, 108-110; various Dublin directories
      throughout the nineteenth century.

In 1819, two years after his father's death in London, William Henry Curran wrote a biography, in two volumes, of his late father, John Philpot. His sister, Sarah, had died some years previously (3 May 1808) and because of that he felt he could make public, in the biography, a letter written by Emmet to John Philpot Curran during the interval between his (Emmet's) conviction and execution. Although John Philpot was held in high esteem by those who opposed the government, especially because of his defence of various United Irishmen (including Wolfe Tone) in trials held during the 1790s, his attitude to the 1803 rising was considerably cooler. It certainly would not have been unaffected by the murder of his friend, although political opponent, lord Kilwarden. As well as that, letters discovered on Emmet's person revealed his relationship with Sarah. These, in turn, led to a raid being made on the Curran residence, The Priory in Rathfarnham. There more letters were found. According to William Henry, his father had not been aware of the relationship that had been growing between Emmet and Sarah; he merely thought Emmet's visits to his house were because of his own celebrity status. However, shortly before the rising he began to have his suspicions. At that point 'he ... recommended to his family not to allow what was at present only a casual acquaintance to ripen into a greater degree of intimacy'.

Immediately after the failed rising, it was thought that Emmet could easily have made his escape to another country but remained because of his affection for Sarah and, according to William Henry, his desire 'to receive her personal forgiveness for what he now considered as the deepest injury'. The correspondence from Sarah, which was found in Emmet's possession at the time of his arrest, together with letters found in Curran's house at the time of the raid, were used in evidence at Emmet's trial. Curran was none too pleased to have himself and his family drawn into the turmoil caused by the rising. It was because of this that Emmet wrote him a letter in which he explains why he had corresponded with Sarah after the failure of the rising – the correspondence that was used in evidence against him at his trial; he was perhaps hoping that it would soften his attitude towards Sarah. This was the letter that William Henry later inserted into his biography of Curran; he noted that it was neither signed nor dated. In it, Emmet wrote:

'That I have written to your daughter since an unfortunate event has taken place, was an additional breach of propriety, for which I have suffered well; but I will candidly confess, that I not only do not feel it to have been of the same extent, but that I consider it to have been unavoidable after what had passed; for though I will not attempt to justify in the smallest degree my former conduct, yet when an attachment was once formed between us – and a sincerer one never did exist – I feel that, peculiarly circumstanced as I then was, to have left her uncertain of my situation would neither have weaned her affection nor lessened her anxiety; and looking upon her as one, whom, if I had lived, I hoped to have had my partner for life, I did hold the removing of her anxiety above every other consideration. I would rather have had the affections of your daughter in the back settlements of America, than the first situation this country could afford, without them.'

In the event, Sarah was sent away from her home to live in Co Cork soon after Emmet's execution.

Emmet had written his final letter, at 12 o'clock on the day of his execution, to his long-standing friend Richard Curran which was largely about his love for Richard's sister Sarah. Reading this letter, William Henry observed that 'the firmness and regularity of the original hand-writing contain a striking and affecting proof of the little influence which the approaching event exerted over his frame. ... He met his fate with unostentatious fortitude'.[74]

The subsequent fate of Sarah Curran was to become the subject of much curiosity giving rise to various myths. This, no doubt, was helped by Thomas Moore who romanticised her death but took liberties with the facts surrounding it in his song: 'She is far from the land where her young hero sleeps'. In fact, Sarah died in Hythe in Kent and was buried, not as she wished at The Priory in Rathfarnham because her father refused to allow it, but in Newmarket in Co Cork.[75]

Perhaps the most lasting image of Emmet held by Irish people was that associated with his famous speech from the dock. For a variety of reasons, however, there is no authoritative version of this speech and this has led to much controversy. An aspect of this can be seen in a conversation which took place long after the trial between William Henry and Peter Burrowes, the leading barrister who defended Emmet and recorded by Thomas Moore in his Journal; they were discussing the part that William Plunkett, one of the counsels for the crown, played during the trial. During the conversation, reference is made to the printed version of the speech in which Emmet is made to call Plunkett 'that viper'; Burrowes was, however, quite supportive of Plunkett suggesting that he could not have refused the government brief. It was agreed that Emmet did not, in fact, refer to Plunkett in that manner and William Henry explained how it

---

74   Boase, *Modern English biography,* i 789; William Henry Curran, *The life of the Right Honourable John Philpot Curran, late Master of the Rolls* (2vols, London 1817) ii 224-24, 234 -38; L Stephen & S Lea (ed), *Dictionary of National Biography* (London 1908) v 336-38; Geoghegan, *Robert Emmet,* 30.

75   Ibid 23-24, 35-36.

had found its way into the printed version of the speech. Leonard McNally had assisted Burrowes in defending Emmet and his son had taken down the speech during the trial; afterwards he had spoken to Emmet who, at that stage, spoke disparagingly about Plunkett. This, according to William Henry, was subsequently inserted into the speech by McNally.[76]

William Henry was one of Thomas Moore's friends. On 8 June 1818, when Moore was at the height of his popularity – his very successful *Irish Melodies* had been published some years previously – he was entertained at a dinner held in his honour at Morrison's Hotel in Dublin. The dinner was chaired by lord Charlemont and attended by 'some of the highest of the land, as well as the most gifted'; William Henry was listed among the latter as were Daniel O'Connell and Peter Burrowes. At a more personal level, William Henry visited Moore at his home in England; on one occasion while staying overnight Moore sang and told stories to him and other guests. However, on the following day Moore wrote in his journal: 'took Curran [out to dinner] with us – this young man's likeness to his father in voice and manner very disappointing – one expects every instant the flashes that used to follow this manner and they never come. His book (i.e. the biography of his father) too promises more than one finds in him'. The comparison with his father is probably unfair when one remembers the impression that he (his father) made on those who met him – including his enemies. One such enemy wrote 'I have heard four orators, Pitt, Canning, Kirwan, and Curran ... perhaps Curran was the most striking, for you began by being prejudiced against him by his bad character and ill-looking appearance, like the devil with his tail cut off, and you were at last carried away by his splendid language and by the powers of his metaphors'. Many others praised his eloquence too including lord Byron who said of him 'I have heard that man speak more poetry than I have ever seen written'. It must have been difficult for William Henry to measure up to such a standard.[77]

In 1827, through his friendship with lord Cloncurry, he became involved in what to us now seems to be a very eccentric plan to build a ship canal through the centre of Ireland from Galway to Dublin; it was, of course, Cloncurry's plan. A meeting was held to promote the idea with Cloncurry playing a leading role but William Henry was also among the speakers. Much effort was spent in

---

76 Dowden, *Journal of Thomas Moore*, iv 1382-83; Geoghegan, *Robert Emmet: a life*, 227, 244-54.

77 Terence de Vere White, *Tom Moore, the Irish poet* (London 1977) 27; Fitzpatrick, *Life, times, and contemporaries of Lord Cloncurry*, 324-25; McDowell, *The Irish administration 1801-1914*, 109; Dowden, *The Journal of Thomas Moore*, ii 494-95; Stephens and Lea, *Dictionary of National Biography*, v 339.

trying to get support from the government but to no avail. Many derided the whole idea and eventually it was abandoned. It is not clear to what extent William Henry supported the plan in practical terms. He may just have been indulging his friend Cloncurry in speaking in favour of it; there is no evidence that he would have invested in it financially.[78]

In the following year, 1828, he became closely connected with political events in the run up to Catholic Emancipation. Early that year a new prime minister, the duke of Wellington, came to power; his was a hard line Tory administration which at that time opposed emancipation. He appointed the marquis of Anglesey as lord lieutenant in Ireland with the expectation that he would reflect his views on the matter. But Anglesey's exposure to the subject as it applied in Ireland was to have the opposite effect; he would soon become a supporter of emancipation. An important part of Anglesey's exposure came through a small private cabinet which he had put in place; it must therefore carry most of the credit for his volte-face. This 'kitchen cabinet' consisted of William Henry, Anthony Blake (a Roman Catholic), lord Cloncurry and George Villiers. Because of Anglesey's new attitude he was recalled to London.

In the meantime agitation for emancipation was growing in Ireland with the election of Daniel O'Connell at the Clare by-election during the summer giving it an extra boost. A monster demonstration was planned for Tipperary which it was thought would bring about the issuing of a proclamation. Because of its undesirability, lord Cloncurry, with the approval of Anglesey, took William Henry along with him to meet O'Connell at the Catholic Association meeting rooms to persuade O'Connell to call off the demonstration. While there, O'Connell invited Cloncurry (and presumably William Henry) to come in to a meeting then in progress. The invitation accepted Cloncurry addressed those present. This, however, won for Anglesey a rebuke from Wellington and probably played a part in his decision to recall him. Soon afterwards Wellington himself reluctantly and slowly came around to the view that emancipation had to be conceded if rebellion was to be avoided. It remained to bring around the king and other strong opponents before the act got the royal assent in April 1829.[79]

Some years prior to this meeting with O'Connell, William Henry had written an article which included his description of O'Connell in his role as a barrister (July 1823). This together with other articles written over a period of

---

78 Fitzpatrick, *Life, times, and contemporaries of Lord Cloncurry* 365-69; Cloncurry, *Personal recollections*, 288-92.

79 Gardiner & Wenborn, *The History Today companion to British history*, 798-99; Cloncurry, *Personal recollections*, 330-33, 394-96; Ó Tuathaigh, *Ireland before the famine*, 68-73.

time he brought together in two bound volumes which were published in London in 1855 while he was living in Clonskeagh; the volumes were entitled *Sketches of the Irish bar with essays, literary and political.* It is quite likely that the work prior to publication was done when he retired as Commissioner of Insolvent Court. The article on O'Connell is interesting for the light it shines on him but also on the style of William Henry's writing. In it he describes for an English readership O'Connell as he appeared in the Four Courts; the following is an extract:

> 'There you will be sure to see him, his countenance braced up and glistening with health and spirits – with a huge, plethoric bag, which his robust arms can scarcely contain, clasped with paternal fondness to his breast – and environed by a living palisade of clients and attorneys, with outstretched necks, and mouth and ears agape, to catch up any chance-opinions that may be coaxed out of him in a colloquial way ... You perceive at once that you have lighted upon a great popular advocate, and if you take the trouble to follow his movements for a couple of hours through the several Courts, you will not fail to discover the qualities that have made him so – his legal competency – his business-like habits – his sanguine temperament which render him not merely the advocate but the partisan of his client – his acuteness – his fluency of thought and language – his unconquerable good humour –and, above all, his versatility'.[80]

William Henry's support for O'Connell continued after emancipation; this can be seen by events in the Union Club. A gentlemen's club founded in 1837 it was not overtly pro-Union despite its name. However, when O'Connell and his sons joined they soon took over its running; that gave the club a more anti-Union hue. Details of this change are not clear due to missing Minute Books but by 1840 the club had changed its name to the Stephen's Green Club. William Henry was elected on to its first committee suggesting that in 1840 he was still an O'Connell supporter.[81]

Many years earlier (1817) his father, John Philpot, was buried in London despite his expressed wish, recorded in his son's biography of him, that he be laid to rest in Ireland. Thomas Moore was one of those who attended his funeral. Some years later a movement began in Dublin to have his remains repatriated. Replying to a request in 1834 by the Committee of Glasnevin Cemetery to do

80   W H Curran, *Sketches of the Irish bar with essays, literary and political* (2vols, London 1855) i 156-57.

81   Smith, 'In the beginning', 37-38, 185.

this, William Henry explained the circumstances surrounding the London burial and acknowledged that it was meant to be temporary. This the Committee interpreted as agreement and preparations were made to bring the body home. Permission was received from the Consistorial Court to have it exhumed, after which it was transferred back to Dublin where it was received by William Henry and a member of the Committee. It was first held in the mausoleum at Lyons, lord Cloncurry's home, and later moved in strict privacy and in the dead of night to Glasnevin where it was buried by torchlight – William Henry had refused a request that there be a grand funeral procession to the cemetery. This refusal did not arise from any negative feelings towards his father's memory; it was merely his view of what was appropriate at such a re-burial. The respect for John Philpot can be seen in the magnificent monument that was erected over his grave. It carried the simple inscription 'Curran' and among the three trustees for the fund raised to pay for it and for another memorial to him in St Patrick's cathedral was a Clonskeagh man, John Richard Corballis.[82] William Henry died at 9 Fitzwilliam place on 25 August, 1858 in his 69th year.[83] He had lived for the last twelve years of his life at Friarsland.

MOUNT DILLON, LATER MOUNT CARMEL MONASTERY, NOW THREE SEPARATE PROPERTIES: ISLAMIC CENTRE, CARMELITE MONASTERY AND ST KILIAN'S GERMAN SCHOOL

Mount Dillon was located across the road from Friarsland (location no. 17 on map). A substantial sized property it is now divided into three separate properties as noted above. Although the configuration of the road in the general area has changed due to its being widened, the main entrance to the original property was located on Roebuck road before it turns left at the point where it meets Goatstown road. A brown gate with a cross on its top is still to be seen at the approximate location of the original entrance. In Taylor's map of 1816 this entrance and the long curving driveway up to the house are clearly visible although it does not actually name the house.

As regards the origins of the house, the first piece of evidence to be examined relates to Thomas Dillon. He was born at Mount Dillon according to one source, the reliability of which is uncertain, in 1778.[84] That date, however, is

---

82 de Vere White, *Tom Moore*, 195-96; William J Fitzpatrick, *History of Dublin Catholic cemeteries* (Dublin 1900) 26-31.

83 Boase, *Modern English biography*, i 789.

84 This source is a website: http://familytrees.genopro.com/honeywood5/SSBB/default.htm

supported by another source the reliability of which is unchallenged. It is a schedule of documents held in the archives of the Carmelite monastery Roebuck road; this monastery has been, for nearly 130 years, located in Mount Dillon. The schedule indicates that a certified copy of a reversionary lease between Nicholas, lord baron of Trimbleston and Thomas Dillon was drawn up on 12 October, 1799.[85] It is most likely that that copy was made upon Thomas Dillon reaching his majority i.e. his 21st birthday. That being so, the year of his birth would have been 1778, the date given in the other source.

A map of county Dublin prepared by John Rocque in 1760 clearly shows Mount Dillon located in the Roebuck area. However, it gives no indication that a substantial house is present there. It is possible, therefore, that the house in which he was born was built at some time between these two dates i.e. 1760 and 1778. That, however, has to be viewed in the light of the statement of Lewis from which it has been inferred that, apart from Roebuck castle, only J E Hyndman's house existed in the area c. 1787.[86] Perhaps Thomas Dillon was born, not in the house at Mount Dillon but somewhere in the area and the house was built not many years later.

It has not been possible to find out anything certain about the origin of his family although one may surmise that it was of some substance since the name of the location includes the name Dillon and that had existed before the house had been built. The Dublin directories of the time are concerned with people and affairs of the city only and Mount Dillon would, at that time, have been considered to be in the countryside. A trawl through these for the years 1770 and 1780 as well as other sources for the period indicates that there were a substantial number of Dillon families in Dublin many of whom would have had the means to build a house of the size of that in Mount Dillon; among them were businessmen, surgeons, attorneys, barristers, physicians, bankers and descendants of the 1st earl of Roscommon but unfortunately no evidence could be unearthed to connect any of them with the property.[87]

---

85   Archives of the Carmelite monastery, Roebuck road, Dublin. Item 1 of Schedule of Documents.

86   Lewis, *Topographical dictionary*, 519.

87   *The Gentleman's and Citizen's Almanack* compiled by Samuel Watson, Bookseller, for the year of Our Lord 1770, 1780; *Wilson's Dublin Directory* for the year 1770. For the lineage of Sir James Dillon, 1st earl of Roscommon: [http://www.stirnet.com/ HTML/genie/british/dd/dillon03.htm]; Maureen Wall, 'The Catholic merchants, manufacturers and traders of Dublin 1778-1782', *Repertorium Novum* Vol 2, No 2 (1960) 298-323: 308; Cullen, *Princes and pirates*, 20.

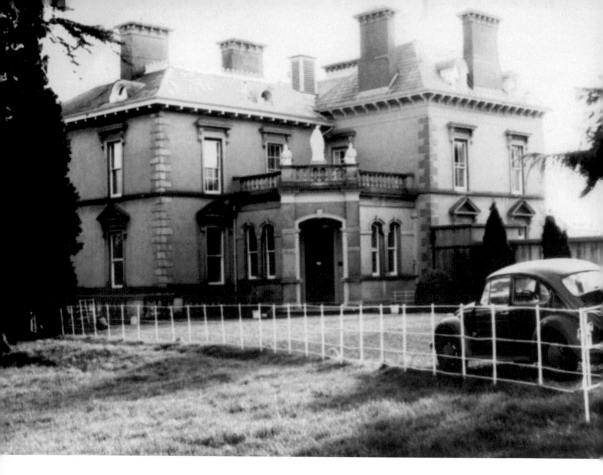

Mount Dillon house after it had been converted for use as a Carmelite monastery

Thomas Dillon and his wife Marcella[88] had only one child that survived infancy, Mary Anne Agnes Dillon (born in 1810, died on 11 November, 1851). On 9 April, 1834 she married, in Paris, Arthur Francis Southwell, (born 6 February, 1789, later lieut-colonel, died 17 February, 1849 most likely at Mount Dillon). They had six children: Thomas Arthur Joseph Southwell, 4th viscount Southwell, born 6 April, 1836 (according to one source at Mount Dillon), lord

---

88 The following inscription is found in the graveyard of Taney church 'This stone was erected by Thomas Dillon, Esq., of Mount Dillon, Roebuck and Marcella, his wife, in memory of their sons Cornelius and Thomas, who died in their infancy' (Ball & Hamilton, *The parish of Taney,* 33). It is from this that the name of Thomas' wife is found. That it was Marcella is confirmed by the fact that his first granddaughter, born to his daughter Mary Anne Agnes Dillon Southwell, was called Marcella. The gravestone informs us also that other children had been born to Thomas and Marcella but did not survive infancy.

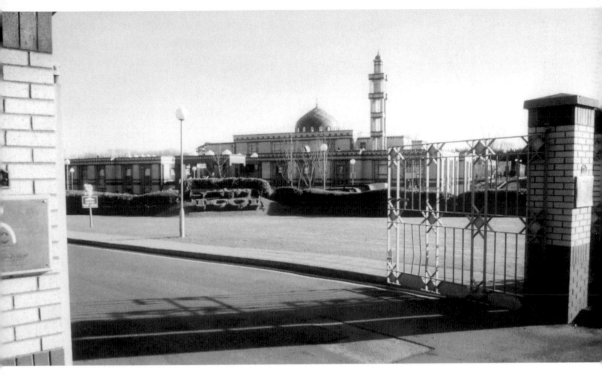

Islamic Cultural Centre, Roebuck road, Clonskeagh (*Photographer: Matt Walsh*)

lieutenant and *custos rotolorum* [Keeper of the Rolls], co Leitrim, died in Tekel Castle, Surrey, England on 26 April, 1878 and buried 3 May 1878 in a vault beneath the pro-cathedral, Marlborough street, Dublin; the hon. Charles Francis Xavier Southwell (born 1839, died unmarried in 1875); the hon. Marcella Maria Agnes Southwell (died unmarried 1901); the hon. Jane Mary Matilda Southwell (married 1860 to John David, baron Fitzgerald, had 10 children, died 1910); the hon. Mary Paulina Southwell (born 1841 probably at Mount Dillon as her parents were living there at that time, married field marshal Sir (Henry) Evelyn Wood, GCB, GCMG, VC, had 6 children, died 1891; Wood was a brother of Katherine (Kitty) O'Shea who, after divorce, married Charles Stewart Parnell); the hon. Margaret Mary Southwell (probably born at Mount Dillon, married 1869 Charles Standish Barry, of Leamlara, co Cork, had one child, died 1916). The titles carried by these children were granted by Royal Licence on 25 September 1860, the precedence of the son and daughter of a viscount. The eldest son inherited the title of viscount after the

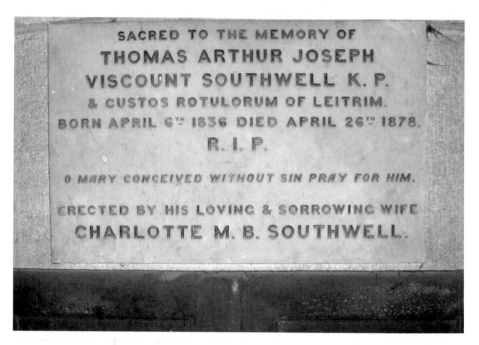

Burial vault under the pro-cathedral, Dublin, of Thomas, 4th viscount Southwell, Mount Dillon, Clonskeagh

death of his uncle Thomas Anthony, 3rd viscount Southwell, in 1860.[89]

The first resident of Mount Dillon whom we meet in the Dublin directories is listed in 1833; he is the Rev John Prior. He could, of course, have been living there earlier as he was a curate in nearby Donnybrook in 1828 and afterwards perpetual curate in Taney, the parish in which Mount Dillon was located, from 1830-34, from which curacy he resigned on the grounds of ill-health. In fact, Roebuck is given as his address in the *Post Office Annual Directory* for 1832 but Mount Dillon is not mentioned. He was born in 1803, the son of Dr Thomas Prior, vice-provost of Trinity College, Dublin and ordained in 1827. In 1833, he

---

89   Peter Townend (ed), *Burke's genealogical and heraldic history of the Peerage, Baronetage and Knightage* (104th ed, London 1967) 2343. For information about place of birth and burial of Thomas Arthur Joseph Southwell see 'http://familytrees.genopro.com/honeywood5/SSBB/default.htm'. His place of burial and date of birth & death is confirmed by the plaque over his burial vault under the pro-cathedral in Marlborough street. For Wood's relationship to Katherine O'Shea: Beckett, 'Women and patronage in the late Victorian army', 474.

married for the first time Sophia, daughter of John Odell of Carriglea, county Wexford. Later he would become rector and vicar of Rathcormack (Cloyne) 1851-3 and finally, rector of Kirklington in Yorkshire (1853-67) the ancestral home of his second wife Sarah.[90]

A number of years after the death of her husband, Sarah and their children were authorised, by Royal Licence on 30 August 1886, to add the name Wandes-forde to their name, thus initiating the Prior-Wandesforde lineage of Castle-comer, Co Kilkenny. Her father had begun a programme of rationalization on his estate in Castlecomer and this became quite controversial. This was further exacerbated by the apparent actions of his son-in-law, the Rev John Prior, who was accused of involvement in evictions and of introducing religious tracts which created resentment. This, after all, was the time in which there was a major evangelical revival within Irish Protestantism; a revival which generated an intense effort to distribute religious material among the Catholic poor throughout Ireland. The controversy, thus stirred up, fuelled local agitation for Tenant Rights. His daughter, Sarah Prior, also became involved in controversy; she and the parish priest of Castlecomer came into conflict over the leasing of a school site and about how the Bible should be taught. Her successor, Captain R H Prior-Wandesforde, however, had a much better relationship with the people of his locality even to the extent of being elected by them as a District Councillor for Castlecomer.[91]

Rev Prior was succeeded at Mount Dillon by another Prior, Rev Dr Thomas, who is listed as living there until 1839. It is not clear if or how he was related to Rev John. Then we find the hon. major (and later, lieutenant colonel) Arthur Southwell in residence; he is listed until the end of the 1840s to be followed in 1850 by captain George Daniel, RN, in 1858 by John D Garde, solicitor and in 1868 by major-general Cunynghame CB. From 1873 to 1875 lord Ventry resided there. After lying vacant for two years, the Carmelite nuns moved in with Mrs Dunne (as nuns were then addressed by some) as Superioress in 1878; her name was Charlotte Dunne and as first prioress she was known in religion as Sr Mary Joseph Magdalene de Pazzi of the Sacred Heart of Mary. Thereafter the property ceased to be called Mount Dillon; it was changed to Mount Carmel.

The property had stayed in the original family until 1 December 1857. The reason we can say this is that, as we have already seen, Arthur Francis Southwell,

---

90   *The Post Office Annual Directory* for 1833; Leslie & Wallace, *Clergy of Dublin and Glendalough,* 990; Ball & Hamilton, *The parish of Taney,* 76-7.

91   Tom Lyng, *Castlecomer connections: exploring history, geography and social evolution in North Kilkenny environs* (Castlecomer 1984) 315-16; Ó Tuathaigh, *Ireland before the famine,* 58-59.

who died in 1849 at the age of 60 and had been in residence there from 1841, was the husband of Mary Anne Agnes Dillon, granddaughter of the man who had built the house. As well as that, Sarah, the wife of Rev Prior who had been living there before Arthur had returned, was a fourth cousin, once removed, of Arthur. Finally, the original lease of Mount Dillon was assigned to John Davis Garde by lord viscount Southwell, the older brother of Arthur Francis, then deceased, on 1 December 1857.[92]

The continuity of family residence in the house seems clear: Thomas Dillon was born in Mount Dillon in 1778; up to 1834, his daughter Mary Anne Agnes Dillon lived there from the time of her birth in 1810. In the previous year the Rev Prior, perpetual curate at the local parish church of Taney was in residence there. Three years later, in 1836, he married Mary Anne Agnes Dillon-Southwell's distant cousin, Sarah. Meanwhile another Prior, Rev Dr Thomas, had moved in. We do not know whether Mary and her children remained there or moved with her military husband wherever his duty called him. Directories of the time referred generally to the male head of a household; they occasionally refer to a woman as well but only in exceptional cases.[93] Just a few years later, in 1841, Mary's husband, Arthur Francis, is listed as being back in residence there; he died in 1849, she in 1851. In between years, in 1850, captain George Daniel RN arrived; he remained there until 1856. There is no available evidence of a family relationship between him and the Dillon or Southwell families; in fact, the

---

92   Townend, *Burke's Peerage*, 1923, 2342, 2343 (Sarah and Arthur were cousins because they shared a common ancestor Robert Southwell of Callow. The level of the relationship is established as follows: on page 2343, Arthur Francis Southwell's ancestors are traced through the Southwells – i) 2nd viscount; ii) 1st viscount; iii) 2nd baron; iv) 1st baron; v) Richard Southwell of Callow. Then on page 1923 (among the Ormondes) the ancestors of Sarah, wife of Rev John Prior, are traced through i) her father, Charles Harward Butler-Clarke-Southwell-Wandesforde; ii) his mother, Lady Frances Susan Elizabeth Wandesforde, wife of the 17th Earl of Ormonde; iii) her mother, Agnes Elizabeth, wife of John, Earl of Wandesforde; iv) her father, John Southwell; v) (on page 2343) his father, Richard Southwell of Enniscourt; vi) (on pages 2342-3) Richard Southwell of Callow); Assignment of Original Lease to John D Garde: Schedule of Documents in Archives of the Carmelite monastery: 1. Co-Part. Lease of Mount Dillon – Lord Viscount Southwell to John Davis Gaide [*r* Garde]; 2. Orig/ Lease of Mount Dillon – Lord Viscount Southwell and an[othe]r to John Davis Grade [*r* Garde]. Both are dated 1 December 1857.

93   See the reference to Mrs Todd as well as Rev Dr Todd at Vergemount house in *Thom's Directory* for 1850. This Mrs Todd was most likely Dr Todd's mother as Dr Todd was unmarried.

evidence would suggest that he was merely a tenant of the Southwells perhaps due to a military connection with the then late lieut.-colonel Arthur Francis. The property was still in Southwell hands as late as 1 December 1857, as we have seen, when the lease was demised to John Davis Garde. On that date, therefore, the Dillon and Southwell connection with the property ceased.

However, before moving on to Garde and Mount Dillon it may be noted that Arthur Francis Southwell seemed to be active in Catholic social circles in Dublin after his return to Mount Dillon. That, at least, is what is suggested by a notice in *The Complete Catholic Directory, Almanac, and Registry for the year of Our Lord 1847*. In that, a marriage notice goes as follows: '30 August 1846. In the Metropolitan church, Marlboro' Street, Patrick Boylan jun, son of Mr Patrick Boylan of Grafton street, Dublin to Augusta Georgiana, daughter of the late col. Alen of Gardiner Street, Dublin. The hon. col. Southwell gave away the bride. His grace, the archbishop honoured the ceremony by his presence.' It may also be noted that captain George Daniell, RN, who was a tenant at Mount Dillon between 1850 and 1856, had got married to Alicia Catherine, eldest surviving daughter of the then Master of the Rolls, Francis Blackburne of Roebuck hall on 23 June 1842. Before marriage he had a very distinguished career in the British navy. From 1810 until 1838 he took part in many sea battles against the French and others in the Mediterranean; he also saw service on the African coast and in the West Indies and received a commission at the coronation of queen Victoria. Since Daniell's death occurred on 2 November 1856 it seems likely to have happened while he was still a tenant of Mount Dillon. It was also during his stay there that Francis Blackburne left Roebuck hall to live in Rathfarnham.[94]

When Garde is first met in the directories (1858) he is said to be a solicitor with offices at 6 Stephen's green. From 1862 to 1865 they give his name incorrectly as John Denis. When this is corrected in 1866 extra information is given; he is then listed as having offices at 14 North Great George's street and being the crown solicitor for Longford and Cavan. He was married to Catherine McVeagh and their eldest daughter, Susan Elizabeth, became the second wife of Edward Perceval Westby of Roebuck castle on their marriage in Taney church on 16 June 1864; his first wife was a daughter of Francis Blackburne of Roebuck hall. Susan Elizabeth Westby's initials, SEW, were ornately carved over the main door of Roebuck castle in the right-hand spandrel where they can be seen to this day. Garde, who had been a churchwarden at Taney church in 1863, died in 1899.[95] In 1868 he was replaced by major-general Cunynghame CB to whom he assigned

---

94 Ball & Hamilton, *The parish of Taney*, 106-8.
95 ibid. III. 152.

the lease that was demised to him by viscount Southwell. While residing there he was knighted and as major-general Sir Arthur A T Cunynghame, KCB he continued to live there until 1872. During this period he was said to have commanded the military in the Dublin area during and after the Fenian rising of 1867. At the end of his stay in Mount Dillon he left to take up command of British troops in South Africa.[96]

For three years afterwards, lord Ventry took up residence there (1873–75) during which time he succeeded in having his family name enhanced to make it sound somewhat grander; it was the type of thing that seemed to be of particular importance to his family in previous generations. He was the 4th baron Ventry, the great grandson of Thomas Mullins of Ballingolin, Co. Kerry who had been created a baron on the 31 July 1800 along with fifteen others at the time that the Irish House of Parliament at College green voted itself out of existence; the creation of peers was a tactic used to facilitate the success of that vote thus making the Act of Union possible.

The first sign of a name change came with the substitution of 'Burnham' for 'Ballingolin', the home in Kerry. The name that was adopted reflected the fact that an ancestor, colonel Frederick William Mullins, was born in Burnham, England in the 17th century. The next effort at changing a name failed however. After the death of the 1st baron Ventry at 'Burnham house' in Kerry, his son and heir, William Townsend petitioned the viceroy to have his title changed from lord baron Ventry to lord baron Burnham 'inasmuch as it [Ventry] is obnoxious to a disagreeable and unpleasant interpretation in continental languages, and would expose memorialist [himself] to ridicule ... when travelling abroad'. Since he kept a residence at Château de la Cocherie, near Boulogne, it seems most likely that he had the French word 'ventre' (stomach, belly) in mind. In the event, the petition was unsuccessful. He died in Dublin in 1837 and was succeeded by his nephew, Thomas Townsend Aremberg Mullins. He managed to get the name Mullins changed, for himself and his descendants, by royal licence in February 1841, to de Moleyns. In doing so, he was following a certain fashion whereby families transformed their names to give the impression that they were of ancient and feudal lineage. He was claiming descent from the fourteenth century Sir John de Moleyns who had been associated with Burnham Abbey in England.

He died at Burnham house, Kerry in 1868 and was succeeded by his son, the 4th baron. This man's grandmother's maiden name was Dayrolles and his

---

mother's Blake, so he was christened Dayrolles Blakeney Mullins in 1828. After he had succeeded to the title, and while he was resident at Mount Dillon, he got by royal licence in November 1874 permission to add Eveleigh to de Moleyns (the name he had since 1841); Eveleigh was the maiden name of an ancestor some 200 years previously. Now the great grandson of plain Thomas Mullins was able to style himself Dayrolles Blakeney Eveleigh-de Moleynes.

He was a substantial property owner in Kerry where, in 1883, he held 93,629 acres worth £17,067 a year. As well as that he was lieut-colonel commanding 4th Military Battalion Royal Munster Fusiliers from 1854-1885; from 1871 he sat in the House of Lords where he was Conservative in politics. What he was engaged at in Dublin, while he lived in Clonskeagh, has not been discovered but it seems clear that he merely rented Mount Dillon for the duration of his stay. As there was no longer a parliament in Dublin it was not as likely that people based in rural Ireland and who held a parliamentary seat, either in the Commons or the Lords, would keep a house there; they were more likely to keep one in London. His principal residence, however, was Burnham house, near Dingle, co Kerry.[97]) After the departure of lord Ventry, Mount Dillon was vacant for two years (1876-1877) before the arrival of the Carmelite nuns. Soon Mount Dillon would become Mount Carmel monastery and its subsequent history is that of the monastery. This is discussed in Chapter 16.

HARLECH

On the other side of the road opposite the monastery we find Harlech (location no. 18 on map). It is at this point that the original entrance to the house once stood although there was another entrance from what is now Goatstown road. This latter entry, through Harlech downs, is the only one that currently survives. When the house was built has not been discovered but neither the Taylor map of 1816 nor the Duncan one of 1821 show it while it is seen to exist in the first printed edition of the Ordnance Survey map (1843). Both entrances, as indicated above, are clearly visible on the Pembroke Estate Survey map of 1866.

Lewis in his *Topographical dictionary* of 1837 did not include Harlech and the first resident to be named as specifically living in Harlech in the directories is William Lewis in 1845. However he had been already named for the two previous years as living in the area without mentioning Harlech. Perhaps the house only

---

97   G E Cockayne, (ed. H White, R S Lea), *The complete peerage or a history of the house of lords and all its members from the earliest times* (London 1959) vol 12, part 2, pp 238-41; Patrick M Geoghegan, *The Irish Act of Union* (Dublin 2001) 121- 28.

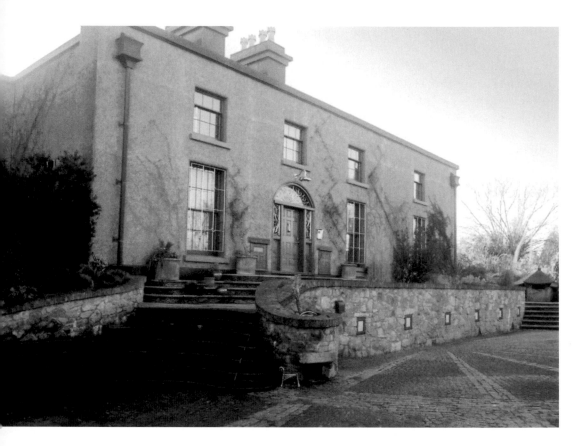

Harlech, now accessed from Goatstown road (*Photographer: Matt Walsh*)

got its name – a very Welsh-influenced one – in 1845. There is even a possibility that a J G Richards had already been living there from 1837 although the only evidence for this is extremely slight – i.e. his name occurs in the same place in a sequence of names in which that of William Lewis subsequently appears. When Lewis is first mentioned he is said to have a city office at 28 College green but we are not told his occupation. In 1845 a William Lewis junior is added and he also had a city office at the same address. Furthermore, we know from later entries that he was a solicitor. If he shared an office with William Lewis, senior, then it is safe to assume that the latter was also a solicitor. In 1846 they changed office to 22 Nassau street and remained there until they cease to be listed as living at Harlech. The rateable valuation of Harlech in 1847 was £178. Mrs Lewis is given as the occupant from 1851 to 1857 with William, junior, living there part of that time.

After the Lewis family left there was a series of short term occupancies until 1863 when it would appear that a family called Murphy took up residence. First there was William Murphy in 1863; he is listed with only a one year break in 1864 until 1868. During this period we learn that the rateable valuation had dropped to £138. After being vacant in 1869, Thomas Murphy is listed as living there from 1870 to 1883 followed by Mrs Murphy from 1884 to 1902. There followed again a few short term occupancies until, in 1909, F Whitney moved in and stayed until 1937. In 1927 the rateable valuation dropped once again to £108 and in 1932 to £106, £5; the latter was a common phenomenon at this time, giving presumably the valuation of an auxiliary house, such as a gate lodge, separately. From 1938 to 1944 Mrs Jeffers lived there. However, after the arrival of M & M Latchmann in 1946 major changes were about to take place. From 1948 to 1960 the entry for Harlech appears in the directories as 'Building Ground, Harlech' still with the same valuation. Quite clearly the building of new houses in the grounds of the house was then about to take place. This is confirmed by the first entry of Harlech villas in the directory of 1952 and of Harlech crescent and Harlech grove in the following year. It was not until 1962/3 that the house itself, Harlech, was once again listed. From that point well into the 1970s it was occupied by James A Walmsley. The house still survives to this day. As well as that, its legacy is to be found in the number of addresses that have been named after it.

HERMITAGE

Across the road from the old entrance to Harlech on the Roebuck road the mansion called Hermitage is found (location no. 19 on map); the Little Sisters of the Poor's Holy Family Home is currently located there. This house and its driveway can be clearly seen on both Taylor's and Duncan's maps of 1816 and 1821 respectively while the house is actually named on the first Ordnance Survey map of 1837. Despite its existence for some years previously, the name of the first resident to be discovered in both Lewis's *Topographical dictionary* and the directories is William C Quin (1836-37). Shortly thereafter The Misses Hendrick lived there for two years. However, in 1840 Mrs M'Caskey took up residence at Hermitage. She is almost certainly the wife of Thomas M'Caskey who, along with his brother William, operated the iron mills which were founded by Henry Jackson at Clonskeagh bridge.

The first M'Caskey found in the sources operating the mills was William; he is listed in the *Pettigrew and Oulton Street Directory* as owning the iron works at Clonskeagh. That was in 1834 which was also the year of his death. According to a tombstone inscription in Taney graveyard he died on 9 June 1834. As his age is given as 62 that would suggest that he was born c. 1772 probably at 22 Church street Dublin where he is described as an iron manufacturer in 1830. By that time, however, he had also taken over the iron mills at Clonskeagh and was living locally since we find that he was a churchwarden at Taney church from 1827 to 1831; later he purchased a pew when the south gallery was erected in 1833. His wife Frances Louisa died on 3 December 1830 and is buried in Taney graveyard. It is most likely that he was living in Hermitage from the time he took over the running of the iron mills at Clonskeagh; the date he took up residence has, however, not been discovered.

The running of the mills was taken over by Thomas M'Caskey most likely his brother although it is possible that it was his son. D'Alton, writing in 1838, says of the mills 'The whole interest in the concern was sold by auction in 1834 and is now the property of Mr M'Caskey, who employs about 10 persons therein'.[98] This Mr M'Caskey was Thomas since William, as we have seen, died in 1834. From 1836 to 1839 there is a record of a Mrs M'Caskey living in Roebuck but, as we have seen, W C Quin and The Misses Hendrick lived at Hermitage during that period. Nevertheless, the location in the directory where Mrs M'Caskey's name is found is in keeping with the position where Hermitage is located. In any case, there is definite evidence that she was living there from 1840. It is possible that, after the death of William M'Caskey and his wife, Hermitage was leased by the other occupants for a few years until Mrs M'Caskey took over in 1840. It is not clear whether she was the wife of Thomas; he is listed as running the iron works in 1840 and 1841 and if he were living at Hermitage one would expect that his name rather than that of his wife (assuming that the Mrs M'Caskey at Hermitage was his wife) would have been listed.

Whatever the truth of the situation was, it seems possible that Hermitage had remained in the hands of the M'Caskey family from the time William had taken up residence there at the latest in the 1820s. There is a record of another William M'Caskey who was one of the treasurers of the school attached to Taney church from 1834 to 1850 but it is not known whether he was related to the M'Caskeys of Hermitage or, indeed, where he lived in the parish.[99] When the iron mills passed from the M'Caskeys to Thomas Portis in the early 1840s it seems that they retained in their possession the cottages which Henry Jackson had caused to be built for the workers at the mill, cottages that were considered to be of superior quality for their time. These cottages then came into the possession of Mrs M'Caskey at some point since there is good evidence that in 1847 she held 'a

---

98   D'Alton, *History of the county of Dublin*, 808.
99   Ball & Hamilton, *Parish of Taney*, 39, 132, 190, 235.

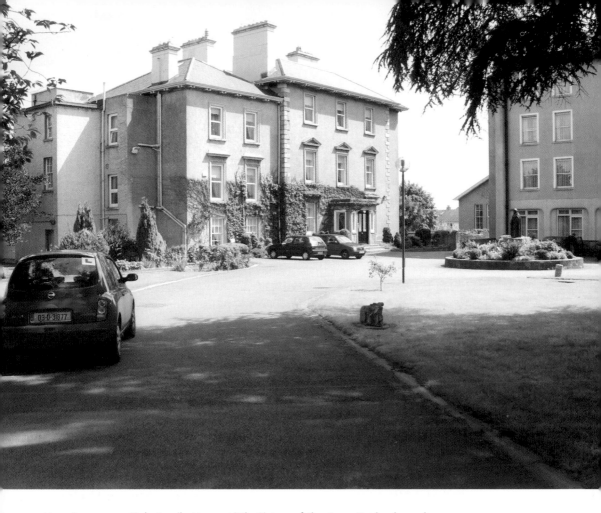

Hermitage, now Holy Family Home, Little Sisters of the Poor, Roebuck road

number of cottages which extended along the Clonskeagh road' with a rateable valuation of £1 to £1-10s; this was a time when the mills had been operated by Thomas Portis for a number of years. That these cottages were in fact those which Henry Jackson had built seems certain from the fact that when they left her possession they became known as 'Henshaw's cottage' and this happened in the same year (1854) that Thomas Henshaw took over the mills from the Portis family. It may be a coincidence but Mrs M'Caskey is known to have taken up residence in Hermitage around the time that her family ceased to run the iron mills. It is only speculation but it is quite possible that her husband died around this period and the James M'Caskey who, according to the evidence, took over Hermitage in 1843 from her was her son; he apparently did not involve himself in the iron business as we are told that he was employed at the Custom House. There he worked, according to *Wilson's Dublin Directory* of 1830, as a jerquer, i.e. a customhouse officer who searches ships for goods that have not been entered on the ship's papers, in other words, smuggled goods. Whether he had climbed the bureaucratic ladder by the time he had taken over Hermitage is not known but it must be considered a strong possibility.

His last entry in the directory is for 1859 and after him we find first William Jameson (1857-58) followed by Henry Jameson who was in residence there for a considerable length of time – from 1859 to 1902. During his time at Hermitage its rateable valuation dropped to £103 and remained at that level during the occupancy of his successor William Robertson until the general increase in valuations which occurred during the First World War. It rose to £146 in 1915. Robertson remained at Hermitage until 1929 and after being vacant for a year Mrs Manseragh (*sic*) moved in. She was joined two years later by Southcote Mansergh. With their arrival a connection between Clonskeagh and the world of opera was put on a special plain since both of the Manserghs had earlier in their careers been top operatic performers.

Southcote Mansergh was born in Hoddesdon, Hertfordshire, the son of Colonel Mansergh, on 27 December 1857. Belonging to an Irish family, he got his early musical training at the Royal Academy of Music in Dublin. This was followed by further training at the Royal Academy of Music in London and later in Florence. The possessor of a fine bass voice, it would appear that he joined the D'Oyly Carte Opera Company in 1881 as part of its choir but soon progressed to leading roles when he adopted the stage name, Charles Manners. Among other achievements he created the part of Private Willis in *Iolanthe* before leaving to join the Carl Rosa Opera Company. It was there he met his future wife, Fanny Moody, whom he married in 1890.[100]

Born in Cornwall on 23 November 1866 Fanny made her debut, according to one source, in 1887[101] and another, in 1886.[102] Be that as it may, her marriage to Southcote Mansergh, aka Charles Manners, was to lead the way to a whole new experience for them. In 1897 (or 1895 in one source) they set up their own company, the Moody-Manners Opera Company and with that a bright new future beckoned. Their first season was at Covent Garden after which the company went from strength to strength. In 1899, the company performed Wagner's *Lohengrin* with Fanny playing the role of Elsa. Further successes saw

---

100 Charles Manners (1882-83): [http://math.boisestate.edu/GaS/whowaswho/M/MannersCharles.htm].

101 Historic Opera-Singers: s. n. [http://www.historicopera.com/thumb_singers_m2_left.htm].

102 According to a collection of opera programmes relating to the Irish tenor, Barton McGuckin, put on a website by Derek Walsh in 1995 [http://indigo.ie/~callas1/mcguk.htm].

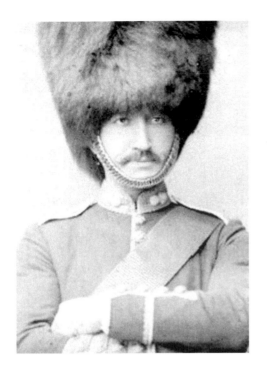

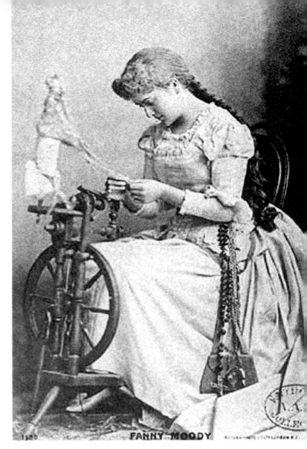

(Above) Photographed in stage costume early in his career, Southcote Mansergh (aka Charles Manners), later of The Hermitage, Roebuck road

(Right) An early photograph of opera singer Fanny Moody (Mrs Southcote Mansergh), last owner of The Hermitage, Roebuck road before it was bought by the Little Sisters of the Poor

the company improve so rapidly that by 1902 Moody-Manners had set up three separate companies, all of which were successfully touring throughout England. In 1902 and 1903 the principal company had a season at Covent Garden while in the following year it was at the Drury Lane theatre. In both 1904 and 1906 it conducted opera festivals at Sheffield with the profits going towards the cost of founding Sheffield University. Although Puccini's *Madame Butterfly* had its first production in England at Covent Garden in 1905, Moody-Manners were the first to perform it in English in 1907 with Fanny playing the heroine and the Irish tenor, Joseph O'Meara, playing Pinkerton. In 1906 Charles mounted a campaign to increase public appreciation of opera and it is principally due to his efforts that the Glasgow Grand Opera Society was founded; it was to become one of the most enterprising amateur opera societies in Great Britain. It is most likely that for this reason the Moody-Manners collection is housed at the Mitchell Library in Glasgow where the city archives are also stored. As part of his campaign to promote opera in Britain, Manners offered prizes for British composers. As well as performing in the various operas put on by the company, Manners acted as its managing director. For a time Moody-Manners' "A" company was the largest opera company ever to tour Great Britain.[103]

However, their tours were not confined to Great Britain. They also toured in North America, South Africa and Ireland. Although no specific dates could be found it would appear that Fanny Moody at least, and perhaps also Charles Manners appeared in Dublin while they were members of the Carl Rosa Opera Company. On 29 March 1875 that opera company made its first appearance in the Gaiety Theatre which had opened only a little over three years previously. This was the first of many times it was to perform operas there; they also performed at the Theatre Royal. On occasion, the company put on new operas first in Dublin before they were produced in London most likely to try them out in the less expensive venue. Not all of these were successful. It may have been with this company that Fanny appeared for the first time in the Gaiety Theatre since her photograph appears in the 1896 souvenir programme published to mark the Gaiety's 25th anniversary. According to Maxwell Sweeney, writing in the souvenir programme published to mark the 75th anniversary of the Gaiety, the Moody-Manners company's first performance in that theatre was in 1914 when its most impressive work was 'Samson and Delilah'. That being the case, it would appear that on previous occasions in Dublin it performed in the Theatre Royal. It is known that it was touring in Dublin in December 1906 as there is a reference in the book, *I hear you calling*, written by Lily McCormack, the wife of John McCormack, that the latter was auditioned by the Charles Manners and the Italian conductor, Ronaldo Sapio in Dublin at that time. McCormack was then at the start of his career and was trying to get opportunities to perform. The audition seems not to have been successful. They argued about money and Manners is said to have been critical of McCormack's acting.

The number and dates of the Moody-Manners performances in Dublin has not been discovered but there was a great demand for opera productions in Dublin in the latter part of the 19th century. This demand was satisfied by touring companies coming from England until around the second decade of the 20th century when amateurs first ventured onto the Gaiety stage and from that humble start the Dublin Grand Opera Society, later Opera Ireland, emerged. These first ventures filled the vacuum left by the demise of the touring

---

103   Eric Walter White, *A history of English opera* (London 1983)372-73.

companies which seem to have faded at the time of the First World War. The Moody-Manners company was wound up in 1916. What Southcote and Fanny did after the ending of the company is not clear. They did not take up residence in Hermitage until 1931. It is possible that Southcote may have assisted the emergence of the new operatic society in Dublin; the annals of the Little Sisters of the Poor when describing their purchase of Hermitage refer to him as the 'head of the Operatic Society' but which society is not stated. It could refer to the Glasgow Grand Opera Society since his papers have been left in Glasgow but there is no evidence to support that. One thing we can be almost sure of is that he would have continued to promote opera among the public at large. He died in Dublin on 3 May 1935, possibly at Hermitage. His wife Fanny lived for another 10 years before her death on 21 July 1945. She had already moved out of Hermitage since the Little Sisters of the Poor bought the house on 30 July 1942 and Fanny handed over the keys on 7 September of the same year. In their annals, the Sisters refer to Fanny as being 'renowned ... for her charitable works'. [104] The subsequent history of Hermitage is found in Chapter 16 in the section which deals with the Little Sisters of the Poor on Roebuck road.

Southcote Mansergh's Irish family connections have not been traced. However, there was a Mansergh family at Grenane house outside Tipperary town from around the middle of the 17th century. One of the descendants of this family, Martin Mansergh, is a prominent activist in modern Irish politics, acting as advisor to the Fianna Fáil party and elected as a TD in the 2007 elections. It is not clear how, if at all, Southcote Mansergh is related to him. One thing, however, suggests that he is related. That is the forename, Southcote. It appears that it was originally a surname which entered the family by marriage and was subsequently used by different generations of Manserghs as a forename. Martin Mansergh follows this tradition since his third forename is Southcote. [105]

---

104 M. B. 'The Dublin public and the stage' in *Souvenir of the twenty-fifth anniversary of the opening of the Gaiety Theatre 27th November 1871* (Dublin 1896) 19-32; Maxwell Sweeney 'The Gaiety story' in *GaietyTheatre 75th anniversary 1871-1946* (Dublin 1946) 9, 15, 23-4; John Ward, 'McCormack on Brighton pier' in *The Record Collector*, 37 (1992) 62-9 reproduced on the McCormack Society website [http://www.mccormacksociety.co.uk/]; White, *History of English opera*, 373 (1916 is given here as the date on which the Moody-Manners company was wound up; other sources say that it ceased to exist with the outbreak of the war); annals of the Little Sisters of the Poor.

105 Kevin Rafter, *Martin Mansergh, a biography* (Dublin 2000) 12-15, 315 n 24.

MOORFIELD (MOOREFIELD)

Moorfield is the next house on Roebuck road to be dealt with. It was located on the other side of the road from Hermitage, a little further on and accessed by a driveway (location no. 20 on map). It no longer exists and indeed, apart from Moorfield cottages, has left no traces in the area. Nevertheless it can be seen to have existed on Taylor's map in 1816 and is mentioned by name on the first Ordnance Survey map of 1837. As well as that Lewis in his *Topographical dictionary* of 1837 tells us that P. Curtis esq. was living there at that time. This is confirmed by an entry in the *Post Office Annual Directory* for 1833 where we find the following: Patrick Curtis, stockbroker, broker of the Stock Exchange Company, secretary to the Hibernian Insurance Company, 42 Dame street, and Moorfield, Roebuck. An advertisement for the company in *The Gentlemen's and Citizen's Almanac* compiled by John Watson Stewart in 1814 informed the public that it was then 'adding to their Establishment the Insuring of lives' and boasted that the company 'was the first of the Kind established in Ireland'. Patrick Curtis was then its secretary. He was still secretary when *Wilson's Dublin Directory* for 1816 and 1817 confirm his stock-broking and insurance business activities including his Dame street address but do not mention Moorfield. That, of course, does not mean that he was not then living at Moorfield; it just means that we lack evidence as to who the occupier of Moorfield was at this early date. Curtis remained at Moorfield until 1836 and on the following year William Haughton, esq. moved in.

Born in Carlow town in 1799 the son of Samuel Pearson Haughton, corn merchant and his wife Mary (née Pim), William set up a successful grain business in partnership with his brother James (1795-1873) at 27 & 28 City quay, Dublin. The latter was to become better known as an activist in a variety of humanitarian causes, in particular in the area of temperance and in the abolition of slavery. A member of the Unitarian congregation and a teetotaller from 1838, he bombarded the newspapers with letters, signed 'Son of a Water Drinker', about the evils of drink; he made common cause with many Catholic clergy including Fr Theobald Mathew and ceased to deal in malt and barley because of their use in the manufacture of alcoholic drink. Although it has not been discovered, this may be the cause why his name ceases to be associated with the City quay business in the 1850s. Thereafter only William is listed there in the directories along with a Wilfred Haughton, possibly another brother. While William was at Moorefield we get the first indication of its rateable valuation - £187 in 1847; it dropped to £138 in 1861. William died in 1877 and Mrs Haughton, presumably his wife remained there until 1885.[106]

---

106 Frances Clarke, "Son of a Water Drinker_ and 'Anti-Everythingarian_' in *History Ireland* 15/3 (2007) 64.

In the following year the new occupant who, as we will see was also a merchant, arrived. He is entered in 1886 as follows: Michael John Clery, esq., JP, co. Limerick, Moorefield (£138). He continues to be listed in this manner but in 1889 we get some further detail. In that year the words 'and Fort Mary, Limerick' are added. Then in 1894, instead of these added words the following were substituted 'and 21 to 27 Sackville street and The Glebe (this name was changed to The Cottage in later years), Athlacca, Co Limerick'. The reference to '21 to 27 Sackville street' immediately tells us that we are here dealing with the owner of Clery's of Sackville street, now O'Connell street.

In order to trace Michael John Clery's connection with that famous shop the directories for the 1880s and 1890s have been consulted. In 1881 we find the entry for 21-27 Sackville street to be 'M'Swiney and Company (Limited) drapers, silk mercers, hosiers, glovers, haberdashers, jewellers, boot and shoe makers, tailors and woollen drapers, upholsterers and general outfitters' and the rateable valuation was £900. In 1883 it is given as 'Dublin Drapery Warehouse' and in the following year that had changed to 'Clery and Company (formerly M'Swiney and Company). In that year, 1884, the residence of Michael J Clery, esq. J P is given as 'Adzar house, Monkstown'. That remained until 1886 when his residence is given as 'Moorfield, Roebuck and Fortmary, Limerick'. One extra item of note at the early stages of Clery's association with 21 to 27 Sackville street is that in 1888 another Clery – Francis W Clery, esq. – is given as being in residence at Moorfield. Who he was has not been discovered but it was not his son whose name was Robert. It could have been his brother as we know that a brother of his was among the partnership which had bought the business in 1883. Francis W Clery continued to be listed as living at Moorfield until 1894. During Michael J Clery's period at Sackville street the description of the business remained substantially as that which M'Swiney had used. The name and description of the business continued into 1897 but in that year Clery's residential address is omitted. This is in line with the entry for Moorfield in the same year: 'Mrs Clery, Moorefield, and The Cottage, Athlacca, Co Limerick (£135)'. This would suggest that at some time around (possibly before) 1897 Michael J Clery had died.

However, according to a book published by Clery and Co, in its centenary year 1983, he died in 1898. This book also gives us some detail on the early history of the store. The outcome of a partnership between two men, Peter Paul M'Swiney and George Delany, who saw a business opportunity in the upcoming International Exhibition of 1853, a new purpose-built 'Monster house' was built in the first half of 1853 on the sites of houses nos. 23 to 28 Lower Sackville street which they had just bought. The business opened its doors to the public a little over two weeks after the Exhibition had opened on 12 May. It has, with some justification, been claimed that it was the first purpose-built department store in the world. Referred to as the Palatial or New Mart it was Delany who had a background in drapery; M'Swiney was involved in politics becoming lord mayor in 1862 and 1875 but he did become chairman of what had become a public company after Delany retired in 1872. The early years of the company were prosperous but an economic depression in 1879 saw the business run into trouble; it was bankrupt in 1882. A short change in direction when it was renamed the Dublin Drapery Warehouse was to no avail and in 1883 it was sold to Michael Joseph Clery for £32,000. A new company, Clery and Co, was set up and an agreement signed in February 1885 indicated the source of the money behind the purchase; William Martin Murphy and his father-in-law James Fitzgerald Lombard, both wealthy business men were Clery's backers. Clery was born in Bulgaden in the Golden Vale in Tipperary but gained his early business experience in Limerick. Although his connection with the business in Sackville street was relatively short (from 1883 to c. 1897/8) his name was retained and to this day it is one of the more prominent titles associated with a business premises in Dublin.

In 1898 the occupant of Moorfield is given in the directory of that year as Robert Clery, esq., Michael J's son. He remained at Moorfield until 1900 the year of his death; in the following year it is listed as vacant. Robert's early death did not, however, break the Clery connection. One of his daughters, Louise, married Christopher Nixon, son of a man we have already met, Sir Christopher Nixon, then living but a short distance away from Moorfield at Roebuck grove. Later, as Sir Christopher Nixon, he was appointed chairman of Clerys in 1931. Unfortunately for him, it was just before the effects of the Crash of 1929 were felt in Ireland. That, together with the "Economic War" with Great Britain, meant that the 1930s were difficult years. In 1940 the company went into receivership, Nixon departed and Denis Guiney took over. The Clery connection was ended; only the name survived.[107]

The new century saw J Ross, esq. move into Moorfield; he had city premises at 12 and 13 Parkgate street. He remained until 1911 when he was replaced by W R Ross who, most likely, was related to him. Interestingly his occupation is given as 'farmer'; he would appear to be the last farmer to live in the area. It does not seem likely, however, that the land he farmed was that which alone was attached to Moorfield; it would not have been extensive enough to sustain a livelihood commensurate with living in a house which was rated at £135. He only stayed at

---

107 Peter Costello & Tony Farmer, *The very heart of the city: the story of Denis Guiney and Clerys* (Dublin 1992) 13-9, 26-35, 38-9, 66-72.

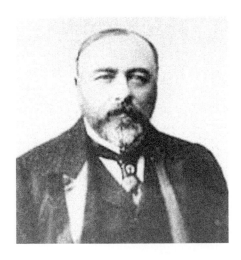

Sir Christopher Nixon of Roebuck grove, now part of UCD campus

Moorfield until 1914 after which it lay vacant for as short while. The next four occupancies were short: from 1916 to 1917 Miss Elizabeth Fayle with city address at 57 Townsend street; 1918 Alex Crockett, inspector, Dept of Agriculture; 1919 Rev J Dwyer Kelly and 1920 Wm Johnston. It would appear that during this period the rateable valuation dropped to £76. It remained at that level while P J Gaynor lived there from 1921 to 1926. However, after Michael Reilly took up residence in 1927 it was changed in 1932 to £74 and £4, perhaps giving a separate rating for a gate lodge. However, in 1936 it rose to £131-10s and remained at that level until J W Kinneen took over in 1943.

Soon the impact of new houses being built in the area would have an effect, first on the level at which its rates were set and afterwards on the very existence of the house itself. In 1945 the rateable valuation dropped to £111-15s, at which level it would remain until the house was no longer in existence. From 1948 onwards for a number of years a new category began to be listed in the directories: 'Moorefield Estate' with 6 new houses said to be already there in 1948. In 1950 it appeared as a separate heading under which various houses were entered. This continued throughout the 1950s although soon some of these were relocated in the directories and placed under the heading of Roebuck road. The house itself was listed separately from Moorefied Estate in 1954 and in the following year it no longer appeared. When Moorefield Estate finally ceased to be listed at the end of the 1950s, the name Moorfield disappeared from the area, apart, that is, from the two Moorfield cottages, already mentioned; they are the only remaining indication on the ground that a house called Moorfield once existed in the area.

ROEBUCK CASTLE

Roebuck castle stands at the other side of Roebuck road from where Moorfield once stood; it is located at a short distance in from that road (location no. 21 on map). The castle left the possession of the long-standing owners, the lords Trimleston, during the tenure of the 14th baron, Nicholas Barnwall. (Their time in Roebuck has been discussed above in Chapter 4.) There is good evidence that already in 1801 it had passed into the hands of Mr James Crofton, an official of the Irish Treasury. It would subsequently pass to his son Arthur Burgh Crofton who, like his father was a Commissioner for the building of Kingstown (now Dún Laoghaire) harbour. Both of their names appear on a monument erected in 1823 to commemorate the laying of the first stone by the then lord lieutenant, earl Whitworth, on 31 May 1817. James Crofton married Frances, daughter of Arthur Stanley in 1797. They had six children; their first son, Arthur Burgh, will be discussed shortly. The second, George, was a lieutenant in the 17th Lancers and died in India. Of their four daughters, two (Anne and Eliza) died young and are buried in Taney graveyard while nothing has been discovered about the other two (Louisa and Frances). James acted as churchwarden on three separate occasions, 1807, 1808 and 1822. His wife Frances died on 8 January 1811 and he died seventeen years later on 5 June 1828; both are buried in Taney graveyard. After his death, Arthur Burgh inherited the castle.

It was during his occupancy that we get the first indication of the size of the property when, in 1847 we find that its rateable valuation is given as £443 suggesting that it was a property of considerable substance. Like his father he took an active interest in his local church since he was a churchwarden in 1829 and 1835. Furthermore he acted as one of the treasurers of the school attached to the church in 1838. On 7 October 1828 he married Catherine in Taney church and together they had five children. In 1842 he became high sheriff of county Dublin and some years later a Justice of the Peace. He died on 29 December 1850. His wife continued to live at the castle for another five years. Why she decided to move has not been discovered but she lived another 27 years; she died on 14 April 1882. With her departure from the castle at date around 1855/56, the Crofton family ceased to own the castle and a new family moved in.[108]

This family was the Westbys, headed at this time by Edward Perceval. He was born in 1830, son of Nicholas Westby (born 1787) and the hon. Emily Susanna Laura Waldegrave (1787-1870); she was the daughter of William Waldegrave, 1st baron Radstock (1753-1825). Edward Perceval's parents lived at Thornhill, county Dublin.[109] He first married, in 1853, Elizabeth Mary Blackburne, daughter of the

---

108 Ball & Hamilton, *Parish of Taney*, 104-05, 190-91; various directories.
109 Ball & Hamilton, *Parish of Taney*, 151-52; some extra detail: www.thepeerage.com/p1333.htm#i13326

then lord chancellor, Francis Blackburne, who for many years up to 1850 had lived at Roebuck hall which is located within walking distance of the castle. Given that they did not move to that castle until about two years after their marriage (when, presumably, it was put up for sale by Mrs Crofton), it is a reasonable assumption that Elizabeth Mary, being familiar with the castle or at the very least with the general area in which it was located, was responsible for that move. Together they had three children but the eldest son, William Francis Perceval, died while still quite young and without issue in 1870. Their second son was Francis Vandeleur, born in 1859 and baptized in Taney church, will be discussed shortly. Their only other child was Emily Jane Laura was baptized at Taney church but nothing else has been found out about her. In 1863 Elizabeth Mary Westby died, four years before the death of her father Francis Blackburne in September 1867.

However, Edward Perceval soon married a second time. On June 16 1864 he married in Taney church Susan Elizabeth daughter of John Davis Garde, whom we have already met when discussing Mount Dillon. There does not appear to have been any issue from this marriage but it was during this period of Edward Perceval's life that he carried out major renovations on the castle. The castle as we see it today is the result of this renovation. He also carried out major work on the gate lodge. On both buildings he has left us evidence of this work which helps to date it. The work on the gate lodge was recorded in an ornate plaque high in the front of the building; it actually carries the date – 1872 – and above it Edward Perceval's initials EPW are ornately carved. On the front of the castle itself, the main door has above it an arching curve within a rectangular space giving scope for two spandrels, one on either side. Within these two spandrels are carved the initials of both Edward Perceval and his wife Susan Elizabeth Westby. Both sets of initials – EPW & SEW – are so ornately intertwined as to be almost difficult to read.

The work carried out on the castle at this time has been described by Bence-Jones as follows: 'E P Westby ... remodelled the castle (in) 1874; giving it an elaborate three storey High Victorian Gothic porch crowned with a steep battle-mented gable, and plate-glass windows with pointed or segmented-pointed heads, some of them set in rectangular surrounds with carving in the spandrels. In the hall, he installed a large and ornate Victorian Gothic chimney-piece of carved stone and marble.'[110]

In 1863 and before this work was carried out, there is evidence that the rateable valuation, which in 1847 was reported to be £443, had dropped to £273.

---

110 Mark Bence-Jones, *A guide to Irish country houses* (London 1988) 244-45.

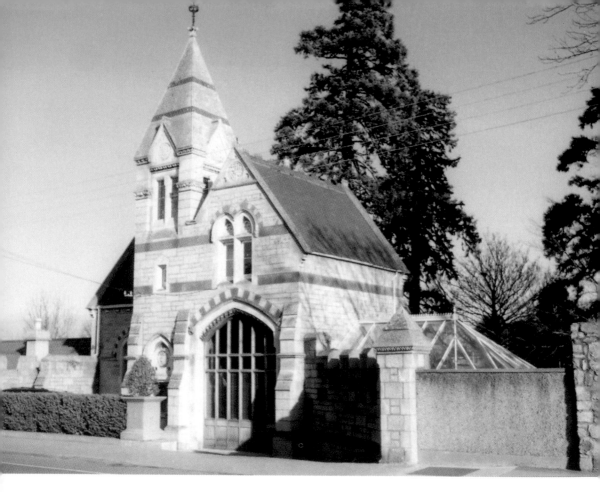

Gate lodge, Roebuck castle (*Photographer: Matt Walsh*)

The reason for this drop is not clear but it will have been noted already that a number of properties had their valuation substantially reduced during certain periods of the 19th century. The Westby family had Clare connections and Edward Perceval had an address in Killballyowen and Roscoe in county Clare. Furthermore, he was a deputy lieutenant and Justice of the Peace for county Clare; in 1854 he became high sheriff for the county. Because of his connection with Roebuck castle he was also a Justice of the Peace for county Dublin. Like the Croftons before him he was an active churchman. He was a churchwarden at Taney church on numerous occasions between 1856, the year when he first took up residence at the castle, and 1875. He died on 23 April, 1893.

It seems likely that his son Francis Vandeleur was living elsewhere when his father died since we find that the castle remained vacant for approximately four years after his death. Francis Vandeleur was probably living in county Clare since he was high sheriff for the county in 1895. When he took up residence in the

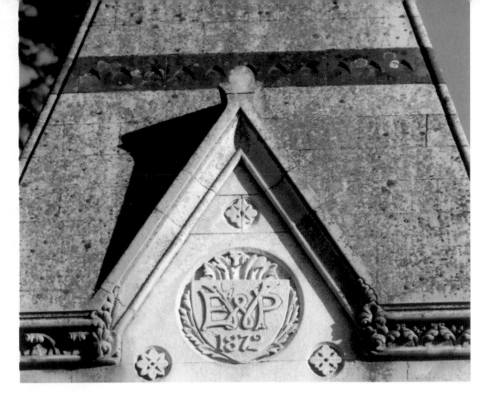

Initials of Edward Perceval Westby together with date of renovation: Gate lodge, Roebuck castle (*Photographer: Matt Walsh*)

(Below left) Initials (SEW) of Susan Elizabeth Westby carved in spandrel on right hand side of main door of Roebuck castle (*Photographer: Matt Walsh*)

(Below right) Initials (EPW) of Edward Perceval Westby carved in spandrel on left hand side of main door of Roebuck castle (*Photographer: Matt Walsh*)

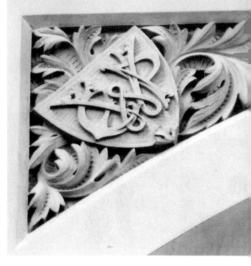

castle in 1897 he was a Justice of the Peace. He was married to Janet Louisa, second daughter of George Orme, esq. of Castle Lacken and they had children. During his time at the castle its rateable valuation rose, like many others during the First World War, from £273 to £328. He continued to live there until 1930 after which his wife is listed as being in residence there until 1943. On 14 September of that year, according to the foundation book of St Brigid's Novitiate at The Hermitage, the Little Sisters of the Poor acquired 'a big property bordering on ours, called "Roebuck castle" that would become the 2nd Home of the Aged in Dublin' and the residents from the Hermitage were transferred to it on 17 May 1944. The subsequent history of the castle is discussed in the section which deals with the work of the Little Sisters of the Poor in Roebuck road.

ROEBUCK HALL

Crossing over Roebuck road from the gate lodge of the castle and a little further along that road we arrive at the access point to Roebuck hall. To get to it in modern times it is necessary to turn into a fairly new development of houses, The Palms, and then quickly turn left (location no. 22 on map). The house still exists but has, for a number of years since, been converted into flats. The date when the house was built has not been found; it is possible that it is visible on Taylor and Duncan's maps of 1816 and 1821 although this is not certain. It is, however, clearly marked and named in the first Ordnance Survey map of 1837 and from the directories we know that the house had been occupied by Francis Blackburne in 1834. In fact, if we follow Ball & Hamilton, he was already in the house in 1827. At that time he was sergeant, a law officer, and during his early years there, in 1830 he was appointed attorney general and in 1841 was raised to the bench. But before that, it is worth noting what D'Alton, writing in 1838, had to say about Roebuck hall. He was generally critical of the area due to the high walls topped with thick hedges, the closed tall gates and concealed gate-houses which he said gave the whole area a sombre unsocial appearance. However, he picked out Roebuck hall as an exception to this but did not expand. From this one must assume that it was possible in 1838 to see Roebuck hall when passing along what is now Roebuck road or, at least, when passing in close proximity to it.[111]

Describing Roebuck hall Bence-Jones has this to say 'A compact late-Georgian two storey house of three bays; recessed centre with Wyatt window and recessed Grecian Doric porch. Wing at rear'. A Wyatt window is a rectangular

---

111 Ball & Hamilton, *Parish of Taney,* 156; D'Alton, *The history of the county Dublin,* 809.

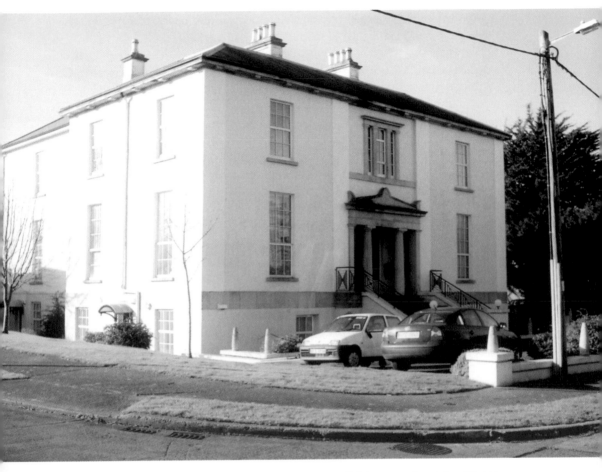

Roebuck hall (*Photographer: Matt Walsh*)

triple window very common in late-Georgian domestic architecture, named after the English architect, James Wyatt (1747-1813).[112]

Following Roebuck hall in the directories from 1834 one can track Francis Blackburne as he moved up through the ranks from attorney general to Master of the Rolls and finally lord chief justice of the Queen's Bench to which he was appointed in 1846. He left Roebuck hall in 1851 just before he was appointed lord chancellor in 1852. He was, therefore, residing at Roebuck hall throughout the period which saw him involved in legal entanglements with various political

112 Bence-Jones, *A guide to Irish country houses,* xxxi, 245.

figures who were prominent in the second quarter of the 19th century; these have been described in some detail in an earlier chapter.

He was succeeded in Roebuck hall in 1852 by Charles Samuel Grey. He worked at the Treasury in Dublin castle where he was Paymaster of the Civil Services; such a title was used to distinguish it from the Military Services. After him at Roebuck hall came Mrs Manders in 1866. During her period there, the rateable valuation was reduced considerably in line with general trends in the area at the time; £263 in 1847 but £130 in 1870. Her successor, Mrs Verschoyle, remained there from 1876 to 1877 accompanied by captain James Verschoyle, probably her son. Andrew Mulligan in 1878 is followed by Francis R M Crozier; a solicitor, he had offices at 19 Dominick street lower where he is also given a country address at Banbridge. At the same address in Dominick street there is listed Thomas Crozier & Son, solicitors and Banbridge; also there is T F Crozier but no reference is made as to what his occupation was.

Next came two more relatively short occupancies, Hugh Sweetman from 1888 to 1897 and Mrs Gresson from 1898 to 1905, before a person of some considerable interest moved in. He is described in the directory entry for the year 1906 as follows: L White King, esq., CSI, LL D, FSA, ICS (ret), professor of Arabic, Persian and Hindustani, Trinity College, Dublin. Later entries would expand on the L in his name to Lucas, give his college address as 37 Trinity College and his club membership as 'Junior Carlton and Kildare street clubs'. In fact the name Lucas had first come into the family as Luke when his grandfather was christened Luke White after a great friend of his father who was known by that name and was a successful Irish publisher and book seller as well as being MP for Leitrim.

Born in Madras, India, in 1856 Lucas White King was brought back to Ireland when he was 8 years old by his parents and left with a grand-uncle. His first school was in Tulla, county Clare. Afterwards he went to Ennis College and in October 1873 Trinity College Dublin. A proficient student, he gained first-class honours in logic and classics and prizes in Persian, Arabic and Hindustani. He graduated with an LL B (later in 1896 gaining his LL D). While still at Trinity in 1876 he sat the exam for the Indian Civil Service which, at the time, ranked second only to the Home Civil Service. Although he did well he sat it again in the following year and did even better. As a result he left for India in September 1878 while still a very young man. His parents were, of course, already in India. His father, who had also excelled at his studies in Trinity College where he studied medicine, had left Ireland to join the Indian Medical Service in 1856 where he spent all of his working life. In his grandson's memoirs he was said to be 'a Fenian and refused to stand up when the band played 'God save the queen' at official functions'. Be that as it may, when Lucas White arrived in India he became, at 22 years of age, assistant commissioner at Lahore and afterwards progressed through other appointments before returning to Ireland on leave in 1890 where he met Geraldine Adelaide Harmsworth whose two brothers became mass-circulation newspaper proprietors, viscounts Northcliffe and Rothermere. Soon after he returned to India she followed him and they were married there. More promotions in the Indian Civil Service followed but he soon began to dislike his time in India intensely; he developed a strong desire to return home to Ireland where he would set up a home. The search for a house and a job in Ireland was put in train even before he retired in 1905.

He applied for and was appointed to the Professorship of Oriental Languages and Reader in Indian History at Trinity College and Roebuck hall was acquired as the home he had longed for so much in India. He had served for 25 years in India and got a full pension of £1,000 per annum as a result. This together with £2,000 allowance a year from viscount Northcliffe and about £300 a year from Trinity meant that the family had an annual income of something like £3,300. As for Roebuck hall, his daughter Enid would in later years recall it being set in eleven acres 'solid and square, late Georgian and built of stone painted cream with a slate roof and granite portico. It was uncompromising, ungraceful'. The furnishing, she recalled, included many valuable Indian carpets and 'oriental china, stone Buddhas, brass figures and embroideries. Our large hall was like a small museum of these things with weapons and musical instruments hanging on the walls as well as Dad's fine tiger skin'. The whole house was lighted by gas; electricity would not arrive for quite a number of years. A substantial array of staff served their needs. His son Cecil in his memoirs wrote 'Though ours was only a middle-class household by the standards of the day, we had a governess, a cook and kitchen-maid, a parlour-maid, and between-maid. We had a coachman, two gardeners and a garden boy. We had two walled gardens in which were a hot-house, a large peach and nectarine house, and a vinery. When we arrived we had two horses ... and four carriages, an open victoria, a landau, a closed brougham and an Irish jaunting-car, the latter in black and yellow, very smart. We had a telephone, at that time unusual for private people in Ireland.' Later, in 1908, a chauffeur was employed instead of the coachman when the first motor-car was acquired, a Darracq, a present from his brother-in-law Leicester Harmsworth, who owned the motor company.

While at Roebuck hall, Lucas White King was a Justice of the Peace and sat on the bench at Dundrum. His work at Trinity College was mostly taken up teaching candidates for the Indian Civil Service. At home he tended his rock garden which he devoted to a collection of Irish ferns while during vacations he went grouse-shooting initially in the Dublin mountains but later in Aberdeenshire. Not long before he retired from Trinity College in 1920 Lucas White received a knighthood. This, according to his son Cecil, was not for his service in India but as a present from viscount Rothermere to Geraldine, wife of Lucas White, when Lloyd George was prime minister and in need of Press support. Some of the items that once were exhibited on the walls of Roebuck hall are now among the archives of Boston University. They were donated to it by Cecil King and included among them is a standard once carried into battle by a Waziri tribesman near the Afghanistan border and what is now Pakistan in the late 19th century. Lucas King, who had brought this home to Roebuck hall, died in 1925. His son Cecil, after a career which saw him become the owner of the Mirror Group of Newspapers and a director of the Bank of England, retired to live in Dublin but not a Roebuck hall which had long left the family. Instead, he lived at Greenfield Park, Donnybrook where he died in 1987.[113]

Subsequent residents of Roebuck hall were William J Kenny (1922 to 1935) and Val Cosgrave (1936 to 1963). In the 1965 directory, Stomac Adhesives Ltd. is given as the occupant of Roebuck hall but Cecil H King in his memoirs says that 'when I saw it some years ago [i.e. before 1969] (it) was used partly for storing Aaron Electricity Meters and partly as a sausage factory. More recently the house has been converted into small flats. The grounds are being covered by new houses and the stables, no longer a sausage factory, are now used for manufacturing an adhesive called 'Stomac'.[114] In the 1965 directory a number of houses with their occupants are listed under the address The Palms and living in no. 28 a man named Val Cosgrave is listed, the same name as that of the last person listed as resident of Roebuck hall. Shortly thereafter the names of the residents of the various flats in Roebuck hall begin to appear in the directories.

ROEBUCK COTTAGE, LATER ARDILLEA (ARDILEA)

Although Roebuck cottage which was later renamed Ardillea (Ardilea) is, strictly speaking, outside the area with which this work is concerned, being located off Mount Anville road, the land associated with it had, in modern times, houses built upon it which are accessed from Roebuck road. These were initially called Ardilea Estate (the first houses built appear under that name in the 1965

---

113   King, *Strictly personal,* 3, 10-19, 25-26; Ruth Dudley Edwards, *Newspapermen: Hugh Cudlipp, Cecil Harmsworth King and the glory days of Fleet street* (London 2003) 12-14, 410-41(see also the unpaginated genealogies of both the King and the Harmsworth families at the start of the book); Hope Green 'Tribal flag gives rare glimpse of Afghan past' in *B.U. Bridge* (Boston University community's weekly paper) vol. 5, no. 10, 19 October 2001.

114   King, *Strictly personal,* 19.

directory) but later given individual addresses such as Louvain, Salamanca, Heidelberg and Salzburg. For this reason it is considered necessary to write a short piece about it (location no. 23 on map).

Roebuck cottage is clearly marked on all the early maps starting with Taylor's in 1816 and the entrance from what is now Mount Anville road is also visible. The name of the first resident that is available to us from the directories is Anthony Dempsey who had a city address in Nassau street. The earliest date we have for him at Roebuck cottage is 1841. He was succeeded there in 1844 by Mr Patrick Brady whose city address was 40 Sir John Rogerson's quay. Captain George Daniel, RN stayed there in 1849 before moving in to Mount Dillon and details about him may be found in the section which deals with that house. For some unknown reason there is no mention of Roebuck cottage in the directories between 1850 and 1856. In 1857 Edmund D'Olier is listed as living there. In 1862 he changed the name of the house to 'Ardillea'; the spelling was changed by him to 'Ardilea' from 1867 onwards and it is still in use to this day. Although it has not been possible to prove it, it does seem likely that it was called after a townland of the same name in county Down which is located beside a river estuary on the bay of Dundrum. In 1862 the part of Roebuck in which Edmond D'Olier's house was located was listed by the compilers of *Thom's Directory* as being part of Dundrum, county Dublin; it was from there that D'Olier's post was delivered. Whether the coincidence of the two Dundrums had anything to do with the name change is not known. According to *Onomasticon Goedelicum*, the name Ardilea is the anglicised version of the Irish *Ard dá Laech*, a name which preserves the memory of two ancient heroes.

As for Edmond D'Olier he would appear to have taken up residence in Roebuck cottage in 1857 and remained there until around 1877; Ardilea was vacant in 1878 and is given as the residence of John Parkes esq. in 1879. Edmond D'Olier was educated in Trinity College, Dublin and later joined the firm of Henry Thompson & Co., wine merchants, which was located in Eustace street. Because of this, the firm then became known as Thompson, D'Olier & Co. He married Maria Louisa, daughter of Isaac Manders of Carthsize, Co. Kildare (there are records of a family of that name, Manders, living in Roebuck at least from the 1840s to the 1870s but it is not clear if Maria Louisa was related to them). Edmond was a Freeman of the City of Dublin and high sheriff in 1864. Like his father, Isaac Matthew D'Olier, he was a director of the Bank of Ireland on a number of occasions (between 1853 and 1887) and governor for one period (1875-77). His grandfather, Jeremiah D'Olier, was even more involved with that bank; not alone had he been a director and a governor but he was a member of the original board at its foundation.

The D'Oliers were descended from a noted Huguenot family which was represented at the famous battle of the Boyne. They had settled in Dublin in the early eighteenth century where they became goldsmiths and bankers and as they progressed in business they attained membership of the prestigious Guild of the Holy Trinity. Jeremiah was made a Freeman of the Goldsmith's Corporation in 1771 and its master in 1781. He was also a Freeman of the City and a sheriff there. A member of the Dublin Society (as the Royal Dublin Society was then known), he was elected to the Wide Street Commission in 1796; D'Olier street was named after him at a meeting of the Commissioners on 1 August 1799.[115]

As already noted, Edmund D'Olier remained at the house now known as Ardilea until 1877 after which it lay vacant for a while before John Parkes moved in around 1878/9. The property which had for a number of years carried a rateable valuation of £139 dropped slightly to £136 in 1895 while Parkes was still there. However, after the turn of the century, Martin Fitzgerald replaced him. Around 1906 he became a Justice of the Peace and remained at Ardilea until his death in March 1927. From the inauguration of the Seanad in the newly founded state he had been a Senator. During his occupancy of the property its rateable valuation was changed to a three part one £38, £138, £6. The next resident of Ardilea, A O'Shaughnessy remained there until 1945. Then after being vacant for a short period R Walker moved in and the last listing of the house was in 1960 when Francis E Walker is given as the occupant. Shortly thereafter the first listing of Ardilea Estate, Roebuck, appears giving the names of a number of its householders. In time this would disappear and give way to specific road names such as Louvain, Salamanca, Heidelberg and Salzburg.

ROEBUCK GROVE, LATER OUR LADY'S GROVE

Roebuck grove, not to be confused with the Roebuck grove (originally Roebuck house) which is now part of UCD's campus, is located on what is now called Goatstown road just beyond its junction with Roebuck road (location no. 24 on map). Although, like Ardilea, strictly outside the area being covered by this study, the fact that it is in Farranboley townland calls for the inclusion of a few words about it. The year in which the house was built has not been discovered but it is marked along with its driveway in both Taylor's and Duncan's maps of 1816 and 1821. The first resident whom we meet in the directories is John Cumming. He was a wholesale bookseller and stationer who had his business premises at 16 Lower Ormonde quay. He was living at Roebuck grove in 1832 but we do not know how long he had already been there, the directories not being

---

115   de Courcy, *The Liffey in Dublin*, 418; Hall, *Bank of Ireland*, 486.

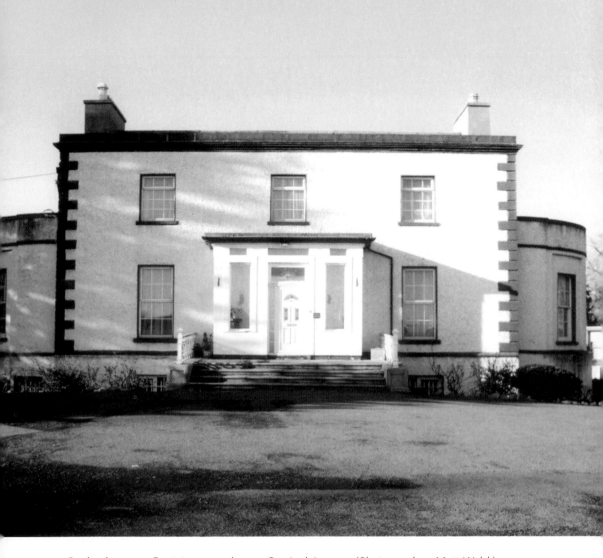

Roebuck grove, Goatstown road: now Our Lady's grove (*Photographer: Matt Walsh*)

of any help in this regard. While he was there we get the first indication of the rateable valuation of the property in 1847; it was £150. He was succeeded in 1849 by a solicitor called Charles Pickering with rooms in the city at 11 Upper Ormonde quay. Prior to moving to Roebuck grove he had lived at Rokeby, Rathgar. As this had a rateable valuation of £35 his move to Roebuck grove would suggest that at the time his business was improving. This is further indicated by the subsequent move of his business from Ormonde quay to 60 Dame street. During his stay at Roebuck grove the rateable valuation dropped, first in 1862 to £135 and then in 1864 to £117. In this latter year his business address changed again, this time to 29 Eustace street. At the end of his stay at

Roebuck grove he was joined there during 1870-71 by William Cuffe Pickering, also a solicitor and possibly his son.

In 1872 Robert Tedcastle took up residence there having previously lived at 7 Herbert road, Sandymount – rated at £28. Like Pickering before him this was an upgrade in living standards. The directory for 1872 describes his business as follows: 'Robert Tedcastle & Co., coal importers and ship agents, 19 & 20 Brunswick street, great, Rogerson's quay and Crofton place, Kingstown'. The reference to 'ship agents' was new for that year but some few years later, in 1878 it would be upgraded to 'ship owners'. In 1879 Robert Tedcastle had left Roebuck grove to live in Marlay, Whitechurch, Rathfarnham while George Tedcastle had taken over in his place. He remained at Roebuck grove until 1881. Thereafter it had some short-stay residents as well as being vacant on occasion until Robert Woods is listed there in 1891.

He had lived previously at no. 5 Vergemount hall and was described in 1891 as being a merchant with business premises at 205 & 206 Britain street, great. He was, in fact, a partner in what was once a well-known Dublin confectionery company called William and Woods. That company first appears in the trade section of the directory of 1884, listed under the heading of 'Confectioners'; it is described there as being a wholesale company with premises at 111 Dorset street, upper. However, according to a company advertisement which appeared in later years it was claimed that it had been founded in 1856.[116] In 1886 the company had acquired premises at 205 & 206 Britain street, great. The Dorset street premises is dropped from the 1890 listing and then in 1891, when Robert moved into Roebuck grove, the name Wood was changed to Woods. Britain street, great, was changed to Parnell street in the 1912 listing and two years later no. 204 Parnell street was added to the company's address. By this time Robert was described as a director of the company. However, in 1915 he was succeeded at Roebuck grove by Keith Woods, possibly his son, described as a manufacturing confectioner with the same business address as Robert had and remained on only a few years.

In 1920, Percy M'Entagart is listed there and remained there until 1937. He appears to be one of the M'Entagart Bros., motor engineers who in 1920 had their business at 10 Leinster street. An advertisement of theirs in 1923 states that they were sole agents for 'Crossley, Citroen, Berliet, etc'. It also stated that their Works and Garage were at the rear of 10 Leinster street. In the following year a similar advertisement said they were agents for Rolls Royce, Crossley, Dodge

---

116   For a copy of this advertisement, see Cullen, *Princes & pirates: the Dublin Chamber of Commerce*, 82.

Bros., Citroen and that their Works and Garage (300 cars) was at Percy place. The advertisements ceased to appear in the directories from 1927 onwards.

Percy was succeeded at Roebuck grove in 1938 by George Archer. He is described as being a family butcher and contractor with premises in Talbot street. During his residency, the rateable valuation of the house was reduced to £108 in 1945. The last person to live at the house before The Congregation of Jesus and Mary bought it in 1963 was T McKeogh. Although it is not certain, it does seem likely that he was the Thomas Keogh who in the directories of the time is described as being an auctioneer and salesman who operated at 23 Blackhall street and 19-20 Blackhall street. It would appear that his business was related to livestock. The period after his residency is dealt with in the chapter on schools, in the section which deals with Our Lady's Grove school.

13

The growth of the suburb

IN THE LAST CHAPTER we noted the extraordinary growth of mansions in the Clonskeagh area beginning around the last quarter of the 18th century and growing to such an extent that the compiler of *Thom's Directory* in 1840 could say of the area that it was 'studded with gentlemen's seats and neat villas'. But alongside that, although perhaps less dramatically and a little later in time, there was another building programme going ahead. This was the building of houses some of which were of quite substantial proportions but not grand enough to attract the appellation of mansion. They did not stand on their own grounds with a driveway sweeping up to the front of the house; they were, nevertheless, a manifestation of the growing reputation of Clonskeagh as a desirable place in which to live. There were two distinct phases in this; the first began early in the 19th century and continued rather spasmodically throughout that century. The second began in the 1920s and soon afterwards gathered pace giving rise to the modern suburb as we know it today.

VERGEMOUNT

The earliest of those in the first phase were called after the house which was located across the road, but secluded from them, Vergemount house. The exact date on which they were built has not been discovered but it is possible to make a fairly accurate estimate of it from the maps of the time and from the entries in the directories. The first to be found in the latter is in 1834, which was the earliest date in which Clonskeagh appears in the directories. As regards the maps, there is no indication in Taylor's map of 1816 of their presence although it has to be remembered that absence from a source is no proof that an item did not exist or occur. However, we are on surer grounds when we look at Duncan's map of 1821. Here we see that the first two houses are marked and we can be confident that the others if they had existed would not have been left out. This gives us a close approximation of the date of construction; that is, starting just before 1821 and continuing in the following years. All were certainly completed at the very latest

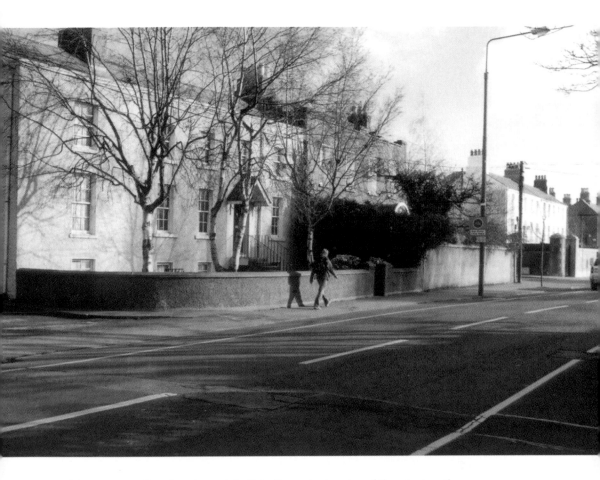

Vergemount, Clonskeagh road: built in the early decades of the nineteenth century
(*Photographer: Matt Walsh*)

by the mid-1830s as both the directories and the first Ordnance Survey map attest.

The only source used to trace the history of these houses has been the directories which tell us who occupied the houses in any particular year. What they do not tell us is who owned the houses; that would require an intensive search of registry that is not required for the purpose of the exercise in hand. Listing all the residents and their years of occupation would make for tedious reading and would not be particularly enlightening. However, it is possible to make some observations of the occupation pattern as it became manifest over the years. Apart from house number 3, all eight houses have had an extraordinary number of residents over the years, many of whom remained for very short periods. This is especially true of the 19th century.

Over the 140 years from 1834 to 1974 house no. 1 had 18 residents, the one remaining longest was Mrs Margaret Fitzgerald (1931-1958) followed by William Boake (1849-66). House no. 2 had 20 residents during the same period. Thomas Griffin was resident for the longest period (1900-1946). Soon after his arrival he gave the house a name 'Ashleigh'. The second longest resident, Dr Peter Denham MB with a city address at 97 St Stephen's green, was first listed in 1947; he is recorded as still living there in 1974. Prior to the residency of these two and just before the end of the 19th century Henry Chamney of the General Prisons Board lived there from 1888 to 1899. These two houses, nos. 1 & 2, are attached to one another and are most likely to be those which are visible on Duncan's map of 1821.

House no. 3 has a completely different residency pattern to the rest of the houses in Vergemount. In the 140 years being examined it only had 5 residents and what is more, the 19th century occupancy was by far the longest of that of any of the houses looked at. James Barton was there from 1834 to 1866 and Mrs Barton from 1867 to 1904, a total of around 70 years. In fact we know that James Barton was there some years previous to the period we are discussing since we find the following in the Nobility and Gentry section of *Watson's or the Gentleman's and Citizen's Almanack* for 1830: James Barton, esq., 9 upper Sackville street and Virgemount, Clonskeagh. 'Government stockdealer' is added to that description in an entry in *The Post Office Annual Directory* for 1832. It is not clear how long his city address remained at 9 upper Sackville street but in 1842 a directory entry gives it as 41 Wellington quay and a few years later at 40 Wellington quay. In 1851 we discover that his occupation is given as 'flour merchant, Ravensdale mill stores, 40 Wellington quay'. We have been tracing James Barton, always with an address at 3 Vergemount but both the change of city address and business (from government stockdealer to flour merchant) must raise the possibility that there are two James Bartons being discussed. If that is the case it seems most likely that they are father and son. As well as that the Mrs Barton who remained in no. 3 until 1904 would have been the wife of James Barton, junior. The next resident of no. 3 also remained there for a substantial period of time – Frederick W Evans (1905-40). It was he who called the house 'Wyverne' later altered to 'Wyvern'. Like houses 1 & 2, nos. 3 & 4 are attached to one another but no. 4 reverts to the general pattern. In the 140 under examination there were 28 different residents living there, the longest being Mrs Moore/More (1906-1937) and the next Arthur Irwin Mahon (1881-97). The latter was a civil engineer and was employed as surveyor to Pembroke Township. While A G Hardy was living there in 1904-05 the house acquired the name 'Lisheen'.

One occupant of this house who is of special interest was William Stoker

MD who was in residence from 1847 to 1849. Dr Stoker was a prominent physician in Dublin city for many years; he was associated with the Dublin Fever Hospital and House of Recovery. He was also the uncle of Abraham Stoker, better known as Bram Stoker, the famous author of the horror novel *Dracula*. In his early life, Bram suffered from some illness which has not been fully explained and he was treated by his uncle William. Since Bram was born in 1845 it seems quite possible that he was being treated at the time that his uncle was living at Clonskeagh. There has also been a suggestion made that his illness and his experience of medicine through his contact with his uncle could have had a seminal influence on his invention of his vampire stories. His three brothers, of course, were also doctors but his uncle William advocated the practice of phlebotomy (blood-letting) for most diseases.[1] Whether Bram ever visited his uncle at Vergemount or not we do not know; if he did he would still have been a very young boy. Incidentally, Bram's brother, the surgeon Sir Thornley Stoker, owned Ely house, in which Alexander Jaffray, an early resident of Clonskeagh, had lived in the previous century.

Houses 5 to 8 are terraced and the first of them, no. 5 had a total of around 20 different residents during the period of almost 140 years between 1835 and 1974; there was no entry for 1834. The person who lived there for the longest time was Mrs Sarah Graham (1918-1941); the second longest was Thomas Collins (1850-70). Until the latter took up residence there was a series of very short term residencies including a period when the house was either vacant or not listed (i.e. 1847-49). The next house, no. 6, fared no better. In the whole period of 140 years it saw nearly 30 different people live there and the longest occupation throughout the 19th century was John Phillips (1865-73); he was a solicitor who worked in the Queen's Bench office. It was also vacant or not listed on a number of occasions. Early in the century saw it used as a 'seminary'; from 1836 to 1837 by Robert Rogers and by Eugene O'Meara in 1838. Mainly due to the long sojourn of the Crosthwait/Crosthwaite family in the 20th century the number of people who lived at no. 7 throughout our period was considerably less than no. 6; around 20 in all. Mrs John Crosthwait (1911-32) was succeeded by Miss Crosthwait (later Crosthwaite) in 1933 and lived there until the late 1960s. Although it has not been possible to establish what, if any, their relationship was to the founder of Vergemount house, John Crosthwait, it does seem quite likely

---

1   Andrew N Papanikitas, '*Droch Fhola*: medical influences in Bram Stoker's *Dracula*, a tale of biological evil' in *Guy's, King's & St Thomas's Hospitals Medical and Dental Schools Gazette*, October 2002 and reproduced in http://www.gktgazette. com/2002/oct/features.asp

that they were in some way related to him. Apart from them, the only other person who spent a substantial amount of time in the house was one Herbert Cooper (1888-1910); his city address was at 27 Molesworth street. House no. 8 adhered to the pattern which, apart from house no. 3, has by now been clearly established; it had around 24 different people reside in it throughout the 140 years under examination. The longest stay was that by Henry William Geoghegan (1876-1906). He was a solicitor, a graduate of Trinity College from which he held an AM and an LL.D degree. His office was at 122 St Stephen's green. At one time a number of people of the same name are, unusually, given as residing with him e.g. Thomas, Harold and Frank Geoghegan (1899-1905). It may be assumed that they were adult members of his family. The other relatively long-time residents of the house were Edward Gerrard (1909-28) and W S Healy who lived there from 1944 until the late 1960s.

When we move to no. 9 we are no longer dealing with the houses on the side of the road which are still visible today. This house was set back from the road and was located close to the Dodder river. The first resident whom we meet in the directories is Patrick Nolan, Dodder cottage (1834-35) and we can clearly see this house, marked by that name, in the first Ordnance Survey map of 1837. It probably got that name from its proximity to the river. However, it was changed when William Henry Brownrigg was in residence (1853-1858); under his name it is called Virgemount lodge. That is the name of the house that appears in the map drawn for *Thom's Directory* for the year 1888. However, that name was not destined to last either for during the residency of Edward Donelan (1890-1917 with a year's interruption in 1895) it changed once more; this time c. 1892 to Rose vale. Of the approximately 25 occupants during the 140 years examined Andrew Ganly, BDS, dental surgeon with rooms at 25 Lr Baggot street was the longest occupant, living there from 1940 until the late 1960s; the aforementioned Edward Donelan was the second longest occupant.

The overall impression gained by the observations of these houses in Vergemount is that they, with the possible exception of the Bartons in no. 3, must have been rented at least for the whole of the 19th century as it is difficult to conceive that the frequent changes of occupants was the result of them being sold. And we have evidence that the houses in another development nearby were rented throughout their 19th century existence. If the Vergemount houses were rented, then the question arises as to who the landlord was. The answer to this has, unfortunately, not been discovered.

The next house, which was given the number 10, was quite different to the others. It was a small house, with a rateable valuation of only £4 in 1895 and was vacant for extended periods of time. It can not have been any more than a ruin, its function during this period seems to have been only to retain its house number. It is first mentioned in 1850 but was vacant the following year. From 1862 to 1868 Joseph Quigley, boot & shoemaker lived there. Much later after being either vacant or not listed for long periods M O'Neill is listed from 1932 to 1938 and the rateable valuation had risen to £11. From 1950 there was a shop there, first a grocery (1950-1954), then a confectioner & tobacconist (1955), then vacant again (1956 to 1965) before being called Mill House (later The Blue Shop) and run by John Thompson as a grocery and newsagent from 1969 into the 1970s. It no longer exists.

The number 11 was not allocated until 1850, the year house 10 (above) was first mentioned. When it first appears in the directory for that year Patrick Costello is given as its occupant. However he had been listed for many years prior to 1850 as follows; *Clonskeagh* – Patrick Costello, vintner and veterinary forge (1834-39); do. veterinary forge (1840-41); do. vintner (1848) with rateable valuation of £14; *Vergemount* – Costello's veterinary institution, £14 (1846-47); Patrick Costello, veterinary institution and vintner, *£14* (1848); There was no entry for the years 1842-45 and 1849. There were no clear lines drawn at this stage as to where Clonskeagh ended and Vergemount began but it is clear that, as time went by, Costello was seen to be more in Vergemount than Clonskeagh. Eventually with this boundary problem resolved his premises were numbered 11 Vergemount in 1850. Thereafter he continued to be listed at that number as either vintner or vintner and horse shoer until 1870 by which time valuation had dropped to £12. From 1871 he is exclusively described as vintner as is Mrs Costello in 1874. Henry Ashton took over in 1875 and was described as vintner, then grocer and later grocer &c. before Mary Ashton succeeded him in 1896 continuing to be described as grocer &c. However, when Thomas Ashton came into possession of the property in 1900 he and all subsequent proprietors are exclusively described as vintners although the final one discussed here, E F Ashton is described as wine, spirit merchant when he took over around 1964/5. By the time he succeeded in the property its valuation had increased to £50. In fact it had previously been steadily rising: Thomas Ashton (1900(£12)-1905(£18)-1915(£24)-1921); Edward Ashton (1922(£24)-1963). One final point of note, there is a record of burial in Taney graveyard of William Ashton of Clonskeagh who died 28 October 1879 aged 24 years.[2]

CLONSKEAGH (CLOSE TO THE BRIDGE):

From the time that Clonskeagh first appears in the directories in 1834 as a main heading, within that main heading is a sub-head also called Clonskeagh which

2   Ball & Hamilton, *Parish of Taney,* 45.

clearly refers to those people who live in close proximity to the bridge. According to *Thom's Directory* there were 352 people living in 67 houses there in the 1840/50s; this dropped to 310 in 54 houses in 1858 and continued at that level until 1907. The latter level of consistency is unlikely so the figures should be taken as being approximate. While these houses can not in any way be considered to be part of what this chapter is about, i.e. new houses and suburbanisation, it seems nevertheless, in the light of the discussion about Patrick Costello in the previous paragraph, that it would be convenient to discuss them at this point. We are at a disadvantage in that there are no house numbers or names to allow us to discuss continuity so the best that can be done is to list the entries in the chronological sequence of their first appearance together with the years in which they are listed. Also since the directories were re-ordered after 1960 and the sub-heading of Clonskeagh disappeared, the chronological sequence below finishes at 1960. Where available, rateable valuation is given.

1834: Mr John Wainhouse; Mr Hugh Motherwell (1834-39); Anthony Murphy, huxter/provision dealer (1834-39); Margaret M'Loughlin, huxter/provision dealer (1834-39).

1839: Patrick Callaghan (1839-41).

1840: Michael Ruth, provision dealer (1840-41); John Lambe, vintner and provision dealer (1840-41); Philip Rynard, sexton of Sandford church (1840-42).

1841: Anthony Murphy, dairy (1841); Patrick Murphy, tailor (1841).

1843: Miss Ger(r)ard, Richview cottage (1843-49).

1847: P Moran, shopkeeper, Clonskeagh bridge (1847-48); Mrs Byrne, vintner (1847-48).

1849: Thomas Bradley, vintner (1849-64); Bridget Bradley (1865-71).

1851: Robert H Kinahan (1851).

1852: Thomas Aicken MD (1852); Daniel Mansergh, Richview cottage (1852-53).

1853: Lawrence Boylan, dairy (1853-54); John B(r)annan, dairy, Dodder view (1853-57).

1855: Patrick Murphy, dairy (1855-69); Chris Dromgold, Palmerstown (1855). (The inclusion of Chris Dromgold, with an address at Palmerstown, may indicate that he owned some property at Clonskeagh although he did not live there)

1856: Thomas Byrne, provision dealer (1856); Mary Kavanagh, provision dealer (1856-78).

1857: Michael O'Neill, dairy (1857-59); do. dairy and car owner (1860-79); do. farmer (1880-91).

1858:   William Andrews (1858); Edward Hodgson (1858); George Jones, Violet lodge (1858-59)

1860:   George Moulds, Violet lodge (1860).

1862:   William Ashton, blacksmith (1862-77); do. *(£3-10s)* (1878-95); Thomas Ashton, do (1896*(£3-10s)* – 1918); do. *(£24)**(1919-31); James Nowlan, provision dealer (1862); Mrs Reddy, laundress (1862); Patrick Sinnott, car owner (1862-73).

         (**this valuation in the exact same as that for Thomas Ashton, vintner at 11 Vergemount but the entry there indicates that he ceased ownership in 1921*).

1871:   James Nolan, cab owner (1871-99).

1872:   John Byrne, vintner (1872); John Sharpe, rope manufacturer (1872)

1874:   John Darby (1874-75).

1875:   James Byrne, vintner (1875-77); do. *(£0-10s)* (1878-81); do. grocer and purveyor (1882-84).

1878:   William Cruice/Cruise, beer dealer (1878-83); do. coal factor and beer dealer (1890-4); do. dairy and beer dealer (1895); Charles Cruise, do. (1896); Eliza Cruise, beer dealer (1897-1918); do. *(£33)* (1919-27); do. without title 'beer dealer' *(£33)*(1928-31).

1881:   Matthew Griffin, manager iron works (1881-1910) followed by Thomas Griffin, do. (1911-32)

1885:   George Griffin, ironmonger (1885); Michael Brophy, grocer and purveyor, res. Rose villa, Roebuck (1885*(£0-10s)*); do. grocer, tea, wine and spirit merchant, res. Rose villa Roebuck (1886*(£0-10)* -91); do. res. Clonskeagh house (1892*(£0-10s)* – 94).

1888:   Thomas Griffin, iron works (1888).

1892:   William Hutchinson, accountant (1892); do. Richview cottage (1893-95).

1895:   Nicholas O'Shea, grocer, tea, wine, and spirit merchant, residence – Clonskeagh house (1895-1912); do. *(£30)* (1913); do. no valuation given, but a new street number, 28 Clonskeagh road, is assigned in 1960.

1900:   Bernard Keogh, sand contractor (1900-31)

1903:   Martin Corless, dairy proprietor, Richview farm (1903-14); do. *(£15, £96)* (1915-36). Note: from 1932 to 1936 John Corless appears with a dairy but both he and Martin Corless disappear from the listings in the same year, 1936. Also note the short appearance of Corless Lodge from 1932 to 1936 during most of which it is vacant; it disappears in the same year as the two Corlesses; it was most likely a house that they renamed but with a valuation of £41 it was of some substance. Could it have been Richview lodge?

1932   (major changes this year; impression given that there had not been a review of the Clonskeagh entries for some time since this is the first year since 1903 that a new entry has been made and others have been omitted. Those omitted are: Bernard Keogh, sand contractor; Eliza Cruise; Thomas Ashton, blacksmith. Some new entries are made especially Mrs Doyle whose property has such a large valuation. Note, however, that Mrs Hennessy's property has the same valuation as that of Eliza Cruise and John Corless is included but separate from that of Martin Corless). New entries are: John Corless, Richview dairy *(£24)*(1932-36); Mrs Hennessy, Beechhill cottage *(£33)*(1932-60); Mrs Doyle, Clonskeagh Bridge *(£88)*(1932-58); Tram cottage – vacant (1932); W Egan, Corless lodge *(£41)*(1932).

1933   Corless lodge – vacant (£41) (1933-36); Tram cottage – Mrs Dunne.

1934   Tram cottage – vacant (1934-36).

1952   Thompson, John – Mill House (1952); do. grocer (1953-58); do. newsagent and tobacconist (1960).

JACKSON'S COTTAGES > M'CASKEY'S COTTAGES > HENSHAW'S COTTAGES

Like the section on Clonskeagh, just discussed, this does not come under the heading of new houses or suburbanisation, but is placed at this point for convenience only. Henry Jackson is reported to have built quality cottages for his workers in Clonskeagh; this would have been around the end of the eighteenth century. It seems most likely that they were located quite near his iron works beside the bridge on the city side. Later, in 1834, the works were operated by William M'Caskey and, after him, by Thomas M'Caskey until 1841; two years later Thomas Portis had possession of them until 1852, then Mrs Portis for a year before finally Thomas Henshaw took over in 1854. It would appear that Jackson's cottages were passed on along with the works as Mrs M'Caskey is reported in 1847 to have held a number of cottages which extended along the road in Clonskeagh with a rateable valuation of £1 to £1-10s. In this year the works were actually being run by Thomas Portis so, perhaps, the cottages were retained in the possession of Mrs M'Caskey as a form of income. They are reported as belonging to her until 1854, the year the works were taken over by Thomas Henshaw. Nothing further is heard of them in the directories after that until 1911 when they are listed under the heading of HENSHAW'S COTTAGES (Clonskeagh road) and are said to be 17 houses with a rateable valuation of £4-10s to £7-10s. Although there is a long gap between the two listings i.e. between 1854 and 1911, it seems most likely that those called Henshaw's cottages are one and the same as those built by Henry Jackson. They would appear to have been located on the right hand side of

Clonskeagh road coming from the city and just before the bridge. They continued to be listed up to 1955 after which there is no mention made of them. If, as one may assume, they were demolished around that time a remarkable link with the late eighteenth century was lost; they would have represented what was considered good accommodation for workers in that period.

VERGEMOUNT HALL

Returning now to the progress of new house building in the area, we get our first reference to this new development, Vergemount hall, in 1857. These houses are not visible from the Clonskeagh road; they are accessed by a narrow roadway immediately after St James's terrace which may be the old entrance to Vergemount house as seen on Duncan's map of 1821. The first resident named in the directory of 1857 is J Macdonnell Royse who was employed at Dublin castle. No house numbers appear until 1865 at which time there were two houses listed with residents: 1. John Teeling and 2. H K White. It was not until 1868 that the next house, no. 3 is listed with George P M'Grath, wine merchant, in residence but with the original two houses vacant. In the following year no. 4 is listed and described as vacant. No new houses are listed for the next five years during which a number of the existing houses remained vacant. In 1875, however, 6 houses are listed with five occupied. Then in 1876 a house that would remain aloof from the numbering system was added. However, it would appear that there was a house on this spot in 1837 as is clearly shown in the first Ordnance Survey map of 1837 (*National Archives*: OS/105E 261.1). When it appears initially in the directories in 1876 it is without a name but later in 1881 it would acquire the name Lever house. It was first occupied by Robert J Mitchell, AM; he was an inspector of registration at the General Registration Office, Rutland square. In 1887 he was awarded with a D Litt from the Queen's University of Ireland and remained at Lever house until 1897. After he left the house name changed to Frankfort and the longest occupant of this house subsequently was J C Loughridge (1909-63). The old name still survives in the name of a cottage built at the end of its garden, Lever cottage.

As regards the six numbered houses in Vergemount hall like Vergemount, already discussed, some of the houses saw a remarkable number of changes in residents with only a very occasional occupant staying for any substantial length of time. House no. 1 had more than 11 different occupants during the 100 years 1865 to 1965 and was listed as vacant on 5 different occasions. The longest-stay resident was George Walmsley (1919-37); from 1930 to 1936 he was assistant traffic manager, Great Southern Railways. House no. 2 had a more stable record with only 7 different residents during the 100 years and being listed as vacant on

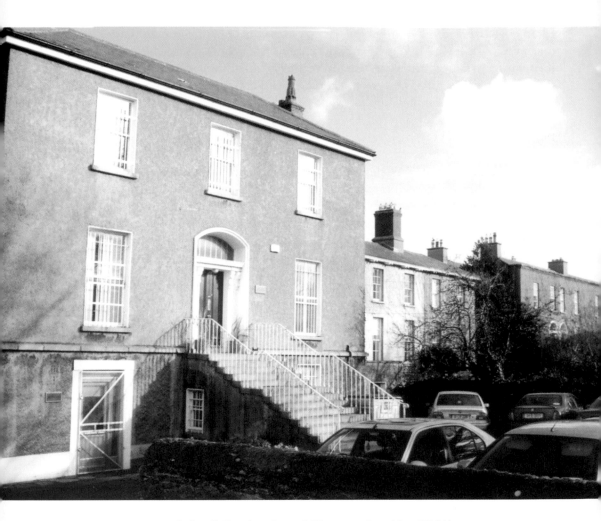

Vergemount hall, off Clonskeagh road (*Photographer: Matt Walsh*)

3 occasions. It was particularly helped in this regard by the long occupancy of Godfrey S Dowd (1905-c.1958) and Julia Dowd remaining there until c1963. The same situation applied to no. 3 where Miss Dora Galwey lived from 1918 to c.1958 followed by Theodia L Galwey who remained on until c. 1963. Miss Galwey owned a secretarial training business with an address first at 104 Grafton street and from 1933 at 33 Dawson street. From 1868 to 1917 house no. 4 had 10 different residents most of whom only stayed between 2 and 4 years and it was vacant on 6 different occasions for a total of 14 years. However, from 1917 Mrs Helen C Pollok lived there until 1928 and after her Miss Pollok or Pollock until

the mid-1960s and possibly beyond. In 1908 a Miss Curran took up residence in house no. 5. Up till the late 1950s, with the exception of 1916/17, there is an entry for a Miss Curran in the directories. Assuming that it is the same person, or a sibling, that would mean that like a number of the Vergemount hall houses the house had acquired a long-stay resident in the 20th century. The final house, no. 6, however, was slightly different; one of the early residents remained living in it for an extended period. First Mrs Alley, in 1888, and then Joseph Uppington Alley in 1889 are listed; the latter continued to live there until 1950. Thereafter, throughout the 1950s, the house is said to have been vacant and there is no entry for it in the directories of the early 1960s. Although it can only be speculation, it seems that the houses in Vergemount hall (apart from Lever, later Frankfort house) were rented in their early years of existence and given the number of occasions on which they are reported as being vacant, it may be assumed that it was not always easy to get tenants and when they were got, to get ones who would remain over a substantial period.

ST JAMES'S TERRACE

The next development of houses to be commenced after Vergemount hall was St James's terrace. The houses on this terrace are the first to be met on Clonskeagh road, on the right hand side coming from the city. They are now numbered 2 to 24 Clonskeagh road, all even numbers and twelve in total. However, the numbers that will be used here are those of the terrace itself i.e. 1 to 12. The first entry for St James's terrace is in 1862; numbers 1 to 8 are listed that year but only two are occupied. Occupancy improved and by 1865 all 8 had tenants. By 1869 four more houses – numbers 9 to 12 – had been built and in that year all four were vacant, perhaps not yet ready for people to move in; two years later, however, they were occupied. It is noticeable that the rateable valuation given to these four new houses was higher than that struck for the earlier eight. Nine years later however (in 1878), it would be reduced for almost all the houses in the terrace. In 1895 it would be further reduced when all but number 12 would have the same rate, £51, assigned to them; two years later number 4 would be reduced to £48. Apart from that, other houses had on occasion theirs adjusted perhaps as a result of their own initiative or that of the owner. Unlike the other new houses in the area, so far investigated, we do know, in this case, who the owner was. This was due to the legal case brought against the Conjoint Boards of Pembroke and Rathmines Urban Council in the first years of the twentieth century concerning its plans to erect an Isolation hospital in the grounds of Vergemount house which was beside St James's terrace. From this we know that the owner of all twelve houses, at this time, was Mrs Boswell. Furthermore, when we observe the early occupancy of the terrace we note that the original occupant of the first house built was James Boswell; he lived at no. 1 from 1862 to 1863. From this it is reasonable to assume that he was the developer and that for at least the next forty years he and his successor/s, represented in 1902 by Mrs Boswell, were the owners of all twelve houses. It has not been discovered how long the Boswells remained landlords of these houses and when, if ever, the houses were sold into private ownership.

An examination of the pattern of occupancy during their early years shows that most houses, with a few noticeable exceptions, were let for relatively short periods and that the number of residents per house from the 1860s to 1974 ranged from 5 to 15. During the same period the number of years that houses stood vacant ranged from 2 to 7. House no. 4 had the best record of occupancy mainly because it had three long-stay residents; Rev Hope M Waddell, Presbyterian minister (1866-95) and, after a year when it was vacant, Spotswood R Bowles, solicitor – office, 2 Westmoreland street, later 18, then 24 and finally 32 Nassau street (1897-1934) – before James B Ganly, auctioneer and salesman, 18/20 Usher's quay took up residence in 1935 and remained until c. 1963. His city address is the same as that of Ganly & Sons, livestock salesmen, auctioneers, woolbrokers, land and stock brokers; they had other offices near the cattle market at 58/59 Prussia street and cattle lairs at 63-65 Prussia street.

After these three occupants Declan D Costello came to reside there c. 1964/5 and was still in residence at the end of our period of examination in 1974. Son of the former Taoiseach, John A Costello, he was elected to the 14th Dail in the Dublin North West constituency for Fine Gael in 1951 and was subsequently elected on 5 more occasions, the last time to the 20th Dail in 1973. During the 1960s he was instrumental in having his party adopt a new political orientation encapsulated in the document *Towards a Just Society*. In 1973, with his party back in government, he was appointed Attorney General and remained in that position until 1977 when he left politics to become a judge of the High Court. He was appointed President of the High Court in 1994 and retired in 1997.

Other long-stay occupants of St James's terrace were: house no. 1 – Mrs Wade (1893-1913) and Richard Wm Nicholls, city address at 35 Poolbeg street (1916-39); no. 2 – A Chisolm Cameron, solicitor, city address at 6 Dawson street (1901-21) followed by Mrs A Chisholm Cameron, (1922-54); no. 3 – H M Wright, BA, & University Club – office, 31 Dame street (1902-42); no. 5 – Herbert Pelham Mayne, AB (Dub. Univ), barrister (1928-54); no. 6 – Newenham Manly (1933-63); no. 7 – Patrick Dunne or Dunn, merchant (1918-c.58) then Cecil Dunn (c.1960-63) and Miss Eileen Dunn (c.1965); no. 8 – the Gordon family (1916-39), mainly Frank V Gordon, solicitor and 5 Clare street, Dublin (1916-38) and Mrs Gordon (1939); no. 9 – the Walker family (1871-95) including James AM, Robert King AB

BE, Thomas Elliott and Mrs Walker at different times and J E Fottrell (1896-1920); no. 10 – Michael Seymour Dudley Westropp (1909-54) followed by Mrs Westropp, (1955-56); no. 11 – The Misses Bewick (1913-39) and the Kelly family (1940 –c.63) including Ambrose Aliaga Kelly (1872-1953), honorary secretary of the Stephen's Green Club (1904-10) and sometime consul for the king of Spain[3] – resident (1940-53), Mrs Kelly (1954-c.58) and Isabel Aliaga-Kelly (c.1960-c.63); no. 12 – the Reeves family (1898-1913) including Mrs Reeves and Jonathan Reeves . This last house had the most occupants during the period and the shortest long-stay resident. In fact, for a period of time (1953-55) it was used as a Boys' Preparatory School and called Brook House under the supervision of W P M Ross, MA MC. It also, like house no. 9, was divided into flats in the late 1950s.

LEVER COTTAGE

Immediately after the last house in St James's terrace there is an entrance road to Vergemount hall. On the other side of that entrance Lever cottage is located. As noted earlier, it got its name from Lever house, later called Frankfort house, which is a detached house in Vergemount hall. It is not known when it was built but the early entrance way to Vergemount house seems, according to Duncan's map of 1821, to be located here and it would have had a gate lodge. In the first Ordnance Survey map of 1837 (*National Archives*: OS/105E 261.1) there is a building at the same spot but no name given. In the map drawn by the Ordnance Survey for *Thom's Directory* of 1888 a gate lodge is indicated as being there but it is not clear enough to determine which side of the entrance it is on. The first reference to it in the directories is for the year 1903. From that year until 1909 it was occupied by Moran and Sons, chimney cleaners and 5 Johnston's court, off Grafton street. It was reported as being vacant from then until it was occupied by J Bedie (1911-18) with a rateable valuation of £10. Thereafter it was occupied by P J Dockery (1922-25), Patrick Killeen (1926-31), Cornelius O'Gorman (1932-39), Patrick Deegan (1940-49) and M Whelan (1950-58). It was omitted from the directories thereafter although it still remains in situ, perhaps because of its low valuation. It is listed in 1974 but no name of an occupant is given.

CLONSKEAGH TERRACE

As we have seen, the first listing for St James's terrace was 1862. Two years later Clonskeagh terrace appears for the first time in the directories. This terrace is now incorporated into Clonskeagh road and the six houses are numbered 55 to

---

3   Smith & Share, *Whigs on the Green: the Stephen's Green Club 1840-1990*, 168.

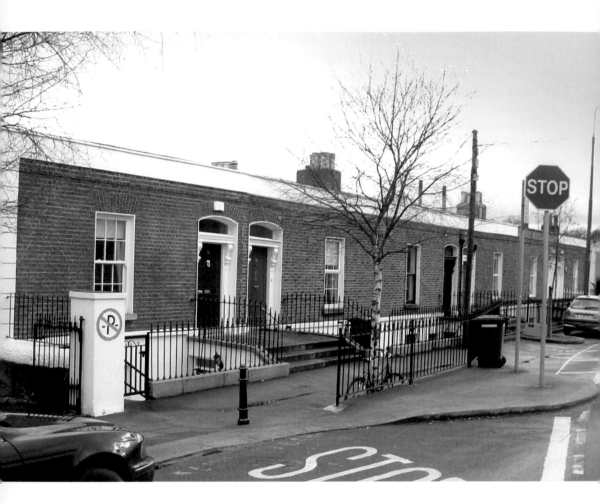

Clonskeagh terrace: first listed in the directories in 1864

65 (odd numbers only); numbers 1 to 6, as originally assigned to the houses, will be used in this discussion. The terrace is located between Ashton's licensed premises and the offices previously used by Smurfits. In its first listing in 1864 all houses are reported but only houses numbered 2 and 6 had occupants; all were occupied, however, by the following year. That does not mean that occupancy quickly stabilized; on the contrary, apart from house no. 4, there continued to be many short-stay residents for a number of years and they were often vacant. House no. 1 did not get a long-stay resident until 1885 when Mrs Thomas Kenny came and remained until 1911; she was succeeded by Thomas Kenny, presumably her son, who stayed until 1937. House no. 2 never had a very long occupancy

until 1926 when B A Treacy moved in and remained until 1951 and was followed by John J McEvoy who was still there in 1974. The person who stayed longest at no. 3 was Mrs Hayes (1910-36); at no. 4 – Michael O'Neill, carpenter (1903-c. 58) followed by Thomas O'Neill (c. 1960-c. 1965); at no. 5 – George Moorhead (1874-1921) followed by Miss Moorhead (1922-34); George Moorhead was a commission agent and had an office at one time at 9 Frederick street, south; at no. 6 – Joseph M Phelan (1918-51); this house was let in flats for a period in the late 1950s.

CONNAUGHT PLACE

The next development of houses to take place was considerably later than the burst of activity that took place between mid-1850s and the early 1860s which produced Vergemount hall, St James's terrace and Clonskeagh terrace. It was almost 40 years before this development – Connaugh place – emerged to be listed in the directories for the first time in 1902. We have noted when discussing the previous three developments that there appeared to be some difficulty in renting the houses for any sustained period of time. That may have been a factor in the length of time that elapsed before another scheme of houses was built. The houses in this scheme are red-bricked and are the first to be met on the left hand side of Clonskeagh road coming from the city; they are now numbered 1 to 13 Clonskeagh road, all odd numbers and seven houses in total. The numbers that are used in this discussion are those of Connaught place itself, i.e. 1 to 7. All houses are listed for the first time in 1902 but only number 1 is occupied. The name of the first resident was Richard James Hartland Mahon, JP, surveyor, GPO, late major East Surrey Regiment. In the following year two more houses had residents – nos. 2 & 3. The next year saw no. 4 occupied while in 1905 no. 3 had become vacant again and no. 7 had yet to find a resident as it still had the following year. It finally got its first occupant in 1908, Miss Murray.

This development does not appear to have been a great success. The first house got its only long-stay resident in the Carnegie family (1914 to c. 1969) including James E E, J Hesketh and later Mrs Gladys Carnegie. House no. 2 saw T C Tobias, barrister-at-law, live there from 1919 until 1937 and was let in flats in the 1950s. J Leslie Harris, solicitor and notary public with office at 6 Lr Abbey street lived at no. 3 from 1919 until 1953 after which it too was let in flats. This was to be the fate of no. 4, already in flats in 1943. Prior to that the longest time spent in the house by anyone was Mrs Annie Jeffers from 1919 to 1933. The next house, no. 5, did a little better; Miss Annie Moore (occasionally Mrs Moore) lived there from 1928 to 1951 before it too was let in flats. However, it did house from 1911 to 1917 the famous Celtic scholar, R A Stewart Macalister, whom we will discuss in Chapter 18. From 1905 until 1920 house no. 6 was occupied by the Griffin family including Robert William AM LL D, John Percy G, Rev A S Garney AB, TCD and H Grattan Griffin. In 1939 Dublin Corporation turned it into a Nurses' Home and it was later Clonskeagh Fever Hospital Nurses' Home. This also happened in 1939 to no. 7. Prior to that, its longest stay occupant was John Muldoon KC who lived there from 1920 until 1938.

BYRNE'S COTTAGES

First listed in 1911, with an entry which records 14 houses, valuation from £3 to £5-10s, on the Clonskeagh road it is not clear if they had just been built or that the directory was now including houses with low valuations for the first time. The exact location of these houses has not been satisfactorily discovered. They disappear from the directories at the end of the 1950s just as Henshaw's cottages do. It is possible that they were on the left hand side of the road, coming from the city, just before the bridge. There were houses located in that spot according to the first Ordnance Survey map of 1837 (*National Archives*: OS/105E 261.1) and these may be the same or successors to these houses. In any case, the shops (nos. 105 to 113) and filling station (no. 115), which now occupy this space just before the bridge, first appeared in the directories in the early 1960s just after Byrne's cottages were de-listed.

CLONSKEAGH VILLAS

These are the 16 houses which are now numbered 73 to 103 Clonskeagh road and located between what used to be Smurfit's office and the groups of shops just mentioned. They first appear in the directories in 1916 and two years later their rateable valuation is given as 'each £7'. These are the last of the houses which were built in the earlier stages of development of the area.

MODERN SUBURBANISATION BEGINS

The first signs of what may be called phase two of the growth of the suburb can be detected in 1927 on what was then called Roebuck road but would later (from 1954) be called Clonskeagh road. After many years with the same entries that year saw new ones; others would follow in subsequent years. Observing the entries in the directories from year to year, a picture is built up of the early developments, the dates of which are accurate enough for our purposes here. One complication attending this process is the tendency some people had to change house names at different periods. Attempts have been made to track these down, in most cases with a considerable degree of confidence in the result.

The first of these new suburban houses were built close to Roebuck house. By 1927 three such houses had been built and occupied. They were: St Teresa's (this changed to Bexley in 1938 and was retained until approximately 1963 when the new occupant, Michael Ua hUiginn, changed it to 'Cruachan'), Luvaun (there are some variations in the spelling of this name) and Roebuck villa, the latter somewhat in off the road. They were then occupied by E J Mullins, Alfred Roberts, builder and W J Webb respectively. In the following year new entries are found: The Arbour, St Helen's, Tambou, Ounavarra (its name was changed to 'Sancta Maria' in 1955; it is now called 'Hollybrook), Envaugh/Invaugh; their occupants at that time were John G Dowling, Bernard Hoey, Patrick Logan, David Patterson and Alfred E Watson respectively. All of these houses are located between Roebuck house and what is now the entrance to Nutgrove park. Building continued in the same general area as it is noticed that in the following year, 1929, that the newest houses listed are immediately on the other side of the same entrance. They are: Roebuck (this name was changed to 'Pro Tempo' in 1934, a name that was retained until 1949; after that the new occupant, Brendan A Woods, changed it to 'Glenbeigh'), The Anchorage and Coolgraney; the occupants in 1929 were Walter J Brown, James F Cherry and Stephen S Kelly.

Soon thereafter, the focus for building shifted down the road towards Clonskeagh bridge and with it the style of house also. In 1931 Woodbourne, built beside the entrance to the long-existing St Bridget's, is listed with the then occupant, Gerald R Irvine. In the following year we encounter other houses close to it although one of them is in the older style and closer to the earlier houses – Beauvais, then the home of Michael Hayden. The others include Somerton, a detached house with a dentist by the name of Herbert J F Green in residence. As well as that two nearby semi-detached houses are listed. In both cases, however, only the name of one half of the building is given along with its owner; St Budeaux (William Partridge) and Lonsdale (Ralph V N Sadleir). It may be assumed that the other half of each of them was by that stage built but as yet occupied. Two years later, that was rectified when we find Inverkeithing (now called 'Muff') with Donald Roy in residence and Montrose (now called 'Heskin') then occupied by H Margey. Also listed in that year are Kilmagar and Annanaar with the names F Lee and James J Comerford, CE assigned to them; Cahircon and Beechview and their residents, E G Roche-Kelly and C Kennedy. Finally the last of the semi-detached houses The Graan and Mayfield with J A McIntyre and M V Buckley are also to be found in the 1934 directory.

By 1934 that particular part of what is now called Clonskeagh road was essentially completed. There would be some later additions e.g. in 1944 'Brookville' (beside Coolgraney) was added and perhaps reflecting the increase in local population a shop, bearing the name 'Cash Stores', was opened around 1939 by Mrs A Sinnott. In 1948 the house 'Redroof' was first listed but this appears to have been the gate lodge to Roebuck house so it can not be considered part of the new development that was taking place.

WYNNSWARD PARK, PREVIOUSLY WYNNSTAY PARK

The year 1934, therefore, saw the virtual completion of what might be called the first phase of suburban development on the Clonskeagh road; the building of what was to be called Richview villas would come later. All of this is what would in modern times be called 'ribbon development'. However, as this first phase was coming to an end a new trend was commencing; this entailed the building of a number of houses on a plot of land secured for the purpose. This was, apparently, hived off from Wynnstay and was initially called Wynnstay park, but changed to Wynnsward park in 1943. The house, Wynnstay, was now listed at this address and remained there until 1954 when it reverted to being listed under Clonskeagh road. It may be a coincidence but the hiving-off took place just as Wynnstay changed from being the long-time (1884-1933) property of the Forster family; in 1934 John O'Hagan Ward took possession of it. Shortly thereafter the reduction in land associated with Wynnstay would be reflected in a lowering of the rateable valuation of the property from £67-10s to £64.

That it was a plot of land prepared for development may be seen by the listing in the 1935 directory: 1.vacant; 2. J A Doyle; 3. & 4. vacant. This does not make it clear whether numbers 1, 3 & 4 represent houses already built and awaiting an occupier or whether they represent plots assigned for houses. However, the fact that number 2 was occupied would suggest that number 1, being attached to it, was already built. In the following year the listing, which includes the rateable valuation of the houses, is: 1.Dr J Doherty (£31); 2. J A Doyle (£28-10s); 3. Wm F Rafter (£28-10s); 4. vacant (£28-10s).

By 1937, no. 4 was occupied by H G Sunderland. The number of houses remained the same, with relatively few changes in occupiers, until the name change occurred around the year 1943. Whether that had anything to do with it or not is unclear but in the following year two new houses are listed as follows: 5. J O'Neill; E B Gordon, En-Dahwin. Further expansion was to follow in 1948 when the following were added to the listing: El Verano: 1. J MacCartney Robbins; 2. R D Bourke; 3. Mrs A Hosford; 4. Col T L Ovens and in 1950 with: D E Smyllie; Arnold P Hadcroft, Olgadene.

A few more houses were added and by 1953 the numbering system was extended to include all fourteen of them, although in retaining the numbers of the houses called El Verano, it was somewhat confusing. By the mid 1960s another house had been added and it would appear that some more were built later on.

VERGEMOUNT PARK

During this period of expansion of Wynnsward park many other developments were being initiated in the general area. New houses were being built along Bird avenue (see below) but a new development, somewhat like that of Wynnsward-park, was commencing at the other side of the Clonskeagh bridge at Vergemount. In 1937 the directory includes Vergemount park for the first time with the following entry: 2. W Codd; 4-16. sites; 18. Vere Heuston. Quite clearly this was a planned development with plots already set out and numbered. At this stage only two houses were occupied but others were likely to be at different stages of erection; perhaps nearing completion as may be inferred from the following year's entry. This goes as follows (with rateable valuations already assigned to some): 1-3. Building site; 2. W Codd (£19-10s); 4. John Orr (£19-10s); 5. Alfred E Holmes; 6. Fred Matthews; 7. Mrs G Lane; 8. Wm J Dowdall; 9. J G Cornish; 10. Richard C Sainsbury, BL; 11. W J Flook; 12. vacant; 13. Cecil O'Shaughnessy (£19-10s); 14-16. Building; 15. Cecil F Sullivan (£20-10s); 17. Alexander St Clair Powderley (£23-10s); 18. Vere Heuston (£23-10s).

Thus, by 1938, 14 of the potential 18 houses were built, 13 occupied, 2 in the process of being built and 2 still building sites. The process of development seemed to slow down at this point since by the following year only one house was added to those already built, number 14, while numbers 1 and 3 remained building sites. By 1940 there were houses, both occupied, on these sites leaving number 16 as the only house still in the process of being built. The whole scheme was complete by 1941 when the following entry is found: 1. Ronald H Brown, BA, LLB, solr. (£23); 2. W Codd (£19-10s); 3. E V Irvine (£22-10s); 4. John Orr (£19-10s); 5. Norman Dymock (£21); 6. Fred Matthews (£22-10s); 7. Mrs G Lane (£19-10s); 8. Wm J Dowdall (£22-10s); 9. J G Cornish (£21); 10. Richard C Sainsbury, BL (£21); 11. W J Flook (£21); 12. E Munnings (£21); 13. Cecil O'Shaughnessy (£19-10s); 14. G S Mathers (£21); 15. Cecil F Sullivan (£20-10s); 16. R H Rooney (£21); 17. Alexander St Clair Powderley (£23-10s); 18. Vere Heuston (£23-10s).

NEW DEVELOPMENTS

In the same year that Vergemount park was completed evidence emerges that on the other side of Clonskeagh bridge work had commenced on two major developments with plots laid out and some houses already built; these two were

Whitebeam-road and Whitebeam-avenue. Both of these schemes were being built on lands that are likely to have belonged to the owner of Clonskeagh castle; its entrance was from Clonskeagh road (then called Roebuck road) and a later development, Whitethorn road, would be built along what appears to have been the driveway to the castle. Not very many years before these new houses were being built, Clonskeagh castle had been sold in 1932 to a new owner, Henry M Whitton, BL having been for more than a century in the possession of the Thompson family. Whether this had any influence on the fact that the lands were now being used for housing is not clear.

WHITEBEAM ROAD

Although Whitebeam avenue was being developed at the same time, for convenience we will first trace the evolution of Whitebeam road from its initial appearance in the directories in 1941; its listing for that year was: 1. S McGloughlin; 3. G Wynne; 5, 7, vacant; 9. P J Daly; 11, 13, vacant; 15. J S East; 17. A J O'Reilly; 19, 21, 23, 25 vacant; 2. P Murphy; 4. S O'Flinn; 6, 8, 10, 12, vacant; 14. Mrs F L Webb; 16, 18, 20, 22, 24, 26 vacant; 28. T O'Keeffe; 30, 32, 34 vacant; 36. K L Somers; 40, 42, 44, 46 vacant.

As will be seen in the later development of the road only part of what would eventually be built had at this stage been completed, assuming that all those described as 'vacant' were in fact houses and not either plots or houses in the process of being built. Of the 13 houses with odd numbers (1 to 25) only 5 were occupied that year and of the 23 houses with even numbers (2 to 46) the same applied. However the following year saw a major upsurge in occupancy; of the 13 with odd numbers 10 had residents as had 17 of those with even numbers. Occupancy of the houses with odd numbers increased by only one in the following year leaving nos. 11 and 13 still vacant while all those with even numbers were occupied apart from nos. 44 and 46 which were apparently still being built. These were still being described as 'building' in 1944 by which time there was full occupancy of all the houses so far built. Both of these were located on the other side of a pathway that leads down to the bank of the Dodder; whether this played any significant role in the choice of where phase one would end has not been discovered.

By 1945 what might be described as the second phase had begun with houses bearing an odd number extended to 37 and those with an even number to 56. A number of these are already occupied as were by now nos. 44 and 46, the last two of the first phase to gain residents. Of the new phase all those with odd numbers were occupied except no. 33 while all those with even numbers, apart from no. 48, were described as vacant. In 1946 it is recorded that all, except no.

56, had got people living in them. This was quite an achievement when one remembers that during this time the second world-war was raging and in Ireland an emergency had been declared. Number 56 was still vacant in 1947 but the house attached to it, no. 58 is now added to the list together with the name of the person living there. There is also an intimation that activity was taking place on the other side of the road as house number 49 is mentioned as is the name of its occupant; there is no reference, however, to any houses between it and no. 37. That would be remedied in 1948 when a number of new houses are included in the list. These were mainly on that side since by then the numbers had reached 53 with all occupied except no 43. On the even numbered side nos. 60 and 62 are added and they together with no. 58 all have residents named.

Building in this road would appear to have stalled at this point as construction approached the front of Clonskeagh castle; there were no additions until, in 1954, the following was added at the end of the list: San Antonio – Blewitt, E; Woodkeys – Davitt, T; Clonskeagh castle – vacant. To these was appended in 1955 Westgarth (colonel A Lancaster) and an occupant for Clonskeagh castle, Dr M McMahon. The year 1957 saw the final phase of building the road underway. The new entries for that year are as follows: 64-70. vacant; 72. G Webb; 74. G R Thompson; 78. W Bates. That year also saw Dr Karl Mullen take up residence in San Antonio in place of E Blewitt. Numbers 64 and 68 were still vacant the following year while no. 76 was listed with G R Thompson in residence. Houses that hitherto had house-names only had numbers assigned to them by 1960 i.e. Woodkeys was now no. 86; Westgarth no. 88. San Antonio no. 90. Clonskeagh castle had as yet no number assigned. Also no. 68 had a resident in that year but no. 64. had no entry beside it. The road was almost complete; there would subsequently be a few additions and some adjustment of the numbering system at the Clonskeagh castle end but nothing of great significance.

WHITEBEAM AVENUE

Although it has been decided to deal with Whitebeam avenue and Whitebeam road separately, building of both of them proceeded alongside one another. In fact, a particular feature of the manner in which some houses were built in the general area would suggest that it is artificial to separate them. This feature occurs where one road or avenue intersects another. At such points semi-detached houses are oriented in such a manner that one half is in one road and the other in the intersecting road/avenue with a numbering system that confirms it. As well as that both Whitebeam avenue and Whitebeam road make their first appearance in the directories in the same year, 1941. The entry for Whitebeam avenue for that year is as follows: 1. vacant; 3. T P Curtin; 5. Mrs M Lytton; 7, 9, 2, vacant; 4. W Erskine; 6. D S McDonald. That is, 8 houses, 4 occupied. There are no reports of any new houses in the following year but the occupancy rate of those already built had risen somewhat; of the eight houses, 6 now had residents. The rateable valuation of those occupied was also given in that year; four had a similar rating of £21-6s while nos. 1 and 2 were rated at £22-8s and £22-10s respectively. It is worth remarking that both of these latter two were part of semidetached houses the other halves being in Whitebeam road (nos. 23 and 25 respectively).

In 1943, however, a substantial number of new houses are recorded. While those with odd numbers remained at no. 9, those with even numbers increased very considerably. Where they had halted at no. 6 for the previous two years they now jumped to no. 34. and, what is more, a great proportion of them had found residents. There were now 22 houses in all and 16 of them had become homes; nos. 7, 9, 16, 22, 26 and 30 were still vacant. Work next seemed to concentrate on the other side of the road since, in the following year (1944) the numbers on that side extended from no. 9 where it had remained for some time to 33 while on the side with even numbers only two new houses are recorded (nos. 36 and 38). The avenue was substantially completed with only one house remaining vacant – no. 15.

WHITETHORN ROAD

The first entry in the directories for Whitethorn road is 1948 when a number of houses were already built and occupied. The entry for that year is as follows: 1. Mallagh, J S; 3. Strachan, Jas. J; 5. Trenwith, T F; 7. Thompson, Ernest; 9. Ledbetter, George; 11. vacant; 13. vacant; 15. McGovern, H J; 17. Cathcart, F M; 19-23. vacant; 2. Thornton, A J; 4. Stuart, George G; 6. Ewen, D C; 8. Cooke, William; 10. Spray, C; 12. Aston, Gordon; 14. Conbeady, A; 16. East, H; 18-24. vacant.

From this it will be noted that, unlike Whitebeam road, the numbering system (and the progress of the building programme) does not start from the Clonskeagh road but from the other end. The reason for this is that building began at the point where Whitebeam road had reached at that time. In fact, no. 53 on that road is one half of a semidetached house whose other half is no. 1 Whitethorn road. Building, therefore, began at that end and proceeded back towards the Clonskeagh road (then called Roebuck road). In doing so, it appears to have followed what had been until then the driveway to Clonskeagh castle. This seems to be fairly clear if one compares the 1837 (and later) Ordnance Survey map of the area with modern maps; both show a curving road approaching the castle. What is more the start of that driveway had what

D'Alton, writing in 1838, described as 'a cumbrous castellated entrance'[4] and this was located on the Clonskeagh road exactly opposite the entrance to Richview. This latter entrance exists to this day – the name on the entrance gate is now 'Richview lodge' – and immediately across the road from it one finds the end of Whitethorn road.

Of special interest is the name chosen for this road. It seems most likely that this was chosen because of its being located in Clonskeagh. As discussed earlier the final element in that name -'skeagh' – is the angilcized version of the Gaelic word '*sgeach*' or '*sceach*' which means 'thorn-bush', 'hawthorn' or 'whitethorn' although in the case of the latter the suffix '*geal*' (meaning 'bright' or 'white') is sometimes attached, presumably to ensure that the whitethorn is distinguished from other thorn-bushes. This suffix is indeed added in the case of the official Irish version of the name of the road; this can be seen on the road nameplate where it is found to be '*Bóthar na Sgeachngeal*'.

The first entry in the directories, in 1948, shows that building was then taking place on both side of the road at a similar rate; twelve houses with seven occupied on the left hand side as one proceeds towards Clonskeagh road and twelve on the right with eight occupied. By the following year building had proceeded rapidly with eight new houses on the left hand side reported; houses were now completed as far as no. 39 but five of these (nos. 31 to 39) remained vacant. On the right hand side even more houses had been completed; fifteen new houses are listed up as far as no 54 but seven of these (nos. 28, 34, 42 and 48 to 54) had yet to find residents. However, all houses that had been reported as being vacant in the first entry in 1948 had been occupied by the following year. Only one new house is reported in 1950; this was number 41. Perhaps building had stalled until vacant houses had been sold. If that is the case, then all but two (nos. 37 and 54) had been disposed of in that year and they were occupied by the following year when building remained stalled. That would soon change, however, as is apparent from the listing in 1952. In that year we are told that all houses on the left hand side were completed as far as no. 59; that meant nine new houses on that side although six of them had as yet no residents (nos. 45, 47, 51, 53, 55, 59). Four new houses, built on the right hand side brought it as far as Clonskeagh road and all were occupied. It took two further years to complete the occupation of these houses; nos. 51, 53, 55 & 59 by 1953, the other two by the following year. At a later date there would be a new house built after no. 57 which would take the number 59 and in the process changing the number of the last house on the left to no. 61.

---

4   D'Alton, *History of the county of Dublin*, 808.

RICHVIEW VILLAS

A feature of building design in all the above three roads in this area which has already been noted (i.e. a semidetached with one half in one road and the other in the road that intersects it) can be seen to continue at the end of Whitethorn road. The final house on either side is semidetached with one half on that road and the other facing on to Clonskeagh road. There they form part of a new development of housing which would become known as Richview villas. However, when the first of these houses appear in the directories there is a duplication of names and numbering. In the 1952 directory the two houses which are attached to the last houses on Whitethorn road are listed as follows: 2. Richview villas –Chapman, Dr T; 3. Richview villas – Byrne, Miss M. However, immediately after that there is a new listing under the heading of Beechview-villas with one entry only. It is: 8. Chapman, Dr Terence. It would appear that this is the same house as recorded immediately before it as 2. Richview villas although subsequent entries cast a doubt on that. It is not clear who was deciding on the name but there was obviously some confusion over what the new name should be. A separate heading of Beechview-villas continued to appear until 1956 but never had more than one entry under it – the original one first found in the 1952 directory. It was most likely due to inertia on the part of the compiler of the directory that it continued for so long. Nevertheless, it confirms the view that no. 8 was not part of the development which saw the others built. Observation on the ground would confirm this as the orientation of this house is different from the rest having its gable rather than its front facing the road. The numbering scheme began to become a little clearer in 1953 when there are two separate entries for Richview villas; one as part of Clonskeagh road as follows: 8. Richview villas –Chapman, Dr T (£43); 3. Richview villas – Byrne, Miss M (£28). The other was a separate listing for Richview villas which was as follows: 1. Sloman, Dr A E (£34); 2. Fox, Chas C (£28). Here it will be noted that the number of Dr Chapman's house is now given as no. 8, the number it held under the heading of Beechview villas. However, number 2 which was the other half of the last house on Whitethorn road is now occupied by a different person. By 1955 all eight houses in Richview are completed and occupied as follows (rateable valuation is included): 8. Chapman, Dr T; 7. Gill, R (£30); 6. Hassell, M K, RA; 5. White, S; 4. Hayes-McCoy, Dr G A (£30); 3. Byrne, Miss M (£28); 2. Fox, Chas C (£28); 1. Walsh, J J (£34). In later years another house would be built beside no. 8.

WYNNSWARD DRIVE

A number of years before Richview villas were built a new development was being set out and constructed further up the Clonskeagh road that was to have unforeseen use in the future. It would in time become the Clonskeagh entrance to the campus of University College Dublin thus proving to be of great importance to people of that area and, indeed, the hinterland of Clonskeagh. For very many years prior to that time there was only one road, if one may call it that, which led deep into what is now the campus, which at that time and for many years before consisted of large tracts of land attached to substantial mansions. That road is already visible on the Rocque map of the 1760s and even more clearly in the first Ordnance Survey map of 1837. It allowed a certain degree of access from Clonskeagh, although to what extent that access was open to the public is not clear. Two particularly important mansions which were accessed along this road were Rosemount and Roebuck house/grove; these together with the families who occupied them were discussed in the last chapter. The road still exists but UCD have put a gate on the entrance to it, and access is strictly controlled. The contrast between that old road which has all but disappeared – at least, it can no longer be described as a road in the proper sense of the word – and the busy, heavily trafficked road that is Wynnsward drive is stark. In fact it is a particularly good example of the dramatic changes that have taken place in the general area in the twentieth century.

Wynnsward drive itself, however, did not appear on the scene until the growth in suburbanisation had become fairly well established in Clonskeagh. In fact it did not appear in the directories until around fifteen years after the other development beside Wynnstay –Wynnstay park (later Wynnsward park) – had first appeared in 1934. Its first listing – in 1949 – was as follows: 1. – 2. Hacienda: Stack, Rev W B; Johnson, B S; Wyatt, W A; Dutton, Lt Commander W L G; 3. Booth, B E; 4. Handcroft, A P. The manner in which the property, here numbered 1.-2. and entitled 'Hacienda', is presented in the listing with four differently named occupants suggests a different approach to that which had previously appeared in the sources. How precisely to interpret it is only slightly improved in the following year by the inclusion of individual rateable valuations; this suggested separate dwellings. As well as that, in that year an entirely new property is included. The listing for that year is: 1 – 2 Hacienda: Dudley, Anthony, solicitor (£20), Coughlan, J; Johnson, B S (£18); Wyatt, W A (£18); Dutton, Lt Commander W L G (£20); 3. Booth, B E (£25-8s); 4. Handcroft, A P (£25-9s); 5. O'Shea, Thomas, Wynnsward house (£26-10s). The individual approach to rateable valuation is dropped the following year (1951), however, when Hacienda, still retaining its unique house numbers 1. – 2. is now reported as having a composite valuation of £76, suggesting that perhaps the property is owned by one person while the individual units were built for renting. In the same year, three new houses are added to the listing: 5. Roy, Edgar (£27); 6. Lambert, Robert D (£27); 7. Ward, M (£26-10s). In subsequent years, the name

'Hacienda' would appear to be used specifically for unit no. 1 while all the other residents appeared, without any specific distinction, as being occupants of no. 2. The composite rateable valuation, however, was always inserted immediately after the name of the resident of no. 1. This situation remained until the early 1960s. Only in the mid-1960s did the situation clarify somewhat although the numbering system still seemed a little eccentric. The listing for 1965 is as follows: Hacienda: 1. Fretton, Clara B; 2. O'Dwyer, Edward.; 3. Sweeney, Patrick F; 4. Hayes, Thomas; / /3. Derrynane -O'Connor, Turlough; 4. O'Neill, A W; 5. Rostrevor – Roy, Edgar H; 6. Richmond – McAuley, Brian; 7. Wynnsward house – Kelly, Maurice. It was around this time that the new entrance to the UCD campus was made thus changing for ever this quiet cul-de-sac as well as allowing the development of a new road which would totally supersede that which had anciently existed perhaps only 50 metres on its southern side.

NUTGROVE PARK

Around the same time as building commenced in what would become known as Wynnsward drive another new development was commencing right across the road from it. Access to it was between two houses which were some of the earliest to be built in the area in the late 1920s. Given the title 'Nutgrove park' for no apparent reason other than the fact that many of the new developments in the general area made use of the name of trees (e.g. whitebeam, whitethorn, maple, laburnum; the latter it would eventually join) its first entry in the directories, for the year 1949 was as follows: 1. Dolan, M F; 3-11. vacant; 13. Lattimore, W; 2-14. vacant. If this may be interpreted as indicating that fourteen houses, seven on either side, had already been built in 1949 but only two occupied then no further building had been completed by the following year. However, occupancy was by then substantially improved since all the houses with odd numbers had by that time got residents but only two with even numbers (nos. 4 & 6) were similarly occupied. It would appear that the rate of building was not getting too far ahead of success in achieving sales. That interpretation would seem to be confirmed by the situation that pertained in the following year when, once again, no new houses were listed as completed. What is more, occupancy remained the same as it was in the previous year.

That soon changed, however, as is apparent from the entries for the following year – 1952. By that year occupancy had improved dramatically and, perhaps because of that, a number of new houses can be seen to have been built, the majority of which also had residents. Most of these were on the side where the houses had odd numbers – the side that had apparently sold best from the beginning of the project. Eight new houses were built there but a peculiarity in the way this happened is that four of them were constructed immediately alongside the existing houses (i.e. nos. 15 to 21 were built after no. 13) while the other four were located at some distance and bore the numbers 31 and 37 to 41. On the other side of the road four new houses were added immediately beside those already there (nos. 16 to 22). By that year only three of the twenty six houses were said to be vacant.

By the following year the gaps, which we have observed to have been left as new houses were built on the side where the houses bore odd numbers and extending beyond, no longer existed; six new houses were listed as having been constructed there (nos. 23 to 29 and 33 to 35). This meant that the development had turned at right angles and gone to the boundary of what would later become another road of houses, Leinster lawn. Development thereafter progressed towards Laburnum road, houses on which were, at that time, being constructed having started from the end where it intersected with Whitethorn road.

By 1953, therefore, Nutgrove park consisted of 33 houses numbered 1 to 41 and 2 to 22 almost all of which were occupied. The names of the residents and the rateable valuation of the houses that year were as follow: 1. Thompson, E (£26); 3. Barry, Edmund (£25); 5. Worthington, Michael (£25); 7. vacant (£25); 9. Mullan, William M (£25); 11. O'Reilly, Michael (£25); 13. Meldon, Anthony P P (£25); 15. J Durrant; 17. Carney, Dr M D (£25); 19. Sanahan, E (£25); 21. O'Sullivan, John Daly; 23. Boylan, P; 25. vacant; 27. Dunbar, A; 29. Smith, E; 31. McKillop, Miss M, MD (£25); 33. O'Halmhain, Padraig; 35. O'Malley, T; 37. Madigan, J (£25); 39. O'Moran, D, BL; 41. O'Connor, J D; 2. Savage, J W (£26); 4. Lenehan, N (£25); 6. McCourt, P (£25); 8. Bowan, Miss J R (£25); 10. Lumley, S M (£25); 12. Guidera, A P (£25); 14. Foran, T (£25); 16. Shorten, J F; 18. Keogh, V J; 20. O'Malley, T (£25); 22. Coakley, O (£25).

Four new houses were listed in 1954 i.e. nos. 40, 42, 43 and 44 and, with that, another feature of the road now became clearer. These new houses which were set at right angles to and opposite the earlier development of Nutgrove park were numbered consecutively starting at number 39 and rising ultimately to no. 48 at which point it met what would later on be the end of Laburnum road. Number 48, however, had not yet been reached in 1955 as only one new house is listed as having been built by that time – no. 28; it too was at right angles to the original part of the development and going in the direction of Laburnum road. By now, however, as we shall see houses on Laburnum road had reached, on one side, the boundary with Nutgrove park and in the following year houses on the two roads finally met and with it the virtual completion of Nutgrove park. In that year, houses were listed as far up as no. 48 on one side and on the other, nos. 24 and 26 (these two houses were built in the manner characteristic of the overall development, already mentioned; two houses attached to one another but facing

different roads) and nos. 30 -38 but still no entry for no. 36. It is possible that
one or two of these houses was not as yet fully completed; all were nevertheless
listed in the directory but some without anything other than the number itself.
That was remedied in 1957 when all 52 houses of the completed Nutgrove park
are listed together with the names of their occupants. A few years later, in the
early 1960s, a new house would be built beside no. 31 and allocated the number
31a.

The stages through which the houses were built are at the root of why the
numbering system ended up in a slightly odd manner – at least as far as no. 38
is concerned. It is, logically enough, located at the end of the houses which bear
even numbers only. However, in another stretch of the road there are houses
numbered initially with odd numbers only e.g. 31 & 33 and 35 & 37; then the
next houses have consecutive numbers e.g. 39 & 40 and so on but missing out
no. 38 in that location.

LABURNUM ROAD

Whitethorn road was effectively completed by the year 1952 when the first signs
of development of Laburnum road become apparent. That road could, of
course, be seen as almost a spur off Whitethorn road since, in a fashion typical
of the area, its first house is attached to a house on Whitethorn road (no. 1 is
attached to no. 52 Whitethorn road). The first entry for Laburnum road in the
directories occurs in 1952 as follows: 1. Barry, Kevin L; 2. Conneady, A J; 4 O
hUallachan, Sean; 6. Gunning, J L; 8. McPhillips, J C. Thus, apart from the
'attached' house, no. 1, development started on the left hand side as one proceeds
away from Whitethorn road; initially it only went as far as no. 8 however.
Progress seems to have halted for a time – there were no new houses listed on
the road in 1953; perhaps the developers were waiting for some houses recently
built on Whitethorn road to be occupied.

By 1954 construction on the right hand side of Laburnum road was well
under way as the evidence for that year indicates that nos. 1 to 23 were already
built with only four remaining vacant (nos. 11, 19, 21 & 23). The road had now
reached the intersection with Maple road; indeed, no. 23 was attached to what
was then no. 8 Maple road. On the other side of that intersection building
continued such that by the following year all of the right hand side of Laburnum
road, as far as the boundary with Nutgrove park, was completed (i.e. up to no.
29). As well as that all the houses, with the exception of no. 19 were occupied;
there was no information given as to the residence status of no. 25. Progress then
halted for a time and when it did resume attention was turned once more to the
left hand side of the road when nos. 10 and 12 were completed by 1957. With

that the older part of Laburnum road was completed. The house numbers and occupants for that year are as follows: 2. Conneady, A J; 4 O hUallachan, Sean; 6. Gunning, J L; 8. McPhillips, J C; 10. Whitton, H M; 12. Leen, K; 1. McDonagh, B; 3. Riordan, H; 5. Gorman, J; 7. Brown, Rev N D; 9. Carroll, J; 11. Halpin, J; 13. Johnston, J; 15. Bell, J E; 17. Trevor, A H; 19. Moore, H; 21. McClay, M; 23. Tomkin, -; 25. Gray, T; 27. Ryan, T; 29. Graham, J W. All had rateable valuation of £25 except no. 1 which was rated at £28.

Not many years later, the rest of the houses on the road would be built. By 1963 houses in a new style had been constructed starting with no. 16 and rising to no. 34 at the other side of the intersection with Embassy lawn, a new road of houses then just emerging. By 1965 no. 36 had been completed bringing Laburnum road to the boundary of Nutgrove park on that particular side of the road. The first occupants of these new houses were: 16. O'Connor, Thomas; 18.Atkinson, John C K; 20. O'Brien, Gerald; 22. Doyle, Patrick; 24. Noonan, John; 26. Kilroy, John; 28. Armstrong, John; 30. Heron, Matthew; 32. Sullivan, Capt John; 34.Culligan, Michael; 36. Bell, Robert. The remaining house, no. 14, would be built in later years.

MAPLE ROAD

Although building in Maple road began around the same time as it did in both Whitethorn road and Nutgrove park and considerably earlier than Laburnum road its progress was much slower than any of these other roads. Tracing the evolution of its progress is a little more difficult than that of other roads as its numbering system changed while the development was still in progress. When it first appears in the directories in 1949 there are only two houses listed, both at the Milltown Bridge road end and on the same side (nos. 1 & 3). By 1952 only one new house had been added (no. 7) but not immediately beside the first two although on the same side of the road. In fact, building would continue on that side, the right hand side as one walks towards Laburnum road, since by the following year another house (no. 5) had been built on the plot between the first two and the one built later. The houses, their residents and their rateable valuation for that year, 1953, are as follows: 1. Anthony, Mrs G V N (£52); 3. Stephens, Brandon, MB, BCh, surgeon (£43); 5. Young, Rev Gordon S, BA (£45); 7. Booth, Robert C (£102).

In the following year the first problem with numbering is encountered. In that year it is reported that no. 8 had been built and occupied. Having an even number coming after those with odd numbers posed a problem as to which house it refers to. Luckily it is also given a house name ('Paray') which is still extant, thus allowing its location to be identified. Furthermore, the progress of

Laburnum park having been traced, confirms that this house is attached to one on Laburnum park (no. 23) which we know had been built by 1954. It was thus the first house built on the left hand side of the road and would eventually be allocated a new number i.e. no. 24. After a brief stay, building resumed on the other side of the road with no. 9 being listed in 1956 and nos. 11 and 17 in 1957. The latter house was in fact attached to house numbered 25 in Laburnum road which we know was already built by the year 1955; it would later be get a different number, no. 19. This had occurred by 1960 since, by that year, three new houses had been built, still on the same side and beyond no. 11 i.e. nos. 13, 15 and 17 thus requiring the renumbering of the last house on that side.

With all the houses on the right hand side completed, building on the other side began – again starting at the Milltown Bridge end. By 1963 nos. 2, 4 and 14 were built and no. 8 had been renumbered no. 18. Within two years the remaining houses on that side had been completed (nos. 6, 8, 10, 12, 16, 18, 20 & 22); there is no information given on the status of the last house, no. 22. This burst of building activity once more caused a change in number of the house originally numbered 8, then 18; it was now, finally, given the number 24.

With the completion of all Maple road by 1965 the list of residents in that year together with the rateable valuations of some of the houses is given as follows: 1. Anthony, William (£52); 2. East, James (£48); 3. Stephens, Brandon, MB, BCh, surgeon (£43); 4. Houwald, Baron Gotz (£52-5s); 5. Young, Rev Gordon S, BA (£45); 6. Lillie, Edwin; 7. Booth, Robert C (£102); 8. Hamilton, J P; 9.Crampton, George (£59-10s); 10. Bamford, Thomas; 11. Hilton, John (£57-5s); 12. Reynolds, Eoin; 13. Hilton, William S (£62-5s); 14. Burke, James (£33); 15. Hill, Allen (£33-15s); 16. Brown, John; 17. Paltridge, Frederick (£33-15s); 18. Hogben, Denis; 19. Bell, William; 20. Weir, Harold (£33); 22. no information given; 24. Donaghy, Edward.

EMBASSY LAWN

From around 1948 the Canadian ambassador lived at St Bridget's on the Roebuck road (later Clonskeagh road). Previous owners of this property have been discussed in the last chapter as well as the fact that St Bridget's well was located within its environs. While he lived there the rateable valuation of the property stood at £90-5s. By 1960 the ambassador had moved out and the entry in the directory that year for St Bridget's is blank apart from the valuation which still remained at £90-5. When it re-appears in the next directory (1962/3) John O'Farrell is given as its occupier but, crucially, the valuation had dropped substantially – it was now £32-5s. In the same year the new road, Embassy lawn, makes its first appearance. These two events are not coincidental; Embassy lawn was built on land attached to St Bridget's, hence the reduction in rateable valuation of the latter. It is also fairly clear that the new road got its name from the most recent use to which St Bridget's had been put – an Embassy.

It is a small road, a cul-de-sac, and almost all of its houses were constructed in the first few years of the 1960s. Their residents appear in the first listing in 1962/3 as follows: 2. Maurice Kent; 3. Joseph Lynch; 4. Michael O'Gara; 5. Martin Dolphin; 6. Walter Alkin; 7. Kenneth Thompson; 8. Fearghus O'Foghludha; 9. Michael O'Rahilly; 10. Desmond Brown. Shortly thereafter the house numbered 1 was built and appeared in the 1965 directory as: 1. Muriel Phillips. The houses were assigned rateable valuations of £27 to £34.

MILLTOWN BRIDGE ROAD

Already when discussing the progress of house building on Whitebeam road it was observed that house number 53 had been listed in the 1948 directory; its rateable valuation is given in the following year as (£22-10s). This is a semidetached house, the other half of which is house number 1 on Milltown Bridge road. That house did not get listed until the road itself was first entered in the directory in 1951. It then appeared with another house as follows: 1. Johnson, Cecil (£22-9s); 3. Van Allst, R B. Two years later the following were added: 5. Mullins, Dr – San Antonio; 7. Devitt, T E – Woodhayo. However, there seemed to be some confusion as these two were also listed under Whitebeam road. This was corrected in 1955 when the list given was: 1. Johnson, Cecil (£22-9s); 3. Kneafsey, Dr; 5. Herd, F. The following year a new house at the other side of the road was added, Dodder Ground, home to the Argentine Legation. The name of this house was enhanced around 1960 when C A Fernandez, Envoy Extraordinary and Minister Plenipotentiary of the Argentine, took up residence; it was henceforth called Dodder Ground house. Two years later we first encounter another house on the road, Dodderbank and its resident, J Arthur Douglas. There would be one or two more houses built in time before this, the shortest road in the general area, was completed.

LEINSTER LAWN

The last substantial development in this area involved a connection between one end of Nutgrove park and Clonskeagh road. However, it would appear to have cut through the grounds of Roebuck house; at least that is the impression one gets from the fact that the result is a separation of what was once the gate lodge of that house (it is now called Red Roof) from the house itself. After the death of Maud Gonne MacBride the house is listed, for the first time in 1955, under the name of

Sean MacBride SC, TD. Whereas the house had been rated at £85, a much reduced valuation – £35 – is now given. This remained until 1965 when it was given as £62. The £35 seems likely to be a typographical error for £85 but the £62 rate may very well reflect a reduction in the size of the ground around the house due to the building of the new road. It is unclear why the title – Leinster lawn – was chosen as it does not appear to have any historical connection with the area; perhaps it was built on what might have been a lawn attached to Roebuck house and there was a building firm listed around that time in Clonskeagh road called Leinster Homes Ltd. The houses on the road were constructed in the first half of the 1960s and appear with their occupiers and rateable valuation in the 1965 directory as follows: 1. Brendan Comiskey £32-10s; 2. Harold Bond £34; 3. William Connolly £34; 4. Jacobus Jansen £34; 5. Frank O'Kelly-Lynch £34; 6. Alan Quinn £34; 7. Conrad Leser £35; 8. Ronald Russell £32-10s; 9. Michael David £34; 10. Derrick Hill £34; 11. Mervyn Keartland £34; 12. Matthew McCormack £34; 13. Philip Parker £34; 14. James Prendergast £32-10s; 15. Joseph Walsh £34; 16. Col. James Cooney £34; 17. Francis A Coffey £34; 18. Eamon Whelan £32-10s; 19. Liam O'Maolchatha £34; 20. (no entry) £38; 21. David Fitzgerald £32-10s; 22. Michael Minch £34; 23. Robert Briscoe £34; 24. Fergus Barron £32-10s; 25. Richard Sweetman £34; 26. Peter F Keogh £34; 27. Michael Coote £36. There continued to be no entry in respect of no. 20 for a number of years; however, we are given a name for the year 1971, Abraham Weinrib

ROEBUCK CRESCENT, FORMERLY WYNNSWARD CRESCENT AND BEFORE THAT CLONSKEAGH ROAD

Before construction of Richview villas, at the bridge end of Clonskeagh road, had begun in 1952 another development along that road had already been completed at the other end. This had made its first appearance in the directories in 1949 and was then called simply Clonskeagh road although the road between it and the bridge was then referred to as Roebuck road. The reason why it should be called by that name under those circumstances is not clear – perhaps it was merely a holding name. Its first listing is as follows: *Clonskeagh road*: 1. Fassenfeld, J W; 2. vacant; 3. vacant; 4. Geller, L; 5. Marshbank, W; 6. Neale, Mrs N H; 7-9. vacant; 10. Baker, H V. From this it can be deduced that all the houses were already built by 1949 but only half of them were as yet occupied. That, however, was quickly remedied as seen in the 1950 entry: *Clonskeagh road*: 1. Fassenfeld, J W (£40-15s); 2. Cooney, Michael F (£40-15s); 3. Haughton, William S, MD, BCh, LM, surgeon (£40-15s); 4. Geller, I (£40-16s); 5. Marshbank, W (£40-16s); 6. Neale, Mrs N H (£40-16s); 7. Morrow, Stanley (£40-16s); 8. Duffy, Patrick J (£40-16s); 9. Brodie, Hugh M (£39-16s); 10. Baker, H V (£40-15s).

The name Clonskeagh road was still in use in 1951 but the following year saw a change to Wynnsward crescent a name that it would retain for only one further year before it was changed once again to its final name Roebuck crescent in 1954. The reason for the latter name change is not clear. The earlier name, Wynnsward crescent, is easier to explain given that there were two developments nearby bearing the name Wynnsward; the nearer one of them, Wynnsward drive, was being built at the same time as this development. However, unlike these two roads which were built beside Wynnstay house, thus giving them a reason to choose the name Wynnsward, it was built at some distance from Wynnstay house. Could this have been a factor behind the change in name from Wynnsward to Roebuck crescent? Whatever the reason was, the development was the last to take place along Clonskeagh road. What had begun around 1927 was completed by 1950 (apart, that is, from later and more modern in-fills).

ROSEMOUNT CRESCENT, PREVIOUSLY ROSEMOUNT AND PRIOR TO THAT ROSEMOUNT ESTATE

Roebuck crescent, just described, may of course not be considered to be a part of what is now called Clonskeagh road; it may be considered to be a separate address that is located between that road and Roebuck road. This is, perhaps, even more so in the case of Rosemount crescent. When this development first appeared in the directories in 1954 it was called Rosemount estate, a name it would retain for many years. The listing for that year was: 1. Buckley, D J; 2. O'Dwyer, J; 3. Nolan, W. 4. vacant; 5. Howell, C G; 6. Gogarty, C; 7. Roger, W F; 8-9. vacant; 10-13. vacant space; 14. Murphy, Rev M G, CC; 15. Murphy, J. Although some of the houses planned for the estate were completed and occupied in that year the reference to numbers 10 to 13 being vacant space would suggest that building was on hold perhaps as we have seen in earlier developments to ensure that building did not outstrip the capacity to sell the houses. This inference would appear to be confirmed by the entry for the following year. Then the houses which were vacant the previous year were occupied and there were now only two 'vacant spaces' reported, nos. 10 and 11. By 1956 houses had been built in these spaces and occupied; the development was complete and valuations ranged between £ 27-10s and £ 34-15s. The name Rosemount estate was still in use up to 1977 when it underwent a relatively small change by dropping the word 'Estate' – such a word had by that time gained negative connotations – and became known simply as Rosemount. However, from 1983 onwards it became known by the name Rosemount crescent, reflecting no doubt the crescent shape of the development; there may, however, have been another reason why the name did not remain simply Rosemount. It seems quite clear why the name Rosemount was incorporated into the title adopted for the development in the first case. It was built on land either immediately adjacent to or in fact part of a property that had for a long time borne that name. That property had been for well over 150 years the home of the Corballis family and latterly through the marriage of a female member of that family, the Woulfe-Flanagans. The address 'Rosemount' in Clonskeagh would automatically refer to this home; its adoption for the name of a new development of houses would have led to confusion at the very least.

ROEBUCK ROAD

There is a problem associated with tracing suburban development on Roebuck road and it is this. What is understood as Roebuck road now was not always the case. It now begins at the Islamic centre and turns sharply left at the next fork in the road but it was once thought to begin at Clonskeagh bridge; what is now called Roebuck road was, at that time, grouped along with properties on the Goatstown road under the general heading 'Roebuck (part thereof listed under Dundrum)'. The sources can therefore be somewhat confusing to decipher. Because of that, what follows may not be fully complete.

The first suburban developments to be detected on the road were two houses which appeared in the directory of 1936. They, together with their contemporary occupants, are: J Brennan, Westray; Peter Joseph Byrne, Tree Tops both with a rateable valuation of £20. These houses today are numbered 116 and 114 respectively. The two Moorefield cottages, close to what would later become The Palms, may not be considered as part of the process of suburbanisation as they were there from at least the early 1900s and were most likely built to provide accommodation for people working locally, most likely in the large house from which they derived their name, Moorefield.

In 1943 two new houses are listed, Urris with J Farley in residence and Glengesh with P Frazer; both were first rated at £18 but were subsequently reduced to £17-10s. Dunerose, which may not be the correct spelling (Dunross?), was first recorded in 1945 with its occupier E Gibney. A list of names were recorded in 1953 under the general location name of Roebuck, some of which were subsequently found to be residents of houses in Roebuck road but are not clearly defined enough at this stage to make any comment on them. However, in the same year Roebuck road was entered in the directories in a manner similar to how it is understood today. In that year, the following were listed under it: Hughes, Vincent P, barrister at law, Culmore (£19); McAllister, M; Drury, M I, MD, MRCPI; Bailey, GWD, Holmington; Greene, Denis, solr., Tinode; Hussey, Misses, Ui Breasail.

It will be noted that the houses we have already detected as having been built in earlier years on that road are not included. This would be rectified in 1955 when the listing was as follows: Nolan, J, Westray (£20); Byrne, Peter Joseph, Tree Top (£20); Clarkson, Mrs, Friarsland (£140); Cosgrave, Val, Roebuck hall (£76-10s); Devitt, J E (£28); Farley, Desmond P, Urris (£17-10s); O'Neill, F, Glengesh (£17-10s); Gibney, E, Dunerose (£20); Hughes, Vincent P, barrister at law, Culmore (£30-10s); Drury, M I, MD, MRCPI; Bailey, GWD, Holmington; O'Carroll, Tighe, Tinode; Hussey, Misses, Ui Breasail; Monastery of the Immaculate Conception, Mount Carmel. Superioress; Sister M Teresa; chaplain – Rev L Shanahan C C (£170); [the following are those newly listed in 1955] Roslyn –Dain, N; Woodville – Ardill, E W; Denvar – Donnelly E; New Trows – Morrissey, J J; Hy Marie – Kelly, T E; Zilmoh – Babington E; Marsden – Dempsey, J; Zennor – Fitzell, W H; Omagh – McNulty, P; Deconade – Scanlan, Miss; Dun Muire – Carey, V; Rosencrin – O'Reilly, M W; Amygale – Jackson, T; Coolevin – Shannon, P; Martin P; Grogan, M; Murphy, P D; Daly, E; O'Reilly, W.

By 1958 a new name had been added: Eiger – Taylor, R; this name would later be changed to Elgin. Confusion was added in 1960 by attempts to introduce a house numbering system, now obsolete, but only some were given numbers: 15. Parkinson, Stanley; 10. Kelly, Thomas (1955 = Hy Marie – Kelly, T E ?); 9. Babington, Thomas (1955 = Zilmoh – Babington E ?); 7. Dempsey, John (1955 = Marsden – Dempsey, J ?); 6. Finn, Michael; 5. Fitzell, William (1958 = Zennor – Fitzell, W H ?); 2. Carey, Vincent (= Dun Muire – Carey, V, 1958); 1. Martin, Ellen; 8. Murphy, Patrick. These include two new introductions: 15. Parkinson, Stanley & 6. Finn, Michael but also two omissions: Deconade – Scanlan, Miss & Grogan, M. It is possible that these are the same houses but with changed occupants.

The new names added in the early 1960s were: Dumfries – Inglis, William (£28-10s); Pembroke – Sheehan, Con; The Elms – Lobo, C J (£19-10s); 4. Lawlor, James D (£21); San Pio – ; 30. Brugha, M; Hillcrest – Searson, James (£30-10s) with the following added by the mid-1960s: St Helen's – Hoey, Maria (£12-10s); Donegal Design Ltd., Friarsland Mill; Colmcille -; Peare, L D & J A; Trusk – McGuckin, Ralph B (£28); San Marino – Brown, Patrick J (£32); Roebuck Hall – Stomac Adhesives Ltd; Mission Hall; Maryville – Reilly, Mary M; 2. – (£22); 3. Corless, Mary. Some of these 'new' entries may be older houses but with a new name or given a house number; the manner in which the houses would ultimately be numbered had not yet evolved. As well as that there would continue to be new houses added, even up to the present day. However, already in the mid-1960s, the road was well integrated into suburbia.

HARLECH GROVE, VILLAS, CRESCENT, DOWNS

Most of the developments on Roebuck road, just discussed, took place on land which would have belonged at one stage to either of two large properties which took their names from the mansions located just off that road, Harlech and Moorfield. Both of these had a long history in the area; one can see them on the first Ordnance Survey map of the area in 1837. However, in 1948 major changes were afoot in relation to both of them. In that year there is an entry as follows: Moorefield Estate: 6 new houses; 1 McAllister, M; Building Ground, Harlech (£106, £5). Although some of their grounds had already been used for houses which faced on to Roebuck road there were now plans afoot for a larger development. However, the detail of that development is not made clear for a number of years as the same entry was continued each year until 1952. In that year we get the first sign of what had been happening when Harlock (later to be spelled correctly Harlech) villas, on the Goatstown road side of the Harlech grounds, is listed with all of its twelve houses occupied. House no. 1 among these, called Electra House, had already been noted as being on what was then called Roebuck road in 1939 when it was occupied by Timothy Murphy.

In 1953 Harlech crescent with 8 houses and Harlech grove with 4 are listed for the first time; both of these are entered from the Roebuck road. Harlech crescent was then only at the start of its development with houses nos. 1 to 9 (odd) and 2 to 6 (even) completed and occupied. Building would continue in the following years. By 1955 21 houses were completed, nos. 1-9 odd, 10-14, 31-41, all occupied (houses nos. 2 to 6 (even) are now re-numbered 10, 11, 12); one new house was listed in 1956 – no. 42; 4 in the following year – nos. 15, 16, 17, 30 and 3 in 1958 – nos. 26, 28, 29- a total of 29 houses. However, some confusion is encountered around 1960 when the numbering system appears to have changed and this makes it difficult to trace the evolution of the crescent. Houses numbers 1 to 9 (odd) are dropped but houses numbered 18, 24, 25 &27 are added, thus giving a system that rises consecutively from 10 to 18 and 24 to 42, a system that would continue well into the 1970s although no. 42 would later also be dropped.

Harlech grove, on the other hand, would continue to have only 4 houses throughout the 1950s; in the 1960s and 1970s it would gain additions, in particular business premises. Finally, Harlech downs would arrive at a much later date.

BIRD AVENUE

In the Rocque map of the county of Dublin in 1760 Bird avenue does not appear discernible as a road. However, this map is not considered to be very accurate.

Nevertheless, it is difficult to believe that a road would be missed out if such existed. It is possible, therefore, that what was in place at that time was a track of some type. There certainly would have been some need for a connection between Dundrum road and Roebuck road since there was a substantial bridge in place at Clonskeagh whereas, apart from the pack-horse bridge, traffic along the Dundrum road going towards the city through Milltown would have had to cross the Dodder by way of a ford at Milltown. This would, and did, lead to danger given the Dodder's propensity for flooding. We know from the first Ordnance Survey map of the area, surveyed in 1837, that the entrance to one of the mansions in the area, Casino – now the residence of the Marist Fathers – was from a point where the church now is on what was called Bird avenue in that map; its present entrance (from Dundrum road) would have been a back or service entrance at that time. Similarly according to the same map, the entrance to another mansion, then called Farranboley cottage but in 1974 called The Manor, was accessed by a driveway at a point nearly half way down Bird avenue. On the other end, the large house that eventually took the name Gledswood house also had an entrance at some distance up Bird avenue from that end; also the mansion, Oak lawn, now Farranboley house, had its entrance at the same point along the avenue but on the opposite side. These entrances are most clearly seen on Duncan's map of 1821. The driveways, at both ends, may well have provided the beginnings of the avenue; at least they would have helped to develop whatever had been there prior to the building of these mansions.

The origin of the name Bird avenue has not been found but since it appears in Ball and Hamilton's book (p221) as Birds' Avenue it may very well have been called after a family with that name, a name that is not uncommon in the Dublin area although no one bearing it, who lived in the Clonskeagh, Roebuck or Windy Arbour area, has been found in the historical sources. A more probable origin of the name may be the presence on Taylor's map of the area, drawn in 1816, where a house called Bird House can be seen on the Dundrum road a short distance on the Dundrum side from the point where Bird avenue intersects with that road. The name already exists from at least the early 1800s when in reality it must have been only a country road although the presence of large houses using it as an address would probably have led to it being maintained in a manner somewhat more in keeping with such houses than just any ordinary country road. This state of affairs continued well into the twentieth century. The first sign of the arrival of suburbia is found in 1935.

In that year the following houses or shops are recorded (some of these house-names would be changed in subsequent years): 1. John Byrne, grocer; 2. Miss J Quinn, newsagent and tobacconist; Avondale – A Marshall; Rienroe – Edwin Squire; Rockdale – John Hughes; Woodside – P J Caulfield; Thildonick – B.

Martin; Kilary – W J Stacey; Enfield – T Lattimore; St Catherine's – T P Gunning; Attanagh (later called'Casa de Porres' and later still 'Westmead'?) – Joseph Dowling. The last six of these would appear to be together, of the same design and located on the Clonskeagh side of what was the entrance to the College of Surgeons sports ground, now 'The Maples'. The three previous to these are on the other side of the same entrance but not together. The number of houses recorded in this first entry would suggest that building had been underway for a few years prior to 1935.

In the following year new entries were as follows: Bird lodge (later called 'Scotia house') – Harry Johnson; Birdville – Patrick Byrne (both of these are off Bird avenue behind Farrenboley house); Agathos – C Norman Jeffares; Millbrae (later called 'Lisnaskea' and later still 'Winamac') – Miss S King; Croneyhorn – J W Bowes; Coolnaholna (later called 'Woodlands') – John Ryan (these four houses are together, of the same design and immediately after Rose Cottage); Mayville – Anthony Gunning (this appears to be the sixth house in the scheme of four houses just mentioned; the fifth appears in 1937 as: St Clare – M H Lennon); Erneville – Philip McManus, VS.

Apart from St Clare's, already mentioned, there were more new houses recorded in 1937: Ballinahoun (this is likely to be a new name for 'Rienroe' which is already recorded but now drops out of the listing) – O'Donoughue of the Glen; Cois Coille – A J (*r.* T) Lucas; Alverno – John Hughes; Varredene – T Fortune (all of these are on the Windy Arbour side of the entrance to 'The Maples'); Clovely – A J Stringer; Littlecroft (sometimes spelled 'Littlecourt')– Thomas O'Byrne (two houses together, of the same design and on the other side of the above entrance). There were no new entries for 1938 but the following year saw a substantial number: Aberdour – J V Lochtie; Seskin – T Nevin; Gaultier – G L Dobbyn (these three seem to have been on the Windy Arbour side of the entrance to 'The Maples'); Rylston (now called 'Arisaig'?)- A R Russell; Ivanhoe – G Colley (both together, close to Clonskeagh end); Failte – Edward Power (at Clonskeagh end); Geraldine (later Glasheen, Glenfin, Glasin) – Patrick Taylor; Hollywood (later Villa Rita, later still Ard Muire/ Ard Mhuire) – Miss A Quinn; Dornford – Mrs Dunne (on other side of Bird avenue at Windy Arbour end). More houses in that area were recorded in 1940: Elfin (*r.* Enfin) – Arthur McCullagh; Cambrai (later Lisavane, Luzon, Legare, Lezayre/ Lez Ayre) – P J O'Gorman. Also entered that year was Ainsdale (later Valpan)- E C Kerr. Again, in 1941, the Windy Arbour end saw more houses listed: Iona – Mrs B Heaton; Rathbrist – D. Roe, St John's – M A Alexander but also on the other end of the avenue: Manhattan – F Dowds and Waldean – James Stalker. Two houses were added in 1942; at the Windy Arbour end: Scartin – M McSweeney and at other end: St Joseph's (later 'Agartala')– J J Mulligan. No new houses were recorded in 1943, 1944 or 1945.

The end of the emergency, associated with the second world war, saw one new house recorded in 1946. However, this broke new ground in that it had a house number assigned, not a house name; an assigned number indicates that it is the first of a planned series of houses, perhaps with building plots having been allocated although, in the event, the number did not survive. These plots were most likely to have been on the other side of the avenue to that on which building had so far been concentrated; that side had been virtually completed a few years previously. The new entry for 1946 was: 5. Keogh, Bernard J. However, 1947 saw the completion of the two houses between Iona and Rathbrist at the Windy Arbour end: Croin Bay (later Cronebane) – Dermot J Dargan and Springfield – R Oakley while in 1948 three new houses were recorded: Ardmore – J Hamil; Rockbawn – R Casey; Eldorado – J J Hogan. Rockbawn is beside Farranboley house but it is not clear where the other two were located, though they appear to have been at the Clonskeagh end. They may have been on the plots referred to above; in any case, work on these was slow as it was not until 1951 that some results appear when four houses were recorded as having been built, two on either side of what would become the intersection with Beechmount drive – on the Windy Arbour side: (later no. 37) Dingley Dell – Braham, A Riobárd AIIS; (later no. 41) P J McDonald; on the other side: (later no. 45) K J Page; (later no. 43) C S Gallen.

Complications are met in 1952 when Beechmount drive (in 1952 called Ardnabel road for reasons which will be explained later) is first listed. Included along with its original 16 houses and their residents are 12 that in fact are on Bird avenue, a fact that would be recognized in 1953 when they are reassigned to that address. These new additions are therefore close to the point where Beechmount drive intersects (they are here given the numbers that they would eventually get on Bird avenue) –on the Windy Arbour side: 31. E J Byrne; 33. J P Mullally; 35. R Bushnell; 39. J G Forbes; – on the other side: 47. M G Byrne; 49. T Kavanagh; 51. C J Moran; 53. A O'Kelly. The inclusion of Bird avenue houses under Ardnabel road (later called Beechmount drive) was not the only complication met in 1952; in that same year a new listing is found in the directory called Gleswood (*sic*) close. The ten houses and their occupants given would appear for the following two years under the heading of Gledswood estate. However, it would transpire in 1955 that these houses were in fact located on Bird avenue where they appear in the directories for that and subsequent years. Furthermore, the numbers allocated to them were also changed that year to fit in with the numbering scheme of Bird avenue. Thus instead of being listed as no. 1 to no. 10 Gleswood (*sic*) close and later Gledswood estate the following appeared in 1955 with their Bird avenue house numbers: 55. T Stewart; 57. R J Merhelan; 59. B McDonagh; 61. H Peelo; 63. H Wilkinson; 65. E W Smythe; 67. S E O'Neill;

69. J C Burns; 71. J Kennedy; 73. D R Bailey. (These numbers would be changed slightly some time later c.1960 from the existing 55-73 to 57 – 75; a new house would be built bearing the number 55). Weymouth lodge with E W Smyth as occupant was listed in 1954 and Linden Lea with Leslie Kearon in residence in 1955. Building had now reached the entrance to Gledswood house, which, incidentally, had been divided into three properties around 1952: Leslie Kearon, solicitor (£40); E White (£35); H R Polden (£35). The valuation of the three new properties came to the same total as that previously assigned to Gledswood house.

In the following year the as-yet unadjusted numbers 75 to 83 were entered but nothing about them was specified while no. 85 had apparently been built as its occupant was given: J Medcalf. The same numbers, 75-83 are entered without any detail again in 1958 but separately new entries, given with house names only, would have included at least some of those numbers: Avonlea – H E Camier; Glenazzana (the spelling is not certain)– (Gerald) Duffy; Rockview – (John) Barnett; Loyola – Flynn, -; Pantiles – Gerard Lane. To these was added Dunnose house in 1960 with Desmond Medcalfe in residence. In that year Bonnington –Lovell Parker is noted; it is not clear whether this is a renaming of an existing house or a new one.

This brought the building of houses on Bird avenue almost to an end. The new Catholic church had been built during the latter years of the completion of the avenue; it was built on lands previously owned by the Marist Fathers. Curiously, up to this point there had been no entry in the directories of what may have, in fact, been the oldest extant house on the side of the avenue, Rose Cottage. It is not found in the directories until well into the 1960s after all the other houses have been completed; the person listed as living there at the time is Margaret Cullen. It has not been possible to find out but there is possibility that this cottage may have been in some way linked to Casino, later the residence of the Marist Fathers; however, it was not its gate lodge.

GLEDSWOOD AVENUE, CLOSE, DRIVE AND PARK

As was noted when discussing Bird avenue some of its houses were first called Gle(d)swood close and Gledswood estate before being listed as part of Bird avenue. The proximity of the new houses to Gledswood house is quite obviously the reason why the name Gledswood was chosen although, in this particular case, later dropped. However, Gledswood would also be used in the names chosen for other developments surrounding Gledswood house. In fact both 'close' and 'estate' would be reused again for different areas but the second use of Gledswood estate did not survive.

In 1952 when building was going ahead at a quickening rate on Bird avenue a new listing under the title Gledswood park is encountered as follows: 2. Murphy, M; 4. Broderick, B; 6. Fitzgerald, M; 8. Morgan, J; 10. Byrne, P; 12. Sturt, W; 14. Boylan, D. In the same year another development in the area also appears – Gledswood drive. Some of the houses listed under it, however, were destined in the following year to be re-allocated to Gledswood park, some to a new Gledswood close while the name Gledswood drive would disappear to re-emerge elsewhere in 1954. Gledswood park in 1953 has the following listed: 2. Murphy, M; 4. Broderick, B; 6. Fitzgerald, M; 8. Morgan, J; 10. Byrne, P; 12. Sturt, W; 14. Boylan, D; 1. Fitzgibbon, T P; 3. Roche, J; 5. Coogan, J P; 7. Quinn, J; 9. Robeson, J; the last 5 being those which had appeared the previous year under the address Gledswood drive. The others which had similarly appeared were included in the 1953 listing of Gledswood close (bearing nos. 2, 3, 4, 5, 6, 8, 9): 1. Jones, R; 2. O'Sullivan, R; 3. Moffat, P; 4. Lloyd, Mrs E; 5. McHugh, T G; 6. Booker, E W; 7. Norton, J W; 8. McGarry, M. 9. Salmon, T.

There were three new houses added to Gledwood park's listing in 1954 (nos. 13, 15 & 17) but none to the close as it was essentially completed. Meanwhile Gledswood avenue had received its first listing in 1953 when it was reported that, apart from building lots nos. 11 to 17 (odd), there were houses already built with odd numbers 1 – 45; of these nos. 35 to 39 and 43 to 45 were still vacant. As for the even numbers, except for lots 24 and 26, houses were already built from no. 4 to no. 40 with nos. 32 to 40 still vacant. By the following year, 1954, considerable progress had been made in the avenue when all houses with odd numbers, were now occupied with only nos. 11 to 15 (odd) still remaining as lots; similarly, there were houses with even nos. 2 to 42 built and occupied with only nos. 24 & 26 still to be built. By 1955 no. 15 had been built and occupied; however, it would not be until the end of the 1950s that houses would be erected on the remaining lots although it is not clear when or if house no. 11 was built.

The year 1954 also saw the re-emergence of the name Gledswood drive with the following entry: 25. Molloy, E; 26. Norton, G; 27. Staves, A R; 28. Turner, R; 29. Holohan, M; 30. Brophy, L; 31. Herbert, Miss E M; 32. O'Reilly, M; 33. Dover, J E; 34. Lynch, M; 35. Fitzmaurice, R M; 36. Smullen, L, chemist; 37. vacant. In 1955 J Feeney, victualler would set up business in this last property, no. 37. The situation would remain apart from some change in occupants until, for some unknown reason, the same list of properties is found in the 1960 directory under the name Gledswood estate. However, they appear once again under Gledswood drive in the 1962/3 edition. Eventually, however, a number of these houses would be reassigned to their proper address on the Roebuck road when that road was finally defined in a manner that was to survive up until the present time. The numbers that were hived off from Gledswood drive were nos. 25 to 33;

these numbers were retained by them at their new address of Roebuck road. The result of this hiving off was that Gledswood drive would be essentially confined to business properties – nos. 34 -37 with nos. 38 and 39 added later although no. 39 was apparently dropped in the mid 1970s.

We have already noted that three new houses were added to the listing of Gledswood park in 1954; the next year saw a much greater increase when it was reported that 32 new houses had been built: nos. 28-52 omitting no. 34 (even) and 19-61 omitting no. 11 (odd). Although nos. 54 – 80 (even) and 49-51 (odd) as well as no. 55 are listed there is no entry after them suggesting that they remained numbered building plots. All the houses built so far with the exception of no. 45 were occupied. The building rate continued strongly as in the next year, 1956, the listing contains 23 new houses: nos. 34, 54-82 (even), 45, 49, 51, 55 and 63-75 (odd) while the vacancy in no. 45 is filled. However, nos. 11, 16-26 (even) and 77-81 (odd) remained missing from the numbering system. Nevertheless, Gledswood park was, by that year, virtually completed with houses being assigned a rateable valuation between £17 and £27.

BEECHMOUNT DRIVE (PREVIOUSLY ARDNABEL ROAD)

We have already noted, when discussing Bird avenue, that when Beechmount drive was first listed in 1952 it was called Ardnabel road. The reason for choosing this name seems to be quite clear. It was built on grounds that were originally associated with (or on an access road, originally a carriageway, to) the house then called Roebuck Manor but known from 1876 to 1948 as Ardnabel. When it was first listed it contained 28 houses but, as already discussed, 12 of these were in fact on Bird avenue and were to be re-assigned to that address the following year. In that year, Ardnabel road appears shorn of these 12 houses but also with a new name, Beechmount drive; the reason for the name change is unclear. The listing for that year (with their 1952 house numbers in brackets) is: 2. (13.) O Cahdhain, Máirtín; 4. (14.) Fogerty, John M; 6. (15.) Maher, T A; 8. (16.) Stritch, G S; 10. (17.) Carr, J; 12. (18.) Mundy, D J; 14. (19.) Murray, F A; 16. (20.) Grogan, W G; 1. (28.) Normoyle, J J; 3. (27.) Hegarty, G J; 5. (26.) Verso, William G; 7. (25.) O'Kelly, J J; 9. (24.) Foody, P; 11. (23.) Hyland, T; 13. (22.) Vaughan, G H; 15. (21.) Sadleir, J W.

In 1956 nineteen new houses were added to this listing when nos. 22-34 (even) and 25-47 (odd) were added together with their occupants. These new houses were beyond the point where Gledswood park then intersected; it, as we have seen, had been completed by that year. These names of the occupants were (some have no first names given; that found in the 1957 directory is given where this happens): 22. P Early; 24. M Bergin; 26. E Vaughan; 28. J Delany; 30. P

Despard; 32. V McQuirk; 34. J McQuirk; 25. S Hill; 27. M Haddock; 29. J Devine; 31. G Jackson; 33. J Walsh; 35. P McNamee; 37. M Downes; 39. P Cleary; 41. B Fagan; 43. A Stafford; 45. M Gallagher; 47. A McMahon. Later, a new development around Roebuck Manor would intervene between these newly added houses and those already on Beechmount drive. It was called Roebuck lawn and in 1974 it was said that 8 new houses were then under construction.

ST COLUMBANUS AVENUE, PLACE, ROAD

These roads are called after one of the most famous of Irish saints with some people arguing that he deserves to be acknowledged, along with St Benedict, as the patron saint of Europe. Most of his writings that have survived are those he wrote outside of Ireland especially at Bobbio in Italy where he died in 615 AD. He is still remembered in Italy where his monastery became the most famous in the north of that country; even to this day, it is called there 'the Monte Cassino of the north'. The Latin he wrote was of a very high quality; he learned it in Ireland and he is, in fact, the earliest Latin scholar known by name in that country. He corresponded with the famous pope Gregory the Great and he had a major impact on the church in Europe during his life.[5] He was truly one of the most famous Irishman of his day; to have one's place of residence bear his name is indeed a great honour.

The first listing of these three new developments which are called after him is in the directory for the year 1953 but the information contained is quite sparse. St Columbanus avenue we are told consisted of 52 Corporation houses but no detail is given of who the occupants were. St Columbanus place has the simple entry 'Houses building' while St Columbanus road is said to have 29 Corporation houses but, like the avenue, no detail of the residents is given. A good deal of extra detail is given in the entry for the following year. Then St Columbanus avenue is said to consist of 56 Corporation houses and the names of most of the occupants are given but houses with odd numbers between 49 and 55 are omitted. The names of the residents are as follows: 1. J O'Hanlon; 3. R J Stapleton; 5. J O'Neill; 7. J Fitzsimons; 9. M Geraghty; 11. P Gaffney; 13. M Forsyth; 15. T Farrell; 17. J Little; 19. P McGrath; 21. P McAdam; 23. E Crofton; 25. J Pepper; 27. B Sheridan; 29. M Cummins; 31. A Doyle; 33. J J Freeley; 35. W Curtis; 37. T Buckley; 39. T Dologhan; 41. T Kershaw; 43. J Coffey; 45. D P Taylor; 47. P Doyle; 2. C Bermingham; 4. D Walsh; 6. A McGovern; 8. C Kelly; 10. N Redmond; 12. J Murphy; 14. P Brown; 16. P McGahey; 18. W Timmons; 20. ———; 22. P

---

5   Michael Richter, 'Columbanus (c. 540-615)', Seán Duffy (ed), *Medieval Ireland: an encyclopedia* (New York & London 2005) 100-101.

McMahon; 24. R Doyle; 26. H O'Neill; 28. M Higgins; 30. V Langton; 32. A Fairley; 34. J Walsh; 36. N Dunleavy; 38. J Grimes; 40. P Devlin; 42. T Milton; 44. J Crabbe; 46. B Burke; 48. N Sheppard; 50. N Stenson; 52. E Ryan; 54. E Grant; 56. P Kavanagh.

The house building in St Columbanus place noted in 1953 had now progressed considerably as in 1954 it is noted that there are 50 Corporation houses there and the names of the occupants of 48 of them are given. They are: 1. P Collins; 3. C Crawford; 5. L Fitzpatrick; 7. J McNamee; 9. J Daly; 11. R Fahy; 13. P Kelly; 15. W Bracken; 17. W Kelly; 19. H Dunne; 21. M Dunne; 23. M Chambers; 25. D O'Kelly; 27. B Pope; 29. R Kavanagh; 31. ———; 33. A Ford; 35. D Mahoney; 37. T Byrne; 39. K Lyons; 41. P Fannin; 43. E Cromer; 45. A Doyle; 47. M Cummins; 49. K Loughlin; 2. E Brown; 4. P Brady; 6. C Clarke; 8. C J Darcy; 10. J Morgan; 12. J Murray & T Murphy; 14. M O'Boyce; 16. J Byrne; 18. S Bryan; 20. M Stokes; 22. M Lynch; 24. P J Dowdall; 26. J Melia; 28. E Boyce; 30. G Lawlor; 32. W Mackey; 34. L Quinn; 36. S Breslin; 38. T Alford; 40. W Wright; 42. P Mullen; 44. B Ketch; 46. ———; 48. F Murray; 50. T Sharp.

Likewise, St Columbanus road had expanded very considerably by 1954; it is now said to consist of 152 houses although houses with even numbers 138 to 152 are not mentioned. This situation would continue for a number of years and, although some more houses would be built later, the name of the first occupants as found in the 1954 directory are now given: 1. R Harte; 3. M Cunningham; 5. J McLoughlin; 7. G Duffin; 9. J Merrier; 11. J Butler; 13. F O'Brien; 15. N Phillips; 17. R Poole; 19. M Conlon; 21. R Vaughan; 23. J Clarke; 25. G Condell; 27. M Cahill; 29. J Frein; 31. J Kenna; 33. G Geraghty; 35. A Smith; 37. T Grumley; 39. E Tighe; 41. V McCann; 43. E Kelly; 45. J McMillan; 47. E Mulhern; 49. M McCarthy; 51. J Thompson; 53. T Kenny; 55. ———; 57. C McDermott; 59. M Kane; 61. R Gaynor; 63. G Fleming; 65. P O'Reilly; 67. J Byrne; 69. M McDonnell; 71. J Davey; 73. J Cassin; 75. R Staunton; 77. L Nugent; 79. J Byrne; 81. P Keane; 83. N Moyland; 85. P O'Brien; 87. P Smith; 89. C Shortt; 91. J Costello; 93. R Harrison; 95. J Flynn; 97. M Dunne; 99. T Keating; 101. P Reilly; 103. T Devaney; 105. M Carroll; 107. H Byrne; 109. Mrs E Vaughan; 111. P J O'Brien; 113. L Spain; 115. K Brown; 117. J J Dempsey; 119. P McElveney; 121. J J O'Neill; 123. J McGuiness; 125. A Murphy; 127. J Wilson; 129. T Kenny; 131. M Murphy; 133. R Costello; 135. W Coss; 137. P Byrne; 139. J Fox; 141. D Gannon; 143. K Lambert; 145. L Keane; 147. W Blackmore; 149. J Godfrey; 151. T Devereaux; 2. B P Boland; 4. B T Shaw; 6. J Fitzpatrick; 8. P Doyle; 10. E Esprey; 12. R Kidd; 14. T Jordan; 16. P Kavanagh; 18. J French; 20. R Coughlan; 22. E Kealy; 24. J Donohoe; 26. T Newman; 28. R Higgins; 30. W Doyle; 32. M Dunne; 34. M Ryan; 36. T Dolan; 38. S Walsh; 40. P O'Farrell; 42. J Griffin; 44. P Dormer; 46. E Littlefield; 48. ———; 50. E Lumsden; 52. P O'Connor; 54. G Troy; 56. J

Kavanagh; 58. J McCarthy; 60. L Leonard; 62. J Sheridan; 64. J Ward; 66. J Carwood; 68. P King; 70. L O'Brien; 72. T Osborne; 74. M Fitzpatrick; 76. M O'Shaughnessy; 78. W Hand; 80. J Grant; 82. J Keane; 84. G Jones; 86. P Byrne; 88. M Doyle; 90. J Murphy; 92. T Bergin; 94. P Higgins; 96. M Byrne; 98. P Farrell; 100. R McGarry; 102. P Smith; 104. W Hunt; 106. M Smith; 108. P Caddle; 110. J Walsh; 112. P Coyle; 114. P Doyle; 116. F Byrne; 118. L McGuirk; 120. R Reilly; 122. J Cullen; 124. T Ennis; 126. M Doyle; 128. P Mulraney; 130. M Harte; 132. R Gurren; 134. R McGarry; 136. J Hurley.

MULVEY PARK

Two years after the names of the residents of St Columbanus are found in the directories Mulvey park makes its first appearance (1956) although it should be pointed out that there is evidence that houses in the park were blessed by the parish priest of Donnybrook on 14 June 1953 (Mulvey park was transferred from the Catholic parish of Dundrum to that of Donnybrook before the institution of the new parish of Clonskeagh). In the 1956 entry it is stated that there are 180 County Council houses there and it gives the names of most of their occupants; there is no entry after 54 of these so it is quite likely that they were not yet completed. If around 150 were already occupied in 1956 building must have commenced some years beforehand and perhaps some of the houses occupied before 1956. But since the entry for that year is the first given, it is reproduced here; those missing in that entry are given below in the year that they appear in the directories: 1. F McElroy; 3. E Hayes; 6. P Costello; 7. E Whelan; 8. P Byrne; 9. E Broe; 10. P Kavanagh; 12. M Cullen; 13. M Kennedy; 14. E Maher; 15. Mrs A Coleman; 16. J McHugh; 17. J Perry; 18. J Malone; 21. P Garrard; 22. P Courtney; 23. W Colleran; 24. J Maher; 25. P Doyle; 26. P Blake; 27. E Sheridan; 28. C Doyle; 29. P Breen; 30. J Furlong; 31. J Kenny; 32. J Keogh; 33. P O'Donnell; 35. P Hayden; 36. J Fitzpatrick; 37. W Hand; 38. H McNulty; 39. E Hamill; 41 J O'Connor; 45. M Doyle; 46. P Doyle; 47. M Caffrey; 49. M Jones; 50. P Webster; 53. W Brown; 54. J Licken; 55. J Kavanagh; 56. P Barcoe; 57. P McArdle; 58. J Gilbert; 60. P Mahon; 61. M Dowling; 62. M Nolan; 64. P Carey; 65. W Carpenter; 66. P Nolan; 67. T Walsh; 68. F Memery; 69. M Mulligan; 70. A Maguire; 71. P Doolin; 72. J Bermingham; 74. T Keogh; 75. J O'Connor; 77. P O'Regan; 78. J McGarry; 79. M Murtagh; 82. P Collins; 83. P Dowdall; 84. J Kearns; 86. P Ryan; 87. F Flood; 88. E Convoy; 90. J Lynch; 91. M Martin; 92. P Nolan; 93. R Greene; 94. M Baker; 96. J Smith; 97. M Swan; 98. J Kearney; 99. P Daly; 100. F Wyse; 101. M Walker; 102. P Corrigan; 103. W Shorten; 104. J Shorten; 105. M Egan; 106. L McClare; 107. F Whelan; 108. J Hume; 110. M O'Donoghue; 111. F Leonard; 112. M Tate; 113. M Hall; 114. J Boland; 115. M

Checkley; 117. P McCann; 121. J Checkley; 123. M Payne; 125. M Mulhall; 126. P McGrath; 127. J Parsons; 128. L Brinkley; 129. E Roche; 130. R Mongey; 131. A Ellard; 133. J Duffy; 135. P O'Toole; 137. M McGiff; 140. R Mulhall; 141. P Murphy; 142. P Doyle; 143. A McPartlin; 144. J Gahan; 146. F Bradshaw; 150. J Garton; 152. F Beasley; 157. R Kelly; 160. F Doonan; 161. J Cummins; 162. F Corbally; 164. P Tannam; 165. M Flood; 169. M Wyse; 171. W Rowan; 173. K McCoy; 176. J Pogne; 177. R Kennedy; 178. P Farrell; 179. M Hume; 180. K Ryan.

In the 1957 entry 48 of the 54 houses, which had no entries in the 1956 directory, are completed and occupied according to the directory of that year; there are also two new houses added, no's 181 and 182, both vacant. The 48 new occupants given in the 1957 entry are; 2. P May; 4. D McDonnell; 5. L Caffrey; 11. J Hennessy; 19. J McCullagh; 20. T Fitzpatrick; 34. P Murphy; 40. P Kelly; 48. M McCaffrey; 51. T Phelan; 52. J O'Neill; 59. P Burke; 63. J Dunne; 73. P McArdle; 76. E Gaffney; 80. T Kelly; 81. W Gorman; 85. E Kerry; 89. T Mangan; 95. P Begley; 109. M Holland; 116. K Murphy; 122. T Byrne; 124. T Hickey; 132. C Byrne; 134. J McNulty; 136. N Darcy; 138. P Duffy; 139. A Doolan; 145. D O'Rourke; 147. N Closkey; 148. E Doran; 149. W Grey; 151. B O'Neill; 153. H McNulty; 154. J Dolan; 155. J Devlin; 156. N Boylan; 158. P Tobin; 159. J Moran; 163. J Masterson; 166. H Doyle; 167. J Brock; 168. J Whelan; 170. N Larkin; 172. P Begley; 174. D Scallon; 175. M Tobin.

Numbers 42-44 and 118-120 remained without entry and 181 & 182 vacant until the end of the 1950s; thereafter the directories cease to give the names of the individual residents. The only information given that is of some note after that is that the rateable valuation of the houses was £3-16s each up to 1960; in the 1962/3 directory it had risen to between £8 and £10-10s.

OLIVEMOUNT TERRACE (WINDY ARBOUR)

Olivemount terrace, Windy Arbour is first listed in 1940 as follows: 1. Martin Byrne; 2. George Heaton; 3. Richard Williams; 4. no entry; 5. Gerard A O'Donnell, chemist; 6. Joseph Headon, butcher; 7. The Misses Kane, draper; 8. John Brady, grocer. The information given in 1941 is somewhat more expansive, with a little more detail such as rateable valuation. It is as follows: 1. John Francis Rogers (£14-5s); 2. vacant (£14-5s); 3. Richard Williams (£14-5s); 4. no entry (£28); 5. Gerard A O'Donnell, chemist (£28); 6. James Brady, victualler (£27); 7. The Misses Kane, draper (£28); 8. John Brady, grocer (£28). It was not until 1946 that no. 2 got an occupant – B Quinn – while no. 4 continued to be vacant. It got its first occupant in 1948 – Thomas Naughton, grocer. In the meantime, a new chemist had taken over in 1945 at no. 5: Miss M M Hunter and a new victualler at no. 5 in 1946: John Merron. There would be further changes; in 1949 no. 8 had become a hardware shop run by Thomas Fallon and a new number was added 9. The Fruit Basket; this disappeared in 1952. It re-appeared the next year with a new number: 1a. Collins, Mrs, M – The Fruit Basket. However, it was delisted in 1957. In 1954 the draper shop at no. 7, having already changed hands, now got a 'Town sub-post office' and was run by Francis McDermot. There would be many more changes in this local shopping area in the remaining years of the twentieth century.

HARCOURT VILLAS (WINDY ARBOUR)

The first reference to Harcourt villa occurs in 1885; Mr James R M'Elroy is given as the sole resident. He is still there in 1887 but it is reported as vacant in 1888. The following year Mr George Wilkinson, who apparently worked in the GPO, had taken up residence there. In 1890 William Edward M'Veigh, captain, ASC is given as its occupant. It lay vacant until Mr Thomas Rooney took up residence in 1893. Its rateable valuation in 1895 was £19. Mr Rooney stayed until 1899 and it was vacant once more in 1900. It was not until 1902 that it found another occupant – Mr Joseph Delaney. He remained until 1909 when Lawrence M'Kenna moved in. Vacant again in 1910 and 1911 until Joseph W Delany was reported to be the occupant in 1912. It is not clear whether he was the same man as was there from 1902 to 1909 or the man with the same name who was listed as a grocer in Windy Arbour from 1891 to 1897 and grocer, publican and billard rooms (owner) from 1898 onwards. In 1915 a second Harcourt villa is reported and it is vacant. The following year Mrs W Reddy had taken up residence in this second house. In 1918 Harcourt villas got a separate listing as follows: 1. Joseph W Delany (£19); 2. vacant. In 1919 the listing was: 1. Joseph W Delany (£19); 2. Mrs Mary Garvin; Jno Connell, Harcourt villa. That would continue until 1933 when house no. 3 (although it is never given that number at this stage) got a new resident – J Judge. In the following year a new name of a house (but no number) and an occupant is added to the listing: Rosario – Jos Doyle. In the following year Joseph W Delany was replaced by John Duff at no. 1 and a new house is added: Breffni stores – E Kelly. Apart from some changes in names, that would remain until 1952 when a somewhat puzzling entry omits no. 2 and adds no's 3 and 4 for the first time. That would be remedied in 1955 when the following is reported: 1. Tierney, Dr John (£19); 2. Doyle, Andrew; 3. Keogh, M P (£19); 4. Duff, John (£19); Harcourt villa – Judge, Miss P; Rosario – Dollard, J (£15-8s); Breffni stores – Hoban, Mrs Mary (£14-7s). By 1960 Harcourt villa had been dropped from the listing but three new houses and their occupants had been added: 5. John Furlong; 7. Edward Byrne; 8. Alexandra McDonnell. Eventually, nos. 6 and 9 were added to the listing and Breffni stores, later *Teac Breffni*, together with Rosario would be entered separately from Harcourt villas. In 1974 the entries were as follows: 1. William Govan; 2.

Joseph Scully; 3. —; 4. Julia Duff; 5. Kathleen Furlong; 6. John Kelly; 7. Mary Byrne; 8. Alexander McDonnell; 9. Myles McGrath. Following on but separate from Harcourt villas are: *Teac Breffni* – Jeremiah Kelleher (£28); Rosario – James Dollard (£35); they are, by this stage, listed in the midst of other business premises.

MILLMOUNT COTTAGES

These make their first appearance in the directories in 1957. The householders given for that year are: 1. – Winstanley; 2. – Hartford; 3. H G Winstanley; 4. D Cahill; 5. M Brennan; 6. J Doyle; 7. S Cruise; 8. T O'Connor; 9. M Smyth; 10. M Boylan; 11. W O'Brien; 12. Mrs Dunne; 13. M Murphy; 14. N Jones; 15. O Mulhall; 16. J Doyle; 17. – Doyle; 18. – Pierce; 19. H Clement; 20. K Farrell; 21. – Jackson; 22. M Redmond; 23. – Ennis; 24. P Ryan; 25. C Sheridan; 26. F Gunning; 27. —-; 28. – Clarke; 29. J O'Brien; 30. A Winstanley; 31. M Vaughan; 32. L Hennessy; 33. Miss O'Rourke; 34. J O'Carroll; 35. S Burke; 36. K Nolan; 37. M Reilly.

MILLMOUNT TERRACE

The first record available of the residents of these houses is found in the 1957 directory. In that their names are given as: 1. J Tully; 2. S O'Connor; 3. J Price; 4. M Jones; 5. J Cruise; 6. J O'Brien; 7. L Moy; 8. – Durnin; 9. M Fanning; 10. – Masterson; 11. M Callaghan; 12. J Lahiffe; 13. J O'Brien; 14. M Hume; 15. —-; 16. J Quinn; 17. M Mooney; 18. – Jackson; 19. E Bradshaw; 20. W Martin.

ST LUKE'S CRESCENT

Like a number of other houses in the general area, St Luke's crescent is listed in the directories for the first time in 1957. The names of the householders for that year given are: 1. E Clarke; 2. T Murphy; 3. M Kearney; 4. J O'Connor; 5. G Moran; 6. M Rathborne; 7. J Kilroy; 8. P Doyle; 9. J Maher; 10. J Pepper; 11. J Kinsella; 12. J Doyle; 13. M Scanlon; 14. M Stewart; 15. J Murray; 16. G Finn; 17. H Warren; 18. J Quinn; 19. T Healy; 20. K Pepper; 21. R Purdy; 22. R Birmingham; 23. W O'Reilly; 24. M Keogh; 25. P Kavanagh; 26. J Gregg; 27. M Kelly; 28. C A Daniels; 29. R Redmond; 30. D O'Connor.

FARRENBOLEY COTTAGES

The name given to these houses is taken from the townland in which they are located – Farranboley (this is how it is spelled by the Ordnance Survey but it often appears elsewhere as Farrenboley). These houses (70) and the name of their occupants first appear in the directories in 1957; it is not clear how long before that date that they were built. The house numbers go from 1 to 34 and 261 to 296. The names given of these early occupants are: 1. P Byrne; 2. K Murphy; 3. J Phelan; 4. A Bell; 5. M Leonard; 6. F McNulty; 7. B Hanley; 8. J Daly; 9. J McInerney; 10. W Hempenstall; 11. M Traynor; 12. J Doyle; 13. J O'Leary; 14. M Melia; 15. J Waters; 16. R Doyle; 17. E Donnelly; 18. Mrs Madsen; 19. J Cordell; 20. P Fagan; 21. M Mason; 22. J O'Donnell; 23. K Farrell; 24. J McArdle; 25. M Burke; 26. M McDonnell; 27. W Webster; 28. J Ennis; 29. J Irwin; 30. M Turton; 31. F Aungier; 32. M Doyle; 33. R Ryan; 34. P Fleming; 261. E Kane; 262. T McCoy; 263. F McDonnell; 264. W O'Reilly; 265. M Courtney; 266. E Mulhall; 267. R J Gilbert; 268. P Finlan; 269. P Walsh; 270. T Brennan; 271. P Duffey; 272. F O'Neill; 273. Patrick Kavanagh; 274. P Lee; 275. A Black; 276. P Keogh; 277. E Leonard; 278. M Ward; 279. P McGrant; 280. J O'Sullivan; 281. D Holland; 282. M McArdle; 283. J T Courtney; 284. C Smith; 285. P O'Connor; 286. J McDonnell; 287. M Kavanagh; 288. F Cassidy; 289. K Tobin; 290. T Sheridan; 291. J Byrne; 292. J Kenny; 293. C Burke; 294. Mrs M Hogan; 295. J O'Connor; 296. J Curtis.

FARRENBOLEY PARK

This development first appears in the directories in the late 1960s with 37 houses. The residents given in this first listing are: 1. —; 2. Michael McDonnell; 3. Laurence McCoy; 4. John Smith; 5. James Courtney 6. John Deaton; 7. James Holland; 8. Patrick McGrath; 9. —; 10. Matthew Ward; 11. Wm Leonard; 12. Dolores Hand; 13. Elizabeth Dempsey; 14. Patrick Lee; 15. Patrick Kavanagh; 16. John O'Neill; 17. Bernard Duffy; 18. Joseph Brennan; 19. Hugh Walsh; 20. Patrick Finlan; 21. Joseph Gilbert; 22. David Mulhall; 23. James Lenehan; 24. Christopher O'Reilly; 25. George McDonnell; 26. Kathleen Keogh; 27. Michael Kane; 28. Brendan McCreddin; 29. Michael Kavanagh; 30. Matthew Whelan; 31. Margaret Cunningham; 32. Michael Hogan; 33. James Burke; 34. Denis Kenny; 35. Joseph Byrne; 36. Thomas Sheridan; 37. Anne Tobin.

COOLNAHINCH

First listed in 1957, the six houses were then occupied by: 1. C A Doyle; 2. T O'Neill; 3. C Gillan; 4. T Drury; 5. M Gernin; 6. J Leonard.

14

Ecclesiastical history

THE STRUCTURE OF THE ROMAN CATHOLIC CHURCH and that of the Church of Ireland with which we are familiar today – parish, diocese, archdiocese, well defined territorially and vertically integrated – did not arrive in Ireland until the 11th and 12th centuries. What existed prior to that is not very clearly understood; the traditionally accepted view of the central role of monasteries, at least for part of the period between the time of St Patrick and the reforms of the 11th and 12th centuries, has recently been challenged and no clear and widely accepted view of early church organisation has yet emerged from this challenge.[1] That does not mean, however, that there were no churches or ecclesiastical establishments; far from it – there were and they were numerous and research has recently begun to focus on the pastoral care which these provided.[2] However, there is no recorded evidence that any such establishment existed in Clonskeagh despite the fact that the element *Cluain* (Clon) in its name was commonly used by various ecclesiastical establishments throughout Ireland e.g. Clonmacnoise, Clonfert, Clonard.[3] There were, however, two such places located at some point on the river Dodder but their exact location has not yet been identified and cannot therefore be claimed to have any known association with Clonskeagh.[4]

---

1   Richard Sharpe, 'Some problems concerning the organization of the church in early medieval Ireland' *Peritia* 3 (1984) 230-70; Colmán Etchingham, *Church organisation in Ireland: AD 650 to 1000* (Maynooth 1999); for a review of the latter, see that by Dáibhí Ó Cróinín in *Peritia* 15, 413-20.
2   See, for example: John Blair & Richard Sharpe (ed), *Pastoral care before the parish* (Leicester 1992); Etchingham, *Church organisation in Ireland,* passim; Elizabeth FitzPatrick & Raymond Gillespie (ed), *The parish in medieval and early modern Ireland* (Dublin 2006).
3   See discussion on this in Alfred P. Smyth, *Celtic Leinster: towards an historical geography of early Irish civilization A.D. 500-1600* (Blackrock, Co. Dublin 1982) 30.
4   Personal communication from Ailbhe MacShamhráin, Research Fellow, the *Monasticon Hibernicum* Project, based in the Department of Old Irish, NUI Maynooth.

Although not a church or an ecclesiastical establishment there is one place with christian associations which most definitely can be associated with Clonskeagh and, what is more, it can be strongly argued that its origins go back at least to the eighth or ninth century and perhaps even earlier. That is the well dedicated to St Brigit[5], the location of which was in the grounds of a large house originally called Springfield (possibly thus called because of the presence of the well) but changed to St Brigit's in 1843. It is clearly visible on the map drawn up during the Pembroke Estate survey of 1866. It was on the left hand side of the driveway from Clonskeagh road to that house which no longer stands. Local tradition has it that many people came to pray and drink the water at the well. A story is told of an incident where the gates were locked to keep the people out resulted in the well overflowing shortly afterwards. Within living memory, the well was apparently blocked up by the County Council and its water piped to the Dodder in order to allow the area to be developed for housing. According to a local man, Bill Webster, it flows into the Dodder near Clonskeagh bridge – there used to be some cottages nearby and he used to drink the water there. The blocked up well is located behind the northern side of the houses on Embassy lawn.[6]

The origins of the dedication of this well to St Brigit are associated with the Uí Dúnlainge, kings of Leinster; an early king of this dynasty, Fáelán († AD 666) already had close connections with St Brigit's establishment in Kildare before AD 638. From 738 all of Leinster was under the control of three sub-dynasties which originated in three brothers who were descended from Fáelán. One of these, the Uí Dúnchada, controlled much of north east Leinster up to the outskirts of Dublin, their seat being at what is now called Castlelyons, on the Kildare-Dublin border. As a result of the influence of the Uí Dúnlainge there were many sites in south county Dublin associated with St Brigit; this happened most likely in the eighth and ninth centuries. A number of these are in the same barony of Rathdown as is that part of Clonskeagh in which the well was located. In the county Dublin part of the barony there are sites with Brigidine connections in Stillorgan and Shankill, while there are others in the Wicklow part.[7]

---

5   There are variations in the way this word is spelled but, for consistency, Brigit will be the usage employed here.

6   Pembroke Estate Papers: National Archives of Ireland, Private Sources 97/46/ 4/31 (Survey by captain Martin RE in 1866); for recent fate of the well: personal communication from Colette Kennedy, Beech View, Clonskeagh road, Dublin via Fr John Murphy PP, Clonskeagh.

7   Francis J Byrne, *Irish kings and high kings* (Dublin 2001) 150-52; Ailbhe MacShamhráin, 'The Monasticon Hibernicum project: the diocese of Dublin', Seán Duffy (ed), *Medieval Dublin VI: proceedings of the Friends of Medieval Dublin Symposium 2004* (Dublin 2005) 114-143: 128, 136.

Given the clear evidence that exists for the dissemination of the cult of St Brigit by the Uí Dúnlainge and given their dominance in the eighth and ninth century of the area in which Clonskeagh is located, it seems reasonable to argue that the dedication of the well to St Brigit that was located there occurred under their influence and at that time. It is possible, although there is no evidence available to indicate it, that it could have had an earlier cult associated with it and was changed through the influence the Uí Dúnlainge brought to bear on it. That this site should survive for well over a thousand years all the vicissitudes of time, whether of war, penal laws or frowning attitudes of ecclesiastical authorities, and be venerated by the people only to disappear without an apparent whimper at the hands of a local authority to make way for urban development is indeed remarkable.

During the period before the reform of the church in the 11th and 12th centuries, the source of pastoral care for the people of Clonskeagh would have been located at the churches in Donnybrook and Dundrum, depending on which end of Clonskeagh or Roebuck in which they lived. Although the former is traditionally said to have been established by St Broc – hence the name *Domnach Broc* which over time became Donnybrook – recent researchers, who are systematically searching out all the evidence available for pre-12th century churches, cathedrals, monasteries, convents and hermitages have so far named evidence for *Berchán* as the original founder or cult figure for the area. She is mentioned in the *Martyrology of Tallaght* and the physical evidence associated with her consists of a graveyard, an enclosure and a well. A less well authenticated possible source of a cult are 'sons of *Erccán*'; this could be the Irish origin of the place name Kilmacergan in Donnybrook c. 1200 as found in the *Calendar of the state papers relating to Ireland* edited by Brewer and others (note also 'Kylmerekargan' near Donnybrook, which we have already met when discussing Dublin's boundaries). Although *Broc* and *Berchán* appear to be two different people they are most likely to be two different versions of the name of the same person. It was quite common in early medieval Ireland to add *-án* as a suffix to the name of a person who was greatly loved or revered like the founder of a church or a saint. Examples of this, which Ó Cuív categorises as a derived name, are *Colmán* (anglicized as Colman) from the name *Colm* and *Aodhán* (anglicized as Aidan) from *Aodh*; both forms of these names are still commonly in use although the derived form has lost its original intent. Without the suffix *–án, Berchán* becomes *Berch* or perhaps *Berc* which is much more easily pronounced if a syllable is inserted between *r* and *c*, e.g. *Beroc* which is pronounced in almost the same way as *Broc*.

Perhaps of more interest is the first element in the place name Donnybrook – *Domnach*. This word is derived from the Latin name *dominicus (locus dominicus* may be translated as an 'ecclesiastical establishment'), and it has been argued that place-names, in which this element occurs, got their names at a very early period; they appear to be pre-600 AD. Furthermore, they were claimed in the *Liber Angeli* (which may be seen in the Book of Armagh, written in AD 807 and still preserved in Trinity College, Dublin) to be 'in special union with bishop Patrick [i.e. St Patrick] and his heir of the see of Armagh'; that is, they were included in Armagh's early claim to ecclesiastical supremacy in Ireland.[8]

The other church from which pastoral care would have been provided was located at Dundrum and was called *Tech Nath Í*, the saint who founded it being the eponymous *Nath Í*. The name *Tech Nath Í* through the passage of time became Taney. Both it and the church at *Domnach Broc* would have had their sphere of influence which, perhaps, could be considered to be a form of proto-parish. The actual formation of clear territorially defined parishes had to wait until the church reforms of the 11th and 12th centuries were underway. But before that happened, the Vikings, or more precisely the Norsemen, came to the area, first as raiders but later as settlers after which they are usually referred to as Hiberno-Norse. Clonskeagh would have formed part of their territory after they had settled as included in that was the northern part of the Uí Briúin Chualann land. However, there is no known or recorded feature in the area, whether archaeological or place-name, which attests to their dominance of the area; the nearest is at Donnybrook where a pagan burial-mound for about 80 to 90 people – about 10% of whom were women – was discovered in the 19th century. Dundrum, on the other hand, may have one such feature. The name *Amlaib* (Old Norse *Óláfr*) can be found in the place-name *Baile Amlaib*, anglicized as Balally. This may commemorate the Norse king and martyr, *Óláfr* (Olave) to whom a church was dedicated in Dublin in the early 11th century and a relic of whom was kept in Christ Church cathedral. However, according to Ronan, this is not the case. He believes that the original name of the place was '*Baile Mic Amhlaibh*' and that it got its name from a Norse settlement there which was founded by Sitriuc, son of Amlaib [Cuaráin]. That would put the foundation date around the early part of the 11th century. [9]

---

8   Ibid., 132, 136; Brian Ó Cuív, *Aspects of Irish personal names,* Institute of Advanced Studies (Dublin 1986)10; Ludwig Bieler (ed) *The patrician texts in the book of Armagh,* Scriptores Latini Hiberniae Volume 10 (Dublin 2000) 52, 188-89; Etchingham, *Church organization in Ireland,* 83-84; Dáibhí Ó Cróinín, 'Armagh, Book of', Seán Duffy (ed), *Medieval Ireland: an encyclopedia* (New York & London 2005) 30-31.

9   MacShamhráin, 'Monasticon Hibernicum project: the diocese of Dublin'137; Howard B Clarke, 'Conversion, church and cathedral: the diocese of Dublin to 1152' in Kelly & Keogh *History of the Catholic diocese of Dublin,* 31-2, 37, 39; Myles V Ronan, 'History of the Diocese', *Reportorium Novum: Dublin diocesan historical record,* 1 (1955) 27-44: 38.

The reforms of the 11th and 12th centuries heralded a new era in church organisation in Ireland; they saw the introduction of a new structure with dioceses and archdioceses territorially defined. These were first set out at the synod of Ráith Bressail in 1111 and got papal approval at the synod of Kells in 1152. To a large extent they survive to this day in the Roman Catholic church while in the Church of Ireland they underwent a major restructuring in the 19th century although they retained names from the old structure when a number of dioceses were united under one bishop.

Before the large-scale reform was formally inaugurated at Ráith Bressail, Dublin had become the first diocese that could be described as canonical by the norms of the western church of the time. It was founded around the year 1030 towards the end of the reign of Sitriuc Silkbeard, king of Dublin; he had just returned from a pilgrimage to Rome. What is of interest here is that Sitriuc's father, Amlaíb Cuarán († 981), was the first Norse king of Dublin to become a christian although the process by which the Norse people of Dublin became christian would have been gradual and complex as was, indeed, their transition to Hiberno-Norse. Despite Dublin being a canonical diocese for approximately 80 years before such dioceses were introduced into the rest of Ireland, Dublin was not included in the new arrangement agreed at Ráith Bressail. This was probably due to an incipient dispute for ecclesiastical superiority between Armagh and Dublin. It would take almost 40 years before a resolution to this problem would be found in 1148. When it was, the Dublin diocese was not alone then incorporated into the new episcopal hierarchy, it was included in it as an archdiocese. It had thus attained the status of a metropolitan see with authority over a number of suffragan sees, such as Kildare, Leighlin, Glendalough and Ferns, which could trace their origins to centuries before the city of Dublin was even founded. [10]

Hiberno-Norse Dublin had become an important and an integral part of Ireland and not just on the ecclesiastical front. However, within a little over two decades the Anglo-Normans arrived and set up their headquarters in the same

---

10   Martin Holland, 'Dublin and the Reform of the Irish Church in the Eleventh and Twelfth Centuries', *Peritia* 14 (2000) 111-60; idem, 'The twelfth-century reform and Inis Pátraic', in Ailbhe MacShamhráin (ed), *The Island of St Patrick: church and ruling dynasties in Fingal and Meath, 400-1148* (Dublin 2004) 159-77; Aubrey Gwynn, 'Origins of the see of Dublin', in Gerard O'Brien (ed), *The Irish church in the eleventh and twelfth centuries* (Dublin 1992) 50-67; Clarke, 'Conversion, church and cathedral', 34-35; Alex Woolf, 'Amlaíb Cuarán and the Gael, 941-81', in Seán Duffy (ed), *Medieval Dublin III: proceedings of the Friends of Medieval Dublin Symposium 2001* (Dublin 2002) 34-43.

city. At that time, Lorcán Ua Tuathail [St Laurence O'Toole] was archbishop of Dublin. This presented him with acute problems in the political sphere with which he had to cope. In the ecclesiastical area he is known to have improved religious discipline and to have introduced a chapter of Augustinian canons into Christ Church cathedral [the order of canons followed the Arroasian rule and was there until the Reformation] but his relationship with various churches apart from the cathedral is not so well known. However, two items from his period as archbishop, that are relevant to our purpose here, are extant.

First, there is a copy of a charter, dated 1178, in which archbishop Lorcán gives 'half of Rathnahi' to Christ Church (Rathnahi is an alternative name for *Tech Nath Í*, later Taney); second, there is a copy of a letter sent to archbishop Lorcán by pope Alexander III on 20 April 1179. In it he confirms him in his possession of '*medietatem de Tignaî*' ('half of Tignai' i.e. half of Taney). Here we see an early indication of the land owned by the archbishop (it was part of what was called 'the archbishop's manor of St Sepulchre') in the area; some of this bounded the river that flows down through Farranboley, in Windy Arbour and into the Dodder at Milltown. This river, now called the Slang (Slann) or Dundrum river, was called Sachaill or Sacoyle in medieval documents.

In the 13th century the archbishop of Dublin granted some of his possession in Taney to the archdeacon of Dublin in exchange for land at Lusk. This included the church (i.e. church and parish) of Donnybrook of which Clonskeagh was then a part but did not, it would appear, include the land in Farranboley. The archbishop's manor of St Sepulchre still had 80 acres of Taney land there in 1326. At a later period, in 1547, an Inquisition (i.e. a formal inquiry) found that the possessions of the archdeacon of Dublin included, *inter alia,* the tithes that issued from the townland of 'Rebow'; those would have included the tithes which came from Clonskeagh, in the townland of Roebuck. It would appear, therefore, that Clonskeagh would have been within the 'half of Tignai' which was confirmed as being in the possession of archbishop Lorcán by pope Alexander III in 1179 but later passed into the possession of the archdeacon of Dublin. Otway-Ruthven, who carried out a detailed study of the land owned by the church in county Dublin in the medieval period, has placed Clonskeagh, in the parish of Donnybrook, clearly in the archbishop's manor of St Sepulchre at the end of the 12th century. She similarly placed Farranboley, in the parish of Taney, in the same manor. Both of these parishes refer, of course, to the respective civil parishes. The ancient distinction between Clonskeagh and Farranboley, whereby both were first in the archbishop's manor of St Sepulchre but went their separate ways when the former was part of the Taney possessions which were granted to the archdeacon of Dublin in the 13th century while the latter remained in the archbishop's manor, was reflected right up to the time when the new Catholic parish of Clonskeagh was in the course of being erected in 1953; (the distinction, it should be pointed out, survived only in terms of the parish to which they belonged, not in ownership of possessions). Most of that new parish, as will be seen, was carved out of the then parish of Donnybrook but Farranboley, Windy Arbour and Mulvey Park were transferred to it from Dundrum parish which had evolved from Taney.[11]

The history of the church in Clonskeagh during the medieval period and right up to the modern era is to be found in that of Donnybrook and Taney (also Dundrum in the later period). Both of these have already been written, the former by Dr Donnelly, the latter by F E Ball & E Hamilton; it is only necessary here, therefore, to give an overview but with particular reference to that which pertains to Clonskeagh and to the period after which they wrote i.e. only developments in the twentieth century. Prior to the Reformation, there is only one ecclesiastical history of the area; thereafter there are two. This complicates matters.

REFORMED CHURCHES IN THE AREA

The archdeacon of Dublin who, as we have seen, was granted part of the archbishop's manor of Taney, remained as rector of Donnybrook until 1864 when it became a parish independent of Taney by order in council (i.e. the Privy council). He also remained rector of Taney until a similar order, made in 1851, replaced the arrangement with the archdeacon and installed an incumbent. The last such archdeacon, Venerable John Torrens, DD, lived at Richview, Clonskeagh for a few years before his death and another Clonskeagh resident, Francis Blackburne, then lord chief justice of the Queen's Bench, was one of the Privy councillors who signed the order. The list of the archdeacons who had been rectors together with those who replaced them, along with their chaplains and curates, at both Donnybrook and Taney are conveniently given by Leslie

---

11   Ailbhe MacShamhráin, 'The emergence of the metropolitan see of Dublin, 1111-1216' in James Kelly & Dáire Keogh (ed) *History of the Catholic diocese of Dublin* (Dublin 2000) 51-71:59-60; Maurice P Sheehy (ed), *Pontificia Hibernica: medieval papal chancery documents concerning Ireland* (2 vols, Dublin 1962) i 27; Ronan, 'History of the Diocese', 27, 32-7; Leslie & Wallace, *Clergy of Dublin and Glendalough*, 92; A J Otway-Ruthven, 'The mediaeval church lands of co. Dublin', in J A Watt, J B Morrall & F X Martin (ed), *Medieval studies presented to Aubrey Gwynn SJ* (Dublin 1961) 54-73: 54-8, 72-3; Holy Cross Centenary Committee, *Centenary of Holy Cross Church, Dundrum* (Dublin 1978) 32; personal comm. from Dr Charles Smith.

and Wallace in their work, *The clergy of Dublin and Glendalough*. In this a brief history of these parishes in the modern period is also given. The present Church of St Mary in Anglesea road, Donnybrook, was built in 1827 and licensed for Divine Service on 1 April 1830. The old church was demolished and its materials disposed of to the great indignation of many of its parishioners. One of rectors of the new church, Rev Arthur Gore Ryder DD, lived, from 1872 to 1878, at Beechhill during which time he was made a canon of Christ Church cathedral. Shortly before St Mary's got its licence, a new church was built on Sandford road, Ranelagh, quite near the city end of Clonskeagh. In fact there is a record of the sexton of this church, Philip Rynard, living in Clonskeagh in 1842. This church was paid for completely by one man, George Sandford, who lived in England. It was consecrated on 25 June 1826 and was given a parochial district from the parishes of St Peter and Donnybrook in 1858. It remained a Trustee church until 1907 when it was vested in the Representative Church Body.

The new church in Taney was constructed between 1815 and 1818 in which year it was consecrated on 21 June. Some people from the Clonskeagh area contributed to the fundraising for its furnishing: pews were bought in 1816 by Daniel Kinahan, Robert Turbett, George Thompson, James Thompson, James Crofton and Alderman Exshaw. Further contributions were made, when the south gallery was erected in 1833, by Lady Harty and Mr M'Caskey. George Kinahan of Roebuck park presented 'a handsome stone pulpit' while W J Goulding of Roebuck hill erected a 'beautiful painted window in the north gallery' to the memory of William Goulding, formerly MP for Cork (1817-84). Also, a number of people from the Clonskeagh and Roebuck area were church-wardens there: Alexander Jaffray (1793); James Potts (1794); John Exshaw (1795/6); Daniel Kinahan (1787, 1824); George Thompson (1804, 1814, 1817/18); Robert Turbett (1804); James Crofton (1807/8, 1822); Humphrey Minchin (1819, 1820, 1821); Robert Billing (1821); John Maconchy (1823); Joseph McDermott (1825); William M'Caskey (1827, 1831); Arthur Burgh Crofton (1829, 1835); John Goddard Richards (1829); George Kinahan (1830,); John Elliot Hyndman (1833, 1838); James Turbett (1833, 1855); Daniel Kinahan (1834, 1836, 1840); William Lewis (1842); Charles Pickering (1848, 1858); William Stanley Purdon (1850); William Lewis (1853); Edward Perceval Westby (1856, 1859, 1864, 1868, 1870, 1874, 1875); Edmund D'Olier (1859, 1861); John Davis Garde (1863); George Kinahan (1865, 1868); Robert Turbett (1865); John Reilly (1869, 1872, 1873); Henry Darby Griffith (1878, 1879). In 1874 a Chapel of Ease was inaugurated at Mount Merrion and became an independent parish in 1956. The old church, dedicated to St Nath Í, was consecrated on 8 June 1760; it is still used for services after its restoration in the twentieth century.

Apart from the Church of Ireland, there was also a Presbyterian meeting-house in Donnybrook at one time. In fact, a Presbyterian minister was one of the early residents of St James' terrace, Clonskeagh. From 1866 to 1895 Rev Hope M Waddell live at no. 4 and was joined there by another Presbyterian minister, Rev William Robb in 1878. Rev Waddell retired c. 1884. It is not clear, however, whether they served in Donnybrook or not. The evidence for the existence of a meeting-house only relates to the period before the 1850s. There was also a Wesleyan Methodist chapel on Beaver row in the nineteenth century. It is clearly marked on the first printed Ordnance Survey map of the area (published in 1843). The building still exists although it is no longer used for worship. It is on the list of protected buildings set out by Dublin City Council and is located at the rear of house no. 9 on Beaver row. Both of these places of worship would have served their members who lived in Clonskeagh. [12]

POST-REFORMATION CATHOLIC CHURCH IN THE AREA

Turning now to the other side of post-Reformation history, the passing of the act of uniformity, six years after Elizabeth I came to the throne, offered two choices: conform or go underground. For those who chose the latter the first sign of the active existence of their church came in 1615 when a synod was held in Kilkenny under archbishop Matthews who was then in the see of Dublin. As a result, the old parishes of Donnybrook, Stillorgan, Kilmacud and Taney were united as one parish. In 1630 it was reported that forty people attended mass at the Donnybrook church; the priest's name was given as John Cawill (Cahill). A few decades later, after the arrival of Oliver Cromwell, it was recorded in the Fleetwood Survey that the townland of Rabuck was the property of Matthew, lord baron of Trimleston 'Irish papist' and that the tithes, which we have already noted belonged at an earlier time to the archdeacon of Dublin, were now the property of 'the Colledge of Dublin' i.e. TCD. There is no direct reference to the religious persuasion of the people of Rabucke in the census of 1659. Around 1685 there was a priest called Patrick Gilmore attached to Donnybrook and Booter-stown; probably, in 1704, one called Richard Fox and possibly, in 1727, one called Mr Barry. We are on safer ground when we say that Francis Archbold was parish priest in 1729. He lived in Irishtown where, according to the findings of a government inquiry, he had a mass-house but no 'convent ... of fryars or nuns

---

12 Leslie & Wallace, *Clergy of Dublin and Glendalough*, x, 92-95,234-35, 247-49; Donnelly, *Short history of someDublin parishes*, vol i, 25; Ball & Hamilton, *The parish of Taney*, 3, 53-8, 63-4, 93-5, 229, 234-5; *Thom's Directory* for various years. My thanks to Councillor Dermot Lacey for information about the location of the listed structure, the Methodist chapel, on Beaver row.

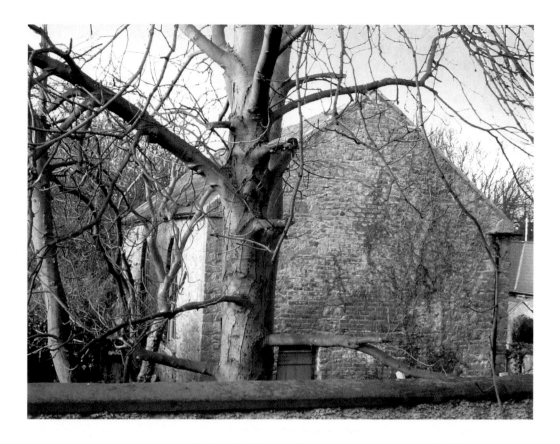

Disused Methodist church, rear of Beaver row: now a listed building

nor popish schoolmaster'. He was succeeded by Dr Mathias Kelly who had entered the Irish college in Rome in 1733, later in 1740 becoming a Doctor of Sacred Theology. He lived at Booterstown leaving a Father Brady as curate for Donnybrook. From the time he was succeeded by Fr James Nicholson in 1775 the records of incumbency begin clearly and a list of the pastors, from his time until Clonskeagh parish was created mainly out of Donnybrook parish, are conveniently set out in the commemorative book produced to celebrate the centenary of the Sacred Heart church in Donnybrook in 1966.

FIRST DIVISION OF PARISH – 1787

In 1787 the parish was divided and Booterstown was separated from Donnybrook; the boundaries between the two remained almost intact at the time Dr Donnelly was writing (1912). Fr Nicholson was now the parish priest of Booterstown and Dundrum and Fr Clinch of Donnybrook, Irishtown and Ringsend. There is no mention at this point about Clonskeagh but it seems most likely, given the subsequent situation, that it was included within the Donnybrook section of the parish. During Fr Clinch's tenure, a new chapel was built in the old graveyard beside the original St Mary's which by now, of course, was Protestant. In 1792 Fr Finn was appointed parish priest and held the position until 1849. He, like his predecessor, was a product of the Franciscan University of Louvain. Living in Irishtown, he completed the chapel begun by Fr Clinch; it was held by lease from lord Downes in trust to a local man, Mr J Madden. In *Thom's Directory* in the 1840s it is described as being 'a plain edifice'. In 1802 Fr Finn presided at Daniel O'Connell's marriage to his (Fr Finn's) second cousin, Mary O'Connell.

At some date between 1825 and 1830 an adjustment was made to the parish boundaries. For years the Swan stream had served as one of these but gradually had become covered in; one of the few reminders today of its underground existence is Swan place, off the city end of Morehampton road. The Grand Canal, opened in 1791, was more visible so it was used as the boundary instead thus incorporating into the parish the territory between the canal and the covered in Swan river; this included an area as far as Lansdowne road. In 1831 a census was taken giving the numbers of Catholics in Donnybrook parish but, unfortunately, being based on the civil parish of Donnybrook it did not include those people who lived in the Taney and Roebuck end of the Catholic parish. Similarly, in a government inquiry in 1833 into the condition of the poor which elicited information from Fr Finn, no specific mention is made of the same end of his parish, apart, that is, from a comment that his parish took in 'a considerable portion of the [civil] parish of Taney – part in the Co. of Dublin, and part in the County of the City'.

NEW CHURCHES BUILT

As the city was expanding outwards beyond the canal, the first public indication that it was planned to build a new church in Haddington road appeared in the *Freeman's Journal* in 1835. Fund-raising had begun and among those who had already contributed £10 each were two men from Clonskeagh, Richard Corballis, Rosemount and John Power, Roebuck house. The latter was voted chair of the fund-raising committee in 1837 since funds were slow in coming in although the building of the church was progressing satisfactorily; though incomplete it was blessed by archbishop Murray, dedicated to St Mary and opened in 1839. It was now the largest and principal church in the parish of

Donnybrook; hence its dedication. Fr Finn, however, who by now had the assistance of curates, remained living at Irishtown. After fifty seven years as parish priest he died on 28 June 1849.

His replacement, Dr O'Connell, the first Maynooth man to hold the position, chose, instead, to live in rented accommodation close to Haddington road church, the completion of which fell to him. As well as that he commenced the building of a boys' school in unused ground around the church with the foundation stone being laid in July 1850 by John Power of Roebuck house, Clonskeagh; Power was, by this time, a baronet. Dr O'Connell had already announced, two months earlier, that it was proposed to build a new church which would be called 'The Church of the Star of the Sea', since the old church in Irishtown was in a state of dilapidation. The foundation stone was laid the following year and it was consecrated in 1853. With the continuing expansion of the parish more curates were assigned to it, one of whom- Dr Moran – was shortly thereafter made a bishop.

The new church at Sandymount was, however, farther away from Ringsend than was its predecessor at Irishtown. The parish priest, therefore, resolved to build a new church closer to it and in 1858 he laid the first stone. It was consecrated by archbishop Cullen in the following year and dedicated to St Patrick. With all these churches having been built in the parish in such a relatively few years attention now turned towards building a new church in Donnybrook. The resident curate there at the time, Rev P J Nowlan, (possibly the Rev P Nolan CC who lived for a time in Clonskeagh, at no. 8 Vergemount) waged a vigorous and successful campaign to have the Donnybrook Fair, which by this time had gained for itself a very unenviable reputation, finally abolished. Plans for the new church began on 12 August 1860 with a public meeting in the old church; at that meeting a substantial amount of funds were contributed, R Corballis of Clonskeagh, according to Donnelly, giving £50. However, it would seem that it was John Richard Corballis (1796-1879) who made the donation, possibly in memory of his father, Richard (1769- 1847), who was dead at the time the contribution was made. He also gave the stained glass windows that are to this day to be seen in the apse behind the main altar on which can be read 'Pray for Richard R Corballis and his deceased relatives'. Fr Nowlan was particularly adept at fund raising, managing to get a clock from the Empress Eugenie of France which raised £1140 in a widely publicised draw. The architects Pugin and Ashlin were engaged, the first stone was laid in 1863 and the church was dedicated by archbishop Cullen, who had just two months earlier got Ireland's first red hat as cardinal, on 26 August 1866, the day on which for so many years previously Donnybrook Fair had been held. The Catholic people of that part of Clonskeagh which was in the parish had now got a splendid new church.

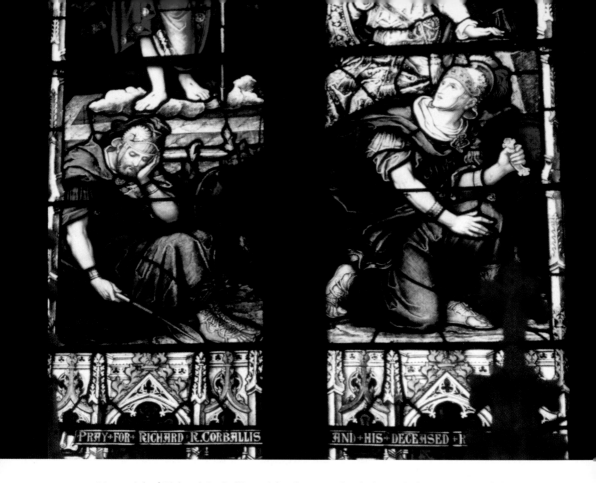

PRAY+FOR+ RICHARD R.CORBALLIS

AND+HIS+DECEASED+R

Memorial of Richard Corballis and family on stained glass windows in apse of the Catholic church in Donnybrook (*Photographer: Matt Walsh*)

DIVISION OF THE PARISH

The expansion of the city, the increase in the numbers of parishioners and the growth in confidence of the Catholic church had seen four new churches erected over a relatively short period of time in the parish of Donnybrook, Irishtown and Ringsend. Now, in 1876, for the first time since Booterstown and Dundrum had separated from it in 1787, the parish itself was divided into three parishes centred on the new churches in Haddington road, Donnybrook and Sandymount; for the time being, the church in Ringsend went with Haddington road as a chapel of ease. After this division the parish of Donnybrook was, naturally, much reduced in size. Dr Donnelly gives the boundaries of the parish as it then stood: '(They) extend citywards as far as Dartmouth square, on Upper Leeson street, and with Clyde road to Balls Bridge proceed up Merrion road as far as the footpath leading to Stillorgan road, thence by a stream to Roebuck, on to the Clonskeagh road as far as Sallymount avenue, and so back to Upper Leeson street'. It is most likely that this stream is the one that can be seen on the right hand side of the path which is inside the door from Roebuck road to UCD land (opposite Harlech grove); the old boundary wall of Mount Dillon, later Mount Carmel and now St Kilian's German school is on the left. That being so, the current parish of Clonskeagh ends at this stream. Another possibility, though less likely, is that it could be the stream which flows under the Roebuck road and through the Carmelite monastery; that, however, would have been through what was then private grounds whereas the aforesaid stream was immediately outside this property and beside a path or road which we have already met when discussing the properties accessed by it – Rosemount and Roebuck house (later Roebuck grove).

The next major division of Donnybrook parish that took place was the erection of the new parish of Clonskeagh after a new church had been built there but because that parish would include a part which was taken from Dundrum parish it is necessary to go back briefly to the separation of Booterstown and Dundrum away from the combined parish of Donnybrook, Irishtown and Ringsend in 1787 and follow their subsequent history.

PARISH OF BOOTERSTOWN AND DUNDRUM

Booterstown and Dundrum constituted a single parish after the division of 1787. Its first parish priest was canon James Nicholson. He had only one chapel, located at Booterstown; he visited Dundrum only at station times. He died in 1794. His successor, Fr John Connolly, was a Franciscan who seems to have been a person of particular interest in that he had contacts with people associated with the stirring political events of the 1790s including lord Edward Fitzgerald. He is reputed to have barely escaped arrest when there was a swoop on the United Irishmen meeting in Oliver Bond's house prior to the rising of 1798. It is not clear how much of this is true; Dr Donnelly thinks the story is apocryphal. When he died in 1811 he was succeeded by canon Michael Ryan. Up to his time there was no chapel or mass in Dundrum but now, with Fr Kelly appointed as a curate, efforts were made to build a chapel. Progress was slow and it was not until the incumbency of his successor, canon Patrick Joseph Doyle, that it was dedicated. After his transferral in 1838 the next parish priest, canon John Ennis, reported that there was a boys' and a girls' school attended by between 65 and 80 pupils in Dundrum and two masses were said on Sundays and one on weekdays. A chaplain was appointed when the Central Mental Hospital was opened in

1850. When Fr Farrell became parish priest in 1873 efforts began to replace the old church, now too small for the numbers using it. The result was a new church dedicated in 1879. Its initial cost was £5,274 but that rose to a final figure of £9,420. It was dedicated by archbishop (later cardinal) McCabe on 6 July 1879.

PARISH DIVIDED – 1879; FURTHER DIVISION – 1943

After the church was built and dedicated, a new parish was created in 1879 – Dundrum and Stillorgan with boundary at the Stillorgan road (Dr Donnelly occasionally refers to this as the parish of Dundrum and Kilmacud; an explanation for this confusion is given below). A census carried out by the first parish priest, Fr Joseph Hickey, in 1881 found that there were 2197 Catholics in the parish. The noted priest, Fr Marmion, was a curate there for some time before retiring to become, ultimately, a Benedictine monk. Only one more parish priest is given by Dr Donnelly after Fr Hickey who died in 1889 – canon Edward Matthews – as he was still in place when Dr Donnelly was writing. However, there appears to have been a parish priest in Dundrum immediately before canon Matthews took up his duties – Fr Fagan. The reason for the confusion in Dr Donnelly's report is due to the fact that an adjustment in the parish boundaries took place during Fr Hickey's incumbency; as a result the parish was reduced in size and it then consisted of Dundrum and Kilmacud only. Fr Thomas Fagan was appointed in 1886 followed by canon Matthews in 1888. After him came mgr. canon Plunkett (1889), mgr. canon O'Donnell D D (1904), Richard canon Duggan (1911) and Francis canon Farrington (1924). During the latter's time in office Mount Merrion and Kilmacud were separated from Dundrum in 1943. After that, a new name for the parish appears – the parish of Dundrum. Fr Dominic Ryan was appointed its parish priest in 1949. In the early 1950s he decided that due to growing numbers of parishioners an extension to the church was needed. All efforts were made to retain, as far as was possible, the existing design of the church and the result was a more than doubling of its capacity without doing damage to the proportions of the building. Fr Ryan was succeeded by Denis canon Keogh in 1959 and it was during his predecessor's time as parish priest that part of the parish was assigned to Donnybrook in preparation for its eventual inclusion in the parish of Clonskeagh that was then planned. [13]

---

13   Donnelly, *History of Dublin parishes,* vol i, 7-8, 12-25, 30-31, 41, 44-46, 49, 51-65, 68, 77-78, 105-23; Simington, *Civil survey,* 261; John Kingston et al, *Parish of the Sacred Heart, Donnybrook* (Dublin 1966) 15, 17, 26-31, 36; Centenary Committee, *Centenary of Holy Cross Church, Dundrum,* 20-22.

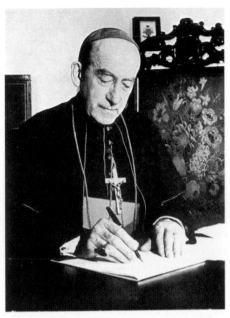

ARCHBISHOP'S HOUSE
DUBLIN 9

24th April, 1966.

I congratulate the priests and people
of the parish of Donnybrook, on the
occasion of their centenary.

Their Church, from being a village
Church, has become a very populous
centre of devotion.

Their parish, distinguished by its
charitable generosity, has now founded
another parish at Clonskeagh.

It is my prayer that, by the inter-
cession of Our Blessed Mother, the
parishioners may continue always
exemplary in their assistance at the
Holy Sacrifice and the reception of the
Sacraments.

+ John C. McQuaid,

Archbishop of Dublin,
Primate of Ireland.

His Grace, Most Reverend John C. McQuaid, D.D., Archbishop of Dublin,
Primate of Ireland.

Archbishop McQuaid and his letter to the priests and people of Donnybrook in which
he congratulates them on the founding of the new parish of Clonskeagh
(*Source: Book celebrating the centenary of the Sacred Heart church, Donnybrook*)

DONNYBROOK PARISH BOUNDARIES ADJUSTED

Just as in the case of Haddington road and Sandymount, it was necessary that a
new church be built in Clonskeagh before it could be hived off from
Donnybrook as an independent parish; for this reason archbishop McQuaid, in
1953, requested its parish priest, Fr Condon, to build a church there. It was also
necessary to make some alterations to the boundaries of Donnybrook parish; so,
on 15 March 1953 archbishop McQuaid transferred Farranboley, Windy Arbour
and Mulvey park to it. By this action, the archbishop, consciously or not,
removed the ancient ecclesiastical distinction between Clonskeagh and Farranboley which had existed since the grant of part of Taney by his 13th century

Clonskeagh, *A Place in History*

predecessor to the archdeacon of Dublin. It should, of course, be noted that Farranboley, as understood in this context, would most likely have coincided with what became the townland of Farranboley; that reaches down as far as the point where Bird avenue meets Clonskeagh road and includes Windy Arbour and Mulvey park. Milltown was also transferred, or more correctly, returned to the Donnybrook parish. It had been part of the parish of Cullenswood, with its church in Beechwood avenue, since being transferred to it from Donnybrook in 1909; this too was in preparation for the setting up of a separate parish of Milltown.

NEW CHURCH BUILT

Events now began to move swiftly. Two new curates were appointed to Donnybrook the day after the parish got new districts; a new curate's house was bought at Rosemount estate, now Rosemount crescent, Clonskeagh some days later. Preparations were made to build the new church on a site donated by the Marist Fathers at the top of Bird avenue. Various events were organised to raise funds; childrens' sports, sales of work, pantomimes, shows, whist drives and many other projects; there was also a system of outdoor collections set up. On 5 January 1954 approval was given for an architects' competition to be put in place for a design for the new church; the result was announced later that year on 5 August. A week later the design submitted by architects Jones and Kelly was formally selected and the following month all the designs submitted went on exhibition in UCD. Two months later, Fr Condon blessed the new site and two weeks after that the foundation stone was blessed and laid; it is still visible under the church's pulpit where its inscription records that the ceremony was performed, at the end of the Marian year on 9 December 1954, by archbishop McQuaid, the parish priest being Timothy B Condon.

Building then got under way; the builders were Messrs Murphy Bros (Dublin) Ltd, Rathmines and the quantity surveyor was Mr Dermot O'Reilly-Hyland. The large amount of ceramic mosaic used in the building was supplied and fixed by Messrs. Ryan and King Ltd., 65 Parnell street; they were also commissioned by L Oppenheimer Ltd., Manchester to fix in position the art mosaic that may be seen on the four main pendentives i.e. the curved triangles formed by the intersection of the dome with its supporting arches each with a representation of the one of the four evangelists; viewed from the main entrance to the church, two of these can be clearly seen over the main altar. The three saucer domes and the apse behind the main altar were also their responsibility. Irish Mosaics Ltd., of Roscommon also worked on the elaborate designs behind the main altar as well as on the gallery mosaic which was assembled from

Venetian glass with a large percentage of gold. Included in their task were the panels surrounding the Stations of the Cross. Sheet copper on the domes was fabricated and fitted by H A O'Neill Ltd., 162 Lower Rathmines road. Suspended ceilings as well as plain and ornamental plasterwork were the work of M Creedon Ltd., South Richmond place, Dublin. The 30 hundredweight bell was supplied by the only bell foundry in Ireland at the time, The Bell Foundry, 42 James street, while the metal furnishings within the church were provided by Gunnings of Fleet street. Interior leaded lights in doors, screens and transomes and exterior fan sashes were supplied and fixed by The Dublin Glass and Paint Co. Ltd., 41 Middle Abbey street. Walton's of North Frederick street and Lower Camden street supplied the church's Lincoln electrical organ. Painting was carried out by Spray Painters Ltd., 138 Capel street and electrical installation was put in place by Bective Electrical Company (Ireland) Ltd., Bective house, Dawson street. The marble altar and the altar railings were the executed by Earley Studios of Ecclesiastical Arts. Finally there were the numerous workers whose names cannot now be retrieved; they too contributed their skills under the general foreman, Mr McNulty, in this very elaborate project. The estimated cost of all the work was £149,000.

DESIGN OF CHURCH

The architects who designed the church describe it as being in the Byzantine style; the distinctive characteristic of this being a dome covering a square space below. The tower, 105 feet high to the top of the dome, creates the impression of control and domination of, in its Byzantine expression, the whole building; it also houses a 30 hundredweight bell. The overall plan of the building is, however, that of a Latin cross. A five light tracery window, executed in stone and glazed with lead lights of varying colour, is a major feature of the front elevation. The church has seven entrances, the main one having a covered loggia outside and three porches inside separated from the nave by mahogany screens and swing doors with access to the organ gallery to the left and the baptistery to the right. The nave ends behind the main altar in a semi-circular apse with semi-dome; this is repeated in the side altars. Inside the three saucer domes in the nave there is a circular panel within each of which there is one of the letters BVM (Blessed Virgin Mary). Side aisles provide good accessibility to seating, confessionals, shrines and to the Stations of the Cross; the latter have their inscriptions in Irish as well as in English. The ceiling is finished in fibrous plaster and the walls are lined with rustic facing bricks. However, the most striking characteristic of the internal appearance is that created by ceramic and artistic mosaics. The mosaic behind the main altar represents the Immaculate Virgin Mary of the

Miraculous Medal to whom the church is dedicated; those behind the side altars feature aspects of the story of the Miraculous Medal. Mosaics are also found, among other places, in the pulpit and on the front and underside of the choir gallery. The main altar, although re-ordered since the architects description was written, is still approached by five steps in black marble riser and white Sicilian marble treads. The altar slab has been brought forward as part of the re-ordering but it still sits on Connemara green columns. The colourful mosaics around the altar complete the Byzantine theme that pervades the whole design.[14]

CHURCH IS CONSECRATED

On Sunday 8 September 1957 the church was dedicated and blessed by archbishop McQuaid. On arrival at the church the archbishop inspected a guard of honour put in place by the South Dublin FCA and members of the Fire Brigade. Among other priests who assisted at the blessing ceremony was Fr Condon, parish priest. He celebrated the Solemn High Mass which followed after the blessing, during which a special choir of Irish Sisters of Charity from Mount St Anne's in Milltown was conducted by Mrs Boylan. General church arrangements were directed by local stewards under the control of Messrs. David Storey, Joseph McInerney, Thomas White and Kevin Somers. That evening a Thanksgiving ceremony was held. After the Rosary, Fr Condon preached and gave Solemn Benediction. The singing of a *Te Deum* concluded the day.[15]

DIVISION OF PARISH

At the time of its consecration the church was, of course, still within the parish of Donnybrook and Fr Condon was parish priest until his death in August 1962. The stress associated with building the church and paying off the mounting debt was, according to some sources, responsible for his death. He was succeeded by Fr C P Crean. While he was in office, in 1965 Clonskeagh and Milltown were split away from Donnybrook and became one parish. In 1966 Donnybrook celebrated the 150th anniversary of its church and on 24 April that year archbishop McQuaid wrote a letter to congratulate the priests and people of the parish and to thank them for their generosity in having founded another parish

---

14   Souvenir, *Blessing and dedication of the Church of the Immaculate Virgin Mary of the Miraculous Medal, Clonskeagh: Feast of the Nativity of Our Lady 8th September, 1957* (Brown & Nolan, Richview press, Clonskeagh, Co. Dublin 1957) unpaginated.

15   'Blessing of new Clonskea church' in *Irish Independent,* Monday, September 9, 1957.

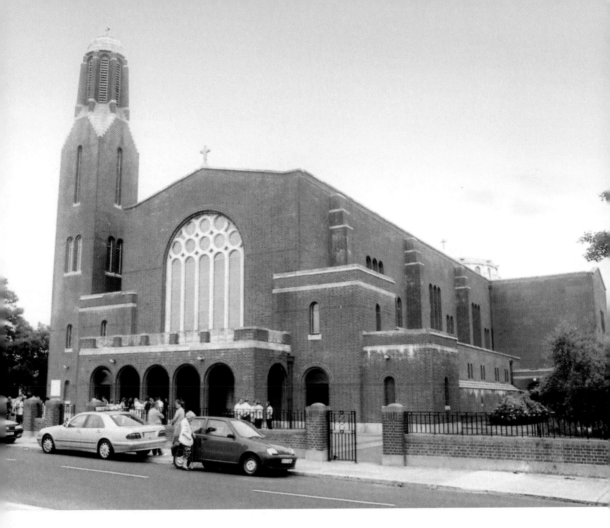

Church of the Immaculate Virgin Mary of the Miraculous Medal, Bird avenue, Clonskeagh (*Photographer: Matt Walsh*)

at Clonskeagh. Subsequently, as the population continued to grow, Milltown was constituted a parish in its own right in 1975. It incorporated within its boundaries parts of the geographical Clonskeagh such as Whitebeam road and Whitethorn road.[16]

16   Clonskeagh church archives, Bird avenue.

15

Schools

THE EDUCATION OF THE CHILDREN of Clonskeagh in the late eighteenth and early nineteenth century saw some differences in approach. It must be remembered that the Roebuck and Clonskeagh of the time was, to quote *Thom's Directory*, 'covered with elegant mansions and demenses', many of its residents obviously quite wealthy. It seems most likely that the children of these people would have got their early education privately from tutors while some would have sent theirs to fee paying schools. We have already noted that in 1807 Richard Corballis of Rosemount sent his young eleven-year old son, John Richard, (probably after he had received his early education from a tutor at home) to the lay section of the Royal College of St Patrick in Maynooth as a boarder. Indeed it would appear that this type of education was being provided for some students in Clonskeagh at a time soon after that date. In the 1830s Rev John Clarke Crosthwaite had a boarding school in Vergemount house; for a few years following that Mr Robert Rogers and later, Mr Eugene O'Meara, had what they termed a 'seminary' at No. 6 Vergemount. None of these enterprises seems to have prospered as they quickly disappear from the sources.

In a later period this type of education would become more widely available for people who could afford it. With the increased expansion of Clonskeagh as a suburb and a growing middle class together with a greater ease of transport many children would travel outside its immediate environs seeking education, something that was enhanced by the advancing demand for secondary education. There were also an extra numbers of schools which offered boarding facilities to which children of the better-off citizens of Clonskeagh could have access. Typical of schools that may have been availed of would be Muckross college, Alexandra college, Gonzaga college and St Columba's college but there were many more.

However, we are here only concerned with the education facilities in Clonskeagh which means, of course, Donnybrook and Dundrum in which parishes Clonskeagh was located. In Donnybrook there were two different types of schools available to Clonskeagh children from the early part of the nineteenth century; a school attached to the Catholic chapel in the village of Donnybrook and schools (male and female) of the Erasmus Smith foundation in what was first called Dodder-bank, Donnybrook and later Beaver-row (from 1869 onwards – although the name Beaver-row already existed in the 1830s and, indeed earlier, as can be seen on Taylor's map drawn in 1816 which also marks the presence of a school there). In the first Ordnance Survey map which was published in 1843 and in the Pembroke Estate Survey map of 1866 it would appear that these schools were located in the first premises one met after passing what later became the tramway depot while going along Beaver-row from Donnybrook towards Clonskeagh; they were opposite the footbridge that crossed the river Dodder but just a little further on towards Clonskeagh.

ERASMUS SMITH SCHOOLS IN DONNYBROOK

Erasmus Smith was an Englishman, born in 1611, who made a substantial amount of money as a merchant and as an army contractor. This money he used to speculate in confiscated Irish land after the 1641 Rising and the subsequent Cromwellian war in Ireland. As early as 1657 he began to devote some of his vast wealth to education in Ireland but an education with an avowedly religious (at this stage Presbyterian) aim. He managed to retain his wealth when the monarchy was restored in 1660 but the schools reflected the changed situation; their religious outlook was now that of the established church with their school-masters licensed by the bishop of the diocese in which they were located. A royal charter granted in 1669 marked the foundation of the Trust fund for his work in education which at that time supported grammar schools in which preparation for entry to Trinity College Dublin was given. Erasmus Smith died in 1681. However, in 1723 an act of Parliament was passed which allowed funds from the Trust to be used to found English (primary) schools. By the early nineteenth century most of the funding was going to these schools. One of their main aims was to convert children to English ways and to the Protestant religion, something which, needless to remark, was resented by the Roman Catholic clergy. This aim (especially the religious one) was, of course, unevenly pursued, some putting it diligently into practice while others were at most lukewarm in following it. It seems likely that the latter prevailed in the Donnybrook since, as we will see, some Catholic children did attend for a time. When one of these schools was being planned, a local contribution was expected to be made. This would be supplemented by a grant of something like £300 from the Trust. Some of the pupils attending such schools would get free education; others might be charged a penny a week to cover school repair costs.

However, the school in Donnybrook was different; it came directly under the Trust itself. It was a large school, founded in 1814 at a cost of £2,063 paid in total by the Trust; it had been proposed by the Treasurer of the Trust, lord chief justice Downes, whose family had lands there (the old Catholic chapel in Donnybrook was built on land leased from the same family as was, most likely, the first Catholic school). All children attending were educated free of charge and, as has already been noted, there were separate boys' and girls' schools. Rules governing the operation of the schools were issued from time to time. One such, in 1820, forbade the employment of Roman Catholic masters; neither were 'Methodists or other Sectarians' to be appointed as masters. From 1827 a system of school inspection was commenced. When the national school system was introduced by chief secretary Stanley in 1831 the established church was largely opposed to it despite the fact that its archbishop of Dublin was one of its supporters. The Erasmus Smith foundation was also against the new system and did not join; it continued to fund its own schools in parallel with the new schools which were then being founded by the established church.

The Trust discontinued its connection with the Donnybrook schools in 1874; soon after (from 1877) they are referred to in *Thom's Directory* as 'National Schools' although, curiously, the directory in its general description of Donnybrook (i.e. the description given under each heading after which detailed listings of streets are given) continued well into the twentieth century to state that 'There are schools of Erasmus Smith foundation' there.

The following are some of the names of those in charge of these Donnybrook schools at various dates during their existence as given in *Thom's Directory* together with assorted details when they can be found. There is a variation in the titles which they have assigned to them over this period. The use of the title 'superintendent' for a time would suggest that the Lancaster Plan of teaching (this method of teaching will be explained shortly) was in use in the school while this title was in use:

> **1838** Mr Thomas Wilson and Mrs Wilson, superintendents; **1848-1860** Thomas L Aldridge and Mrs Wilson, superintendents (Mr Aldridge lived in Donnybrook village, East Fair Green); **1861-1862** Thomas L Aldridge, master and Mrs Frances Bernard, mistress with Rev. Frederick Fitzgerald, superintendent (Rev Fitzgerald was also Incumbent of the Parish of St Mary's, Simmonscourt and teacher of Donnybrook Sunday School. Mrs Frances Bernard lived in Donnybrook village); **1863- 1864** James Morrow, master and Mrs Frances Bernard, mistress with Rev Frederick Fitzgerald, superintendent; **1865-1866** James Morrow, master and Mrs Frances Bernard, mistress (James Morrow lived on Donnybrook road i.e. from Upper Leeson street to

Donnybrook village); **1867** Charles Bryan, master and Mrs Frances Bernard, mistress; **1868-1869** James N Farquhar, master and Mrs Frances Bernard, mistress; **1870-1871** Mrs Frances Bernard, mistress and James Ramsey, master (it may be significant that from this time until 1875, during the period when the schools finished their connection with the Erasmus Smith foundation, Mrs Bernard's name is given ahead of the master's name. She may have become the head of the school during this period); **1872-1875** Mrs Frances Bernard, mistress and John Elliot, master; **1876** Miss Burke, mistress (this is the last entry in *Thom's Directory* where the schools are called Erasmus Smith schools. Reduction to one teacher suggests a falling in numbers of scholars attending); **1877-1885** Miss M A Burke, mistress (title of schools from now on is 'National Schools'); **1886-1888** Miss Barber, mistress; **1889-1891** William Vaughan, master; **1892-1894** George Griffin, sexton; **1895-1935** Samuel McElroy, BA, RUI, teacher and Robert Luke, assistant teacher – sexton (sexton only from 1905); **1936-37** F MacPhilib, teacher and sexton, Robert Luke; **1938 -59** Robert Luke, sexton. It would appear that at least from 1937 when the last teacher is listed in the directory that the schools were in decline. Robert Luke continued on until around 1959 as sexton only, a period of well over sixty years; thereafter the entry in the directories is simply 'National school' with no teacher or sexton named, presumably because it was now just a building. Then, from 1969, it disappears altogether.[1]

CATHOLIC SCHOOLS IN DONNYBROOK

For the greater part of the nineteenth century there was a Catholic school in Donnybrook although there would appear to be some dispute as to its location. Some people have expressed the opinion that it was in Belmont court which is just behind what is now Madigan's licensed premises; this was known as Barrack Yard, as the police barracks were behind where the public house now is. Others think it was at the rear of the Crescent, or near the old chapel and graveyard. Although it is not marked in any of the early 19th century maps, the latter location was, as will be seen, the most likely location. Although it has not been possible to find the exact date of its foundation it is possible to make some reasonable assumptions about it.

In 1830, before he made a visitation to the combined parish of Irishtown and Donnybrook, the archbishop of Dublin, Dr Murray, sent out a questionnaire to

1 Pembroke Estate Papers at the National Archives, Parish of Taney: 97/46/4/31 Map 1; W. J. R. Wilson, *Faithful to our Trust: a history of the Erasmus Smith Trust and The High School, Dublin* (Dublin 2004) 13-28, 39, 67-8, 81-91, 100; *Dublin Almanac* for 1834, 35, 36, 37, 38; *Thom's Directory* from 1848 onwards.

the parish priest about the state of the parish; it should be noted that the parish at that time included parts of Clonskeagh, both on the county and the city sides of the bridge. One of the questions concerned the situation regarding schools in the area. His answer was as follows: 'There are three or four small schools in the parish where parents pay for the education of their children. There is a Sunday school in Sandymount, the Catholics do not attend it. There is an Erasmus Smith school in Donnybrook, but the Catholics have discontinued going there. There are two free schools in Irishtown for boys and girls. The boys' school is supported by a charity sermon and the contributions of the school, but chiefly by a collection made every Sunday through the parish. On an average 80 boys receive instruction in it – the master's name is Christopher Leeson. 70 or 80 children are generally in the girls' school – it is supported by a penny a week from them, which is, however, not insisted on – and in every respect by Mrs Verschoyle who pays the rent and gives a salary to the mistress. Her name is Mary Gravenor. There is a boys' free school in Donnybrook, at which on an average upwards of 70 boys attend. There is also an evening school kept by the same master. This is supported, like that at Irishtown, by its share of the product of the charity sermon – a penny a week from the boys, which many, however, do not pay, but chiefly by some subscribers and a Sunday collection made in that part of the parish. The master's name is Michael Carroll. There is a very good school for girls in Donnybrook and a schoolhouse, at which there are sometimes 120 children. They are furnished with books and every requisite for education, free of any expense. It is supported by subscription from some respectable families in the neighbourhood, many of whom attend frequently and assist in the education of the children. The name of the mistress is Agnes Gaffney'.

There is a possible clue in this statement which may allow us to assume an approximate date for the foundation of the school attached to the Roman Catholic chapel. When the parish priest, Rev C J Finn, states that Catholics have discontinued going to the Erasmus Smith school it is possible to assume that the reason for this was that a Catholic school had been provided for them in the meantime. That would place the foundation date at some point after the arrival of the Erasmus Smith school in Donnybrook in 1814 and probably some number of years after that date. The most likely date would be during the time when the Rev Thomas John Baptist Grosvenor was a curate in the parish between 1825 and his death on 4 November 1827. The reason for this is that this man, before he became a priest and was assigned to Irishtown/Donnybrook, had been a follower of Edmund Rice and was a Christian Brother for a number of years. Furthermore, he had been in charge of the Christian Brothers' school in Hanover street east and, as the plaque erected to his memory in the chapel of Donnybrook after his untimely death noted he had been 'for several years

Superior in the City of Dublin of the Religious Society of Christian Schools' before leaving to become a priest. It is, perhaps, also worth noting that during his time as a priest most of his energy was deployed in the Donnybrook part of the parish.

As regards the type of education which the children received, Joseph Redmond has written 'It is very probable that the Lancaster Plan, which was introduced into Ireland in 1805, was the method of teaching employed. One teacher, or superintendent, with a number of pupil teachers, or monitors, taught one subject all day, and every day, until the pupils had a certain facility with it. English reading came first; this was followed with spelling, and that was followed with writing before any arithmetic at all was taught. It often happened, therefore, that a large number of pupils left school with no knowledge of arithmetic whatever. Illiteracy continued to be widespread until late in the century. In 1871 in a parish population of 13,361 of all denominations, 8,837 could read and write, 1,047 could read only, leaving 3,375 illiterates.'

The parish priest's report for Dr Murray, already discussed, does not identify the location of what appears to be two separate schoolhouses, one for boys and one for girls. However, it seems most likely that they were both on the grounds of the old chapel which had been in close proximity to where the garda barracks now exists i.e. beside the old graveyard. *Thom's Directory* (from 1848 to 1871) simply states that there was a school 'attached to the Roman Catholic chapel'; being 'attached' must mean physically attached not in some way merely 'associated with' (i.e. under the control of) something that would not be necessary to state. Its reference to a school, in the singular, need not rule out the possibility that there were in fact two separate schoolhouses there; although they are not easily read, maps of the period suggest that there was sufficient room there for them. The building of the new chapel in the 1860s (it was consecrated on the 27th August 1866) meant that the old chapel with its schoolhouses attached was made redundant. This is probably the reason why, some years later, a new school was built in the grounds of the new chapel (now sometimes called a church rather than a chapel in public sources perhaps because of the grandeur of the new building in contrast to the plain exterior of the old one).

It is not surprising, given what has already been discussed in Chapter 9 about John Richard Corballis and his involvement with the new national education system and given that he was a wealthy parishioner, that he would provide the funds for the building of this new school. And perhaps it was because he was born in the Clonskeagh part of the parish that he would specifically lay down that the school was for the education of boys from Clonskeagh as well as those from Donnybrook as stated on a plaque erected on the school building. This building still exists and serves as a parish centre.

In 1870 an application was granted for the new school in the townland of Belville. It then consisted of one room only. While funds to build it were provided, as we have said, by J R Corballis the manager undertook to contribute £10 a year towards the payment of the teacher, and to meet the cost of repairs. Pupils were expected to pay one or two pennies a week but many of them were simply unable to pay this. They were, nevertheless, admitted on the authority of the parish priest who was the manager. There were one hundred and eight pupils present on a particular day when the school was visited by an inspector of the Board of Education. One hundred and eight pupils squeezed into one room of approximately 160 square feet gives a fairly clear indication of the problems which beset the teacher of the day as he tried to educate these children. Furthermore the children had to endure such crowded conditions from 10 o'clock until 2.30 pm each day.

It is perhaps the action of J R Corballis, in funding the new boys' school in Donnybrook for boys from Clonskeagh as well as from Donnybrook, that spurred the compilers of the directories to include from 1868 onwards in the descriptive part of the Clonskeagh entry the note 'There is a male and a female National school [there]'. This followed the initial part of the description which stated 'Clonskeagh, a village in the parish of St Mary's, Donnybrook ...'. It seems almost certain that the compiler is referring to the schools which were in Donnybrook although taken in isolation the note would appear to suggest that they were actually located in Clonskeagh. There is certainly no specific reference to schools in the listings which appear under the heading of Clonskeagh. Why this information did not appear earlier in the same descriptions that had appeared for quite a number of years is hard to say; perhaps their appearance in the descriptive section in the Donnybrook entry was thought sufficient. The highlighting of the Clonskeagh use of these schools by the action of J R Corballis may, as we have said, have been the catalyst for the note to be entered when it was. It continued to appear until the last appearance of Clonskeagh as a separate section in the directories in 1907.

In 1892 the parish priest, canon Horris, added one large classroom to the school and that remained the situation until 1964 when the reconstruction work began on the building to bring it into line with modern requirements. The result of this work was that there were then three well-lighted and properly furnished classrooms as well as a teachers' room and the whole building had been provided with central heating. The numbers of pupils attending at that time was 90 and there were three teachers; a considerable improvement on the situation where 108 pupils attended in one room with one teacher in the late 19th century.

It has not been possible to find the names of the teachers of the boys' school in the early period apart from Michael Carroll whom Fr C J Finn mentions in his report to Dr Murray. There is a record of a schoolmaster, James Marren, living at house no. 20 in the village of Donnybrook from 1875 to 1887 but it is not possible to say anything more than that he was probably a teacher at the Catholic school since we know that he was not a teacher at the Erasmus Smith school, the names of whom we know for that time. However, in the more modern period we do know some teachers' names. In 1966 the principal was Mr Henry Browne. He had come from Finglas school in 1944 and succeeded Mr Con Kennedy as principal in 1965. When Mr Kennedy reached retiring age in 1965, he was requested by the parish priest to continue his service beyond the statutory period. The necessary extension having been granted to him by the Board of Education, he continued to serve as assistant principal. Mr Kennedy was a Dublin man who came from the parish of Haddington road, once part of Donnybrook parish. He had started his teaching career, in 1914, as a monitor in the schools of Haddington road parish. In 1917 he began his studies for the diploma at St Patrick's Training College and in 1919 he was appointed junior assistant in Donnybrook where he was to remain for the rest of his career. In 1935, the then principal Mr Kelly, who had held that position for a long period of time, retired and was succeeded by Mr Kennedy. He was principal for the next thirty years until, as we have said, he stayed on after retirement as assistant principal. His exceptionally long association with the school – from 1919 until well after his retirement in 1965– meant that his contribution to education of the youth of Donnybrook, including Clonskeagh, was immeasurable. In September 1980 the boys' school was on the move again. In both of its earlier manifestations it had been built in close proximity to church buildings; at first it was close to the old chapel and later on to the new church where its last principal was Mr Jerry O'Sullivan, a Kerryman. Now it would take its departure to a separate site when it relocated to Belmont avenue where it remains to this day.

As regards the girls' school we have already noted the report given in 1830 by the parish priest, Fr C J Finn, to archbishop Murray in which he stated 'There is a very good school for girls in Donnybrook and a schoolhouse, at which there are sometimes 120 children. They are furnished with books and every requisite for education, free of any expense. It is supported by subscription from some respectable families in the neighbourhood, many of whom attend frequently and assist in the education of the children. The name of the mistress is Agnes Gaffney'.

A few years later a Mr Dillon of Roebuck paid £250 for a house near the old chapel to be used as a girls' school. It has not been possible to identify this Mr Dillon with any degree of precision as there is no one of that name in the appropriate directories of the time. However, shortly afterwards James Dillon Meldon is mentioned; from 1840 to 1841 he is said to have an address called

'Rosemount' not, it would appear, the house of the same name occupied by the Corballis family. In any case, he moved to Casino (at present Mount St Mary's belonging to the Marist Fathers) in 1842 and is listed as living there until 1871. He was a solicitor and his family, originally from Westmeath, also had property in Galway; in fact according to one report, a James Dillon Meldon was from Lackagh, Co Galway and was a Catholic. Whether this is the man who provided the money for the girls' school or not cannot be proved due to lack of supporting evidence.

Apart from Agnes Gaffney, mentioned by Fr Finn in his report, her sister M Gaffney acted along with her as superintendents in the Lancaster Plan for teaching at the school. They were supported by James and Catherine Boyland. In 1835 there were 148 pupils attending and they were taught reading, spelling, writing, arithmetic and needlework. In 1879 the school came under the National Board and when Miss Gaffney retired, in the following year, the school was taken over by the Irish Sisters of Charity. The school was then replaced by a fine two-storey building on a site presented by the Sisters on their grounds in Belmont avenue. During the incumbency of canon Charles Horris (1881-1909) two large classrooms were added. The nuns remained there until 1912 when they handed over the running of the school to lay teachers. In 1966 there were 188 girls and 50 boys under eight years of age on the rolls and a teaching staff of six.

SUNDAY SCHOOL IN DONNYBROOK

It will have been noted from Fr Finn's answer about schools to Dr Murray's questionnaire that there was a Sunday school in Sandymount and that Catholics did not attend it. It may be assumed from this that no such school existed in Donnybrook in 1830. However, there was one there later in the century; from 1848 onwards it is regularly reported in *Thom's Directory*. There it is stated that it was run by the Incumbent of St Mary's parish church in Simmonscourt road. It appears to have had a schoolhouse but its location has not been identified. As for the Presbyterian and Methodist churches, they were both present in Donnybrook; their meeting-house and chapel, respectively, would have served any of their congregation living in Clonskeagh. They would also have provided religious education for their congregations but is not clear where this activity was carried out.[2]

---

2   Donnelly, *History of Dublin parishes,* 24, 27-28; Joseph Redmond, 'The schools of Donnybrook' in Kingston, *Parish of the Sacred Heart, Donnybrook,* 47-51; Kerr, *Emmet's Casino,* 6; various Dublin directories.

SCHOOLS IN DUNDRUM

The first mention of the 'English school' at Taney church is found in 1790. Two years later, the Vestry passed a vote of thanks for a charity sermon preached to raise funds for the school. In the same year Mr Potts of Roebuck, most likely the Mr Potts who lived at Richview, Clonskeagh, was appointed one of two governors of the school which had thirty boys attending. The subsequent history of the school from 1805 onwards can, according to Ball and Hamilton, be easily traced. Among the Clonskeagh treasurers of the school was William McCaskey from 1830 -34 and Arthur Burgh Crofton from 1834-50. In 1838 it was reported that 38 girls were attending school. This continued until a new school was built by lord Pembroke in 1859. According to its lease, it had to remain under Church of Ireland control.[3] As regards Catholic schools in Dundrum a report made by the parish priest canon John Ennis soon after his appointment in 1838 stated that there was a boys' and a girls' school attended by between 65 and 80 pupils in Dundrum at the time, presumably there before he arrived. This school would appear to have been in some rooms at the back of the church. It was necessary to wait until 1944 before a proper school was built. This had twelve classrooms and catered for two hundred pupils. Principal teachers around that time were Mr Andy Walshe and Mrs Buckley; they were succeeded by Mr Pearse Morris and Mrs Harmon. That school grew over the years such that by 1978 there were 26 classrooms and more than one thousand pupils with seventeen teachers for the boys and twelve for the girls. The principals in 1978 were Mr J Foley and Mrs K Deering. With such growth in the numbers attending the school, plans were then afoot to replace it with a completely new building.[4]

MASONIC ORPHAN BOYS' SCHOOL AT CLONSKEAGH

For almost a hundred years the Masonic Orphan Boys' school was located at Richview in Clonskeagh. Its presence over such an extended period is of considerable importance in any study of the Clonskeagh area and requires particular treatment even though the pupils educated there did not necessarily come from the surrounding area. Some of the buildings that were erected during its stay at Richview are still to be seen, now part of the University College, Dublin campus.

---

3   Ball & Hamilton, *Parish of Taney,* 186-91.
4   Donnelly, *History of Dublin parishes,* i. 112-7; *Centenary of Holy Cross church, Dundrum,* 44.

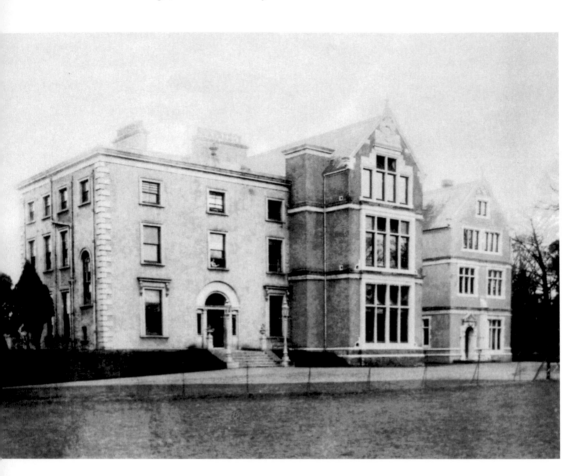

Masonic Orphan Boys' School, Clonskeagh: early 1900s

As for its origins, it was probably the success of the Masonic Girls' school in Ballsbridge, founded in 1792, (it was located where Jury's Ballsbridge hotel now stands) which inspired the foundation of a similar school for boys. The first move was made in 1867 when a meeting of people interested in such a project met to initiate it. Later that year, at a public meeting held on 31 May 1867, the school was founded; a motion was passed 'That a school be established for the support and education of the sons of deceased and deserving members of the Masonic Order under the Irish Constitution, and that a subscription list be forthwith opened for carrying out this benevolent object.' Its first president was the duke of Leinster. However, it also decided that no move to build or purchase a building should be made until the subscription fund had reached £5000. In the meantime, interest on the moneys collected would be used to maintain the boys at an existing school; the one chosen was the Santry Endowed Training school, owned by the Incorporated Society for Promoting Protestant Schools in Ireland, founded by the Church of Ireland. However, conditions there were not considered by the governors of the Masonic School to be satisfactory and the boys' stay at that location lasted only a few years. A sub-committee got to work and after some deliberation it was decided to accept 'for a period of one year' an offer made by Rev A A Skreen, who owned Adelaide hall, Sydney parade. He would maintain, clothe and educate the boys for £40 per boy, per annum; he would be headmaster and his wife matron. The boys moved there in January 1873 and, despite the initial decision, the school remained there for fourteen years. During this period the governors bought out Skreen's interest in the premises, thus gaining their own control over the school. However, there was a problem looming. In the Annual Report for 1884, the following can be found: 'The lease of the present school-house [Adelaide hall] will expire in 1890; but the board confidently expect, with the aid of the brethren, to be in possession of a "new school" long before that time.' Before that Report was written, the governors had already decided that Adelaide hall was no longer suitable and, on 1 November, 1883 a deputation had appeared before the Grand Lodge urging it to seek greater support for the school from the members of the Order throughout Ireland. A member of that deputation, Thomas Fitzgerald, a civil engineer of considerable standing who practiced in Dublin, set about searching for a suitable site for the school.[5]

Fitzgerald was secretary (and the most active member) of a building committee, set up to advance the project. It made two suggestions to the governors in May 1885: a piece of land near Lansdowne road railway station (most likely what is now the Rugby stadium) or Richview in Clonskeagh. The latter, a premises and land, had recently come on the market; it was just outside the city boundary and had a lease of 202 years from lord Trimleston, the ground landlord. Its owner was Charles Barden Hely of Charles Barden Hely, Son & Co, Wholesale and Export Stationers, 17 Dame street, Dublin and the asking price was £4000, excluding the ground rent to be paid to lord Trimleston. The property consisted of a substantial and elegant house (which still exists), a large garden, a wide range of out-offices and twenty two acres, three roods of land. The governors concluded that Richview was the preferable site; in what was then

---

5   J F Burns, *Shop window to the world* (Dublin 1966) 3-12; *The Report of the Masonic Orphan Boys' School of Ireland, Adelaide Hall, Merrion for the year 1884* (Dublin 1885) 4; R E Parkinson, *History of the Grand Lodge of Free and Accepted Masons of Ireland* (2vols, Dublin 1957) ii 223-24.

a rural setting, it was considered to be a healthier location than Landowne road which was considered to be subject to fog. It gave the building committee the go-ahead to complete the purchase. A price of £3500 was agreed with Mr Hely and on May 13, 1885 Richview became the property of the Masonic Order.[6]

In July, the governors unanimously resolved that £500 be lent, from the General Current Account, to the Trustees of the Building Fund to help it in the purchase; money also came in from individuals and lodges throughout the country, some donating as much as £300, others just £1. This allowed the governors to announce in the Annual Report for 1885 (dated March 5, 1886) 'They [the governors] have much pleasure in stating that through the liberality of the brethren, the full purchase has been paid and the amounts borrowed from the General Fund and from the Royal Bank to complete the purchase have been discharged.' The purchase was, however, only the start; much work, both building and alterations, was required to make the property suited to a boarding school. The Report, therefore, goes on to state 'The plans of the alterations and additions have been prepared by Bro. Drew RHA and approved by the board at their February meeting. Tenders for the work have been advertised for, but the building committee do not feel themselves justified in closing with a contractor until a sufficient amount will be subscribed to enable them to pay the usual instalments as they become due.' Nearly £5,000 had been promised by subscribers but almost £1,400 had not yet been paid; a plea was, therefore, made to these people to redeem their promises and allow the work to get underway. A full list of those who had promised sums and those who had or had not paid was annexed to the Report. A sketch of Mr Drew's plans for alterations and additions was also included in the Report.[7]

Money was, however, slow coming in and to add to the building committee's problems work that had not originally been part of the plans had to be tackled. Nevertheless, at the end of 1886 the governors were able to report 'It is a matter of no small gratification that not only has the entire purchase money been paid, but a considerable sum has also been provided towards the making of the necessary alterations. Those alterations are now in progress and it is most confidently hoped that after the summer vacation of the present year, the removal to the new premises will take place.'[8] A decision had been made to

---

6   Burns, *Shop window*, 62-63.
7   *Report of the Masonic Orphan Boys' School of Ireland, Adelaide Hall, Merrion, for the year 1885* (Dublin 1886) 4. Report is dated 5 March, 1886. The Appendix 'Subscriptions to "New School Fund" promised and paid to 20 March, 1886', pp 81ff.
8   *Report of the Masonic Orphan Boys' School of Ireland, Adelaide Hall, Merrion, for the year 1886* (Dublin 1887) 3-4; Report is dated 31 December, 1886.

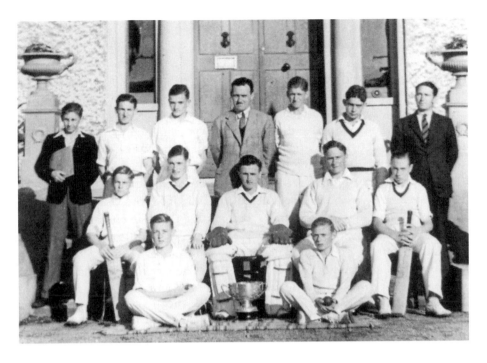

Cricket team of the Masonic Orphan Boys' School, Clonskeagh: winners of the Leinster schools' senior cup 1945

increase the number of students from 35 in Adelaide hall to 60 in Richview; this added to the amount of work that was required to be done there. An extension to the existing house was added to provide a dining hall and two dormitories with bathroom and washing facilities while the out-offices were converted into a schoolroom and a gymnasium. The boys did not move in after the summer vacation of 1887, as confidently predicted, but they did, finally, on 16 January 1888 – after the Christmas vacation. All the improvements had cost around £12,000 and a special appeal met a good response; £10,000 had been raised when the fund finally closed in 1890 and another fund, set up to honour the queen's Golden Jubilee in 1887, brought in £2,500. Apart from the buildings immediately associated with the school, a ball alley was provided and about three acres were allocated for the students to play cricket and football; the rest of the land was used, some for grazing, but mainly to raise the money that was needed to pay the annual head rent so as to leave the school free of this burden. The land used for grazing most likely refers to what was called 'Barney Keogh's field', probably called after a local Clonskeagh man who at some time previously had some title to it. Initially the number of students at the school grew very slowly although demand for places always outstripped capacity. Soon, however, two new dormitories were built; as a result numbers grew to seventy seven. This increase brought other pressures; classroom facilities were found to be inadequate so a campaign to bring about improvements was initiated.

The Century Fund, so-called because a new century, the twentieth, was about to begin, was started and as a result a new school building was erected a short distance south of the original Richview mansion. When completed it was topped by a clock which would become in time a central feature of the school (it is still in place, prominent as it ever was; the building now houses the Richview library of the School of Architecture, of University College, Dublin.). Much of the funding for this building came from Masons in county Antrim and they indicated their close interest in the school when around 400 of them came south in 1897 to pay it a visit. The new building as well as some alterations to existing ones, also paid for by the Century Fund, meant that the school was now very adequately provided for. Apart from the annual cost of running the school, around £28,000 had been spent on Richview between 1887 and 1901; a truly remarkable amount for the time in what was essentially a charitable activity looking after the education of orphans in the era before the welfare state.[9]

With the school now fully set up with all the facilities required, it flourished academically. One issue, however, soon came to the fore. From the outset it had been the policy of the governors that education be provided for the boys only up to the age of 16; at that point they had to leave the school. Secondary education in Ireland at that time was only indirectly funded by the state due to resistance by the churches to its policy of only funding religiously integrated schools. The indirect funding was conducted through an examination board set up under the Intermediate Education Act of 1878. Funds were given to school managers on the basis of success rates of their pupils in public examinations. A progressive headmaster at Richview, James Moore (he had previously taught in both Catholic and Protestant schools; at a later date a new building at Richview would be dedicated to him), seeing the potential for further education in some of his pupils, as a result of performance in examinations, set about the task of getting the governors to change their strict rule relating to the leaving age. In this he had success; in 1908 they agreed that boys who at 16 years of age had passed

---

9   Burns, *Shop window*, 63-71 (two different costs for the original improvements are given: £12,000 on page 63 and £10,086 on page 67, perhaps the latter not including all covered by the former. In any case, it was a very substantial sum for the time); *Report of the Masonic Orphan Boys' School of Ireland, Richview, Clonskeagh, Dublin for the year1887* (Dublin 1888) 3-6; Report dated 31 December, 1887.

either the Junior or Middle grade examinations or were otherwise qualified could remain on in the school, until they were 18 years old, receiving further education to prepare them for competitions such as the Civil Service examination.

Whatever the difficulties James Moore faced in having the strict age rule changed, they were nothing compared to those which he was now about to face. Soon thereafter, the Great War of 1914-18 began and, in Ireland, there was the Easter Rising of 1916, followed by the War of Independence, the Civil War and the emergence of the new state, now no longer in the United Kingdom. Not long after the Great War had begun, Richview started to lose substantial numbers of its teaching staff who joined up for service in France; recruiting replacements was a problem for the same reason. However, one positive side-effect of this was the appointment of the first female teacher. This was so successful that it set a trend for the future with female teachers continuing in her position after she had left Richview. As well as the staff who joined up, around 200 former pupils also answered the call; they served with distinction, many gaining military honours. In the slaughter that characterised that horrific war, fifteen of them lost their lives in Flanders, Gallipoli and elsewhere. Another went down with the *Lusitania,* torpedoed off the Old Head of Kinsale, as he was returning home from America in order to join up. As in so many places, the effect that that war had on those associated with Richview was profound. In characteristic fashion, the memory of those who served in it was commemorated in a practical way; by the building of what was felt to be much needed – a gymnasium and an infirmary. Although a fund to erect these buildings had been subscribed soon after the war, for a variety of reasons they were not opened until 1930. That was only nine years before the outbreak of another horrific war (1939-45) in which 114 ex-pupils of Richview served and eight were killed.

Much nearer home, the Easter Rising in 1916 was to a large extent focussed on the General Post Office in O'Connell street, only three miles from Richview. Despite this, however, the school was physically untouched by any of the destruction that accompanied that Rising; apart from obvious anxiety the only problems endured were associated with getting supplies to keep the boys fed. As for that very basic commodity – bread, then very scarce in Dublin, the school was well looked after by the staff of the bakery, Johnston, Mooney and O'Brien. Later, during the War of Independence and the Civil War, the school carried on without being impeded in any serious way; the only disruption felt was that associated with the travel of the boys to and from the school at vacation time due to the disturbed state of the country.

The emergence of the Irish Free State, however, caused a number of problems for the school since it abolished the Board of Commissioners of Intermediate

Education on 8 June, 1923. State funding was to be no longer based upon the examination performance of pupils; instead it would be on a capitation basis but only when an approved course was followed. In June 1924 the Intermediate Education (Amendment) Act saw the disappearance of the old Junior, Middle and Senior Grades and the introduction of the now familiar Intermediate and Leaving Certificates examinations. Richview adapted well to the new structure of examinations. Under the old system, pupils who performed well in the lower grade examinations were state-funded to go on to the next grade; Richview had developed an arrangement with Mountjoy to cater for these students. This arrangement disappeared under the new system and Richview catered for pupils doing both the Intermediate and the Leaving Certificate examinations. Initial apprehensions about relations with the new Free State Department of Education were not borne out as early reports by that Department about the school were quite complimentary and a good relationship between the two did develop. One particular problem was the introduction of the Irish language into the curriculum. Initially the school successfully faced up to the problem by employing, on a part-time basis, a well-qualified teacher of Irish. However, by 1928 when Irish had become compulsory for passing the Intermediate Certificate, a very substantial number of those presenting for the examination failed because of this barrier despite doing well in the other subjects. This situation lasted until about 1933 when only one pupil failed the Intermediate examination because of going down in Irish. Any inherent antipathy there may have been held towards the language was swept away after the appointment of a full-time teacher of Irish, George W Coghlan, in the early 1930s. The headmaster's report for 1934 indicates that answering at the examinations in Irish was very satisfactory. Thereafter, adjustment to the new political regime was much more straightforward.

Perhaps, somewhat ironically, a greater problem arose for Richview from changes in the law relating to education in the United Kingdom and particularly as it related to Northern Ireland. The British Education Act of 1944 and the subsequent Northern Ireland Act of 1947 brought about radical change; it opened up education to all classes irrespective of their financial position. Up to that time two thirds of Richview's intake of pupils came from the Northern state. Now new competing and attractive options were available to these students nearer to their own homes. Initially there seemed to be no impact on Richview as it continued to have just over 100 pupils, the same number as it had for the previous fifty years. However, by the mid 1960s signs of a decrease in demand for places were becoming apparent.

Given that Richview was a boys' school, it was inevitable that sport would play an important part of its mission. Cricket, and to a less extent, rugby were

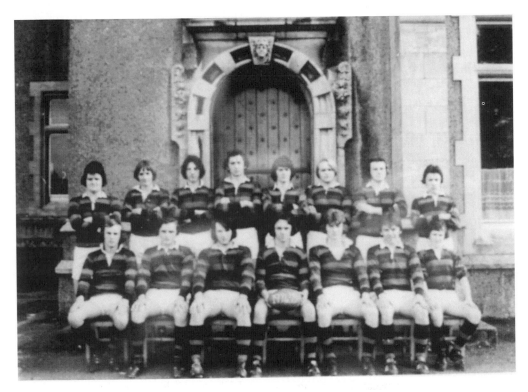

Rugby team of the Masonic Orphan Boys' School, Clonskeagh: senior cup team 1974-75

the games of choice. It would appear that even before the move to Richview, cricket was being played. However, when the move came, the opportunity provided by the great increase in space available gave the game a boost. As early as the 1901 season, the school cricket team was only beaten by one other Irish school. Playing in cup competition sharpened its competence and in 1910, for the first time, it won the Senior Leinster Schools' Cricket Cup, a feat it would repeat fifteen times, while tying once, in the years up to 1966. It was even more successful in the Junior Leinster Cup, won 27 times between the years 1909 and 1966, almost three times as often as its nearest rival, Belvedere, which won it eleven times during the same period.

The school closed in 1981, just short of a century after it had moved to Richview. The buildings and land were sold to University College, Dublin in 1980; the amount of land purchased was somewhat less than that which had been bought for the school in 1885, 17.4 acres against the original 22 acres 3

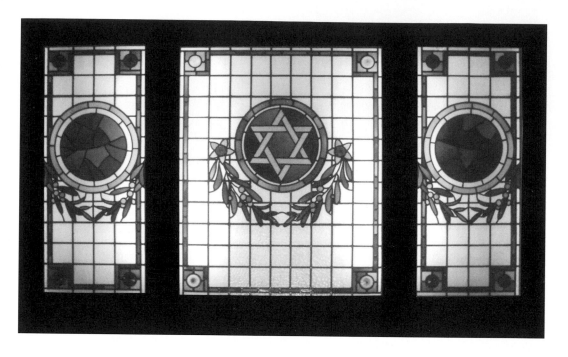

Stained glass window from the Masonic Orphan Boys' School, Clonskeagh now installed in the Library in Freemason hall, Molesworth street (*Photographer: Matt Walsh*)

roods. The buildings became the headquarters of the University College, Dublin School of Architecture. Although much moveable material had been taken to Freemason's hall in Molesworth street where it is prominently on view there remains in Richview many visible signs of the long-term residence there of the Masonic Orphan Boys' school. But perhaps of equal importance is that the original mansion, occupied by James Potts in the latter part of the eighteenth century, still remains intact in all its elegant splendour.[10]

DE LA SALLE SCHOOL

There was a school run by the De La Salle order on Roebuck road from about 1969 to 1980. It was built on land which had previously belonged to the Carmelite monastery and which it then bounded. It was sold to the De La Salle

---

10   Burns, *Shop window*, 85-104, 108-09, 116-17 135-39, 181-82, 225-26; Coolahan, *Irish education: history and structure,* 52-53, 73-76.

brothers at the request of the archbishop of Dublin, John Charles McQuaid. A purpose built school was erected by the brothers and it was used as a primary school for the period which they were there. They had planned to build a secondary school as well but they were refused planning permission. This was apparently the reason why the project was abandoned. The site subsequently passed to Cert Ltd, training centre for the catering business. It used the school building to conduct its training. That organisation remained there until around 1992 after which it was vacant for a short while. In 1994 Muslim schools and colleges are recorded in the directory for that year as being located there. The original De La Salle primary school is now used as an Islamic national school (this latter school is dealt with under the heading of the 'Islamic Cultural Centre of Ireland' in Chapter 16).

OUR LADY'S GROVE

The Congregation of Jesus and Mary run the well-known school on the Goatstown road called Our Lady's grove. This congregation was founded in 1823 by Claudine Thevenet who was born in Lyons, France in 1773. As a young person she had lived through the troubled times associated with the French Revolution; in fact, two of her brothers were murdered during that period. After its foundation, the congregation spread rapidly but it was not until 1912 that its first house was opened in Ireland at Errew House on the shores of Lough Conn. A few years later it moved to the other side of the lake to a large house called Gortnor Abbey. Others houses in Ireland were later founded and a hostel for women students was opened in Galway in 1925. Archbishop McQuaid invited them to open a similar one in Dublin in 1956; this was first located in Sandford road and later for a few years in Milltown. With the expansion of the suburbs in Goatstown/Clonskeagh, the archbishop asked the congregation to provide a school for the children of the area. In 1963 a suitable property was put up for sale; this had been known for many years as Roebuck grove. The congregation bought it and built a school on the site, leaving the original house in place – it is still there today. On 16 May 1966 the new school building was formally blessed and opened by archbishop McQuaid. Although the title was changed to Our Lady's grove, the word 'grove' in the title maintained a link with the historic name of the property.[11]

---

11   *Centenary of Holy Cross church, Dundrum* (1978); Dublin directories.

ST KILIAN'S GERMAN SCHOOL

In September 1972 the Ministry of Foreign Affairs in Bonn sanctioned the purchase of a 9 acre site on Roebuck road from the Carmelite monastery, the aim being to build a new school there for St Kilian's. Prior to that it had been located at St Brigid's house on a 4 acre site at 15 Stillorgan road. The school had emerged from the post-war activities of the 'Save the German Children Society' founded in Dublin in 1945 to provide help for German children who were suffering badly as a result of the war which had just ended. Many of these children were brought to Ireland and were looked after by Irish families. Most returned eventually to Germany but some remained with their foster parents in Ireland. To preserve their mother tongue, German classes were provided for them and out of this came the idea of setting up a German school. The first headmaster was appointed in 1954 and a day school was begun. The school was called after an Irish monk, St Kilian, who preached christianity in Europe in the 7th century and is still honoured to-day in Germany, in particular in Franconia, now part of Bavaria. A special exhibition was organised in Würzburg in 1989 to celebrate the 1300th anniversary of his martyrdom.[12]

The school moved to St Brigid's house in 1957 and a new headmaster appointed. With the extra space available the school expanded and a kindergarten was added. Then a secondary school was mooted as there were then some 60 pupils attending. Although supported by the German government, there was trouble ahead because of its interdenominational and co-educational ethos. In time, however, this was overcome and plans to extend into second level education began again in the second half of the 1960s. The possibility of getting a new school arose but, in the meantime, extra classes were being held in prefabricated classrooms at St Brigid's. By the end of the 1960s the condition of the school and, with the ever expanding numbers of pupils, the limitations of the existing site were a cause for concern. A move to a new site was now strongly considered under the chairmanship of Helmut Clissmann. This resulted in the purchase of the present site at Roebuck road. The site together with that of the Carmelite monastery on which it borders and the Islamic Centre were originally one unit; it was called Mount Dillon before being purchased by the Carmelite nuns in 1878 after which its name was changed to Mount Carmel.[13]

---

12 For the wide range covered by this exhibition and its elaborate extent see: *Kilian: Mönch aus Irland – aller Franken Patron – 689-1989* Katalog der Sonder-Ausstellung zur 1300-Jahr-Feier des Kiliansmartyriums, 1 Juli 1989 – 1 Oktober 1989.

13 For more detail on the history of this site, see the discussion on Mount Dillon.

Initially on arrival at Roebuck road work was begun on the provision of a temporary building. This commenced in April 1973 with seven new prefabs being ready, with only a minor delay, for the start of the school year that September. In the following year the long-planned second level teaching project got underway when, in April, the Department of Education gave permission for pupils to continue to the Leaving certificate examination. In November, the school was officially opened by the then ambassador of the Federal Republic of Germany. A routine inspection carried out in December 1975 for the central department which oversees German schools abroad brought endorsement of progress and a recommendation that further class rooms be built; funding for these came in due course from Germany and they were erected. A school library was added in 1976 and its recently founded orchestra gave its first public performance. A pupils' representative system was set up in 1977 and in June of the following year the first St Kilian's pupils sat their Leaving certificate.

Thoughts were now turning towards getting a permanent school building and an all-weather sports pitch. Then tragedy struck; a fire demolished half of secondary school block on 28 March 1979. However with all hands on deck, the site was cleared and new prefabs were erected in record time. After consultation with the appropriate authorities in Germany, a building committee was set up. It issued invitations in 1980 to a small number of architects to take part in limited architectural competition. The architect selected, Murray Murray Murphy & Partners, Cork, was appointed in December 1981. Some delays were encountered as further discussions were held with authorities in Germany while classes continued to be held in the old prefab building. By 1985, however, construction of the new school was underway and eventually it opened on 8th October 1986. A major milestone in the progress of the school had been reached.

Numbers of pupils now increased even more and also the reputation of the school. Entrance scholarship examinations for the secondary school were introduced and it was decided that there would be separate classes for German and English-speaking pupils at the lower primary level; this would later extend to the higher primary level. Increasing number of classes put pressure on the space available; an extension to the building was needed. With no grant available from Germany, the school set about raising the funds needed. A new extension, supervised by architects Duffy and Mitchell, was added in time for the school year 1994/95. In that year the school had 12 classes at secondary level (6 German, 6 English), 9 at primary (3 German, 6 English) and 3 in Kindergarten. The total number of pupils was 440 and it was felt that it should be pegged at that level (although it would, in fact, expand to around 650). Achievement recorded that year in Leaving certificate and *Deutsche Sprachdiplom Stufe II* (level two in German speaking) examinations was the best to date.

In 2002 the school celebrated its golden jubilee and the president of Ireland, Mrs McAleese attended. The occasion was marked by the official opening of a 9 classroom extension. Throughout those 50 years many dignitaries had visited the school including two presidents of the Federal Republic of Germany. Recently, however, St Kilian's saw a new departure. The *Lycée Français d'Irlande* began to share the premise and as a result, in an agreement between the two schools, it assumed a new name – Eurocampus. This agreement was finalised in May 2005, with both the French and the German ambassadors in attendance. The *Lycée Français* is planning to add more buildings to the school as it expects that there will be an expansion of student numbers in the near future; these buildings are expected to be in place by the start of the 2008/9 school year.

Finally, in May 2006 an agreement was reached between the Department of Education in Ireland and the government of the Federal Republic of Germany on the establishment of a Bilingual Leaving Certificate. Students may now be taught German language and literature using advanced foreign language teaching methods as one subject and history where the Irish part is taught in English but the world and European one is taught in German. If a student passes both of these subjects in the examination, s/he will be awarded this new 'Bilingual Leaving Certificate'.[14]

OUR LADY'S, CLONSKEAGH PARISH NATIONAL SCHOOL

In the late 1940s and early 1950s, with new houses being built or planned for the area around Clonskeagh plans were afoot to erect a new parish to cater for the increase in population that was the inevitable consequence of this expansion. On 15 March 1953 archbishop McQuaid transferred Farranboley, Windy Arbour and Mulvey park to Donnybrook parish as a first step and preparations were put in hand for the building of a new church in the area. A new school was also part of those plans. With that in mind, a site was chosen convenient to the new houses in Farranboley and Mulvey park and near Highfield park.

At the request of archbishop McQuaid in March 1955, the parish priest Fr Condon asked the Irish Sisters of Charity to take charge of this new school; since 1880 they had been in charge of a girls' school at Belmont avenue in his parish of Donnybrook. This they agreed to do and in anticipation of the new school becoming available they set up the first girls' school in the Marian hall, in Milltown. It was located at these premises from 1955 to 1957 and during that time

---

14 St Kilian's school chronicle with added material from the school principal, Mr Rolf Fenner.

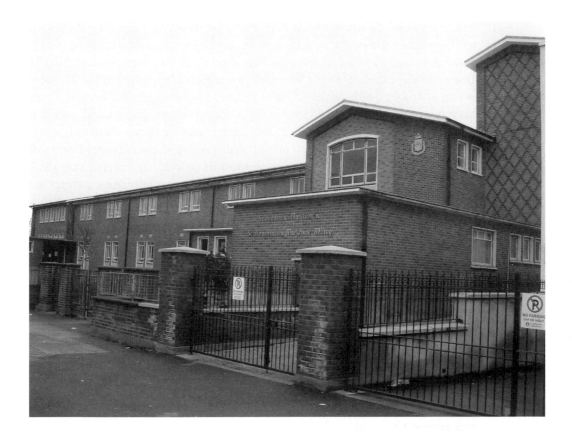

Our Lady's National School, Clonskeagh

the principal was Sister Elizabeth Ann McAteer. In November 1955 what was described at the time as 'an auxiliary infants' school' was also opened at the Marian hall. It is worth noting that at this time both Clonskeagh and Milltown were still within Donnybrook parish. At the same time the boys were being taught at St Gall's national school in Milltown. This school was opened in January 1943 and in 1957 had 231 boys on the rolls. The teachers at that time were Messrs. Joseph Hayes, Matt Griffin, Seamus O'Ferrall, Seamus O'Dowd and Michael Tubbridy. It was a lively institution which had football, hurling and athletic teams.

On 18 March 1956 the site of the new school on St Columbanus road was taken over. Less than a month later, on 15 April, it was blessed and the first sod was turned by Fr Condon PP with other priests from the Donnybrook parish attending; there too were the Mother General of the Irish Sisters of Charity and the architect of the school, Mr J Oliver Murray. His design for the new school was considered to be very striking with large windows, acoustic ceilings, sound-proof classrooms and a fine assembly hall. At the outset it was planned that the girls and infant section would be under the charge of the sisters while the boys would be taught by lay teachers. This indeed was what transpired when the girls were transferred from the Marian hall to the school after it was blessed and opened on 2 September 1957 with the sisters still in charge. As a temporary measure they occupied the boys' school, next door to their own which was not yet completed. The builder, Mr Patrick McGuinness & Co Ltd., 42 and 46/48 Patrick street, Dublin, was still on site. The girls did eventually occupy their own school where the Sisters of Charity continued to teach them until 1987, in which year it was amalgamated with the boys' school. During their time at Our Lady's, there was a succession of principals following Sister Elizabeth Ann McAteer. They were: Sr Teresa Angela, Sr Teresa Ursula Kennedy, Sr Anne Kennedy, Sr Claire Neylan and Sr Bernadette Sweeney.

The boys moved into their new school a little later than the girls; they remained at St Gall's, Milltown, in the meantime. When they and their teachers did move, their first principal was Mr Matt Griffin, who as we have seen, was already one of their teachers in Milltown. Mr Griffin, who played an active part in the Irish National Teachers' Organisation, was succeeded as principal by Mr Patrick McNulty. A writer, Mr McNulty was a well-known contributor to various magazines such as *Ireland's Own*. He continued in that post until 1980 when the position of principal was taken over by Mr Gerard Heneghan, a native of Mayo.

When the Sisters of Charity withdrew from Our Lady's in 1987, following over thirty years of service to the community, the two schools were amalgamated on 2 September of that year. Mr Heneghan was then appointed principal of the newly amalgamated school and remains in that position to this day.[15]

---

15   My thanks to Mr Gerard Heneghan, principal of Our Lady's national school, for information supplied. Some details were also found in the Souvenir booklet produced for the Blessing and Dedication of the Church of The Immaculate Virgin Mary of the Miraculous Medal, Clonskeagh.

16

Institutions: social, religious and cultural

OLIVE MOUNT INSTITUTION OF THE GOOD SAMARITAN

DURING THE MID-VICTORIAN PERIOD, amid appalling scenes of poverty and misery and in the absence of any government social services, it became very fashionable to set up various charitable institutions. A particularly popular type was one for females who were considered to be in great moral danger. One such institution was set up in Clonskeagh, more precisely in Windy Arbour, in 1843 but it does not seem to have survived very long; at least that seems to be suggested by the fact that it ceased to be listed in *Thom's Directory* in the late 1850s (it is listed under Windy Arbour in 1857). To give an indication of what its aims were and how it operated, as well as giving a flavour of the thinking as well as of the language of the time (sometimes very verbose), the following is the description of it that appears in the 1845 directory (italics and letters in upper case as found in the original are preserved):

'The Olive Mount Institution of the Good Samaritan.
Founded AD 1843 by the Rev. B[ernard] Kirby, Under the patronage and support of the people of Ireland.
   'A certain Samaritan being on his journey, and seeing him, was moved by compassion'. St Luke c.10.
This Institution was opened (*without any religious distinction*) to save from vice and degradation the *chaste*, but unprotected female, and to raise from a low estate the fallen and penitent children of the poor – the victims of brutal treachery and cruel abandonment. Those form two classes, hitherto neglected amid domestic ruin on one side, and public apathy on the other.
There are at present in the Institution 135 inmates, who are employed at washing, mangling, and needle-work etc. The Institution is conducted under the superintendence of the Rev. B. Kirby.
The Rev. B. Kirby returns his sincere thanks to the people of Ireland, who so

nobly and generously came forward in support of this work of benevolence, and to the gentlemen who have so zealously devoted their time and labour in collecting subscriptions. He feels confident that the public, who have placed the Institution on its present extensive basis, will enable him to carry out the original intention of extending the number of inmates to six hundred. Donations and subscriptions will be thankfully received by the Rev. B. Kirby, at the Central Office at 15 Arran Quay, Dublin or at the Institution. Washing, mangling, and every description of needle work executed on the most moderate terms.

N.B. – The spiritual wants of the Protestant and the Roman Catholic are attended to with the greatest care and consideration.

The Institution is beautifully situated near Milltown, on the road to Dundrum, and presents an object of attraction from the arch thrown across the gateway, surmounted by a gilded cross. On the two angular mouldings right and left of the pedestal, are two DOVES upon wing, bearing in their mouths branches of OLIVE. This design is perfectly appropriate; the Olive branch being the emblem of peace and reconciliation with God.'[1]

The Rev B Kirby was also Catholic chaplain of the Richmond Female Penitentiary, Grangegorman lane around that time.[2] An interesting aspect of this Institution, and one that may have some resonance that persists right up to the present day, is the name chosen for it. That name, Olivemount, still exists in the area and it is most likely that it is derived directly from the name chosen for the institution founded by Fr Kirby. It could, of course, have existed prior to the founding of that institution but given the explanation found in the 1845 directory, as reproduced above, Fr Kirby seems to have chosen the name himself since it says that the olive represents 'peace and reconciliation with God' and that would appear to reflect the purpose which the founder seems to have had in mind for those whom he wished to have housed in the institution.

CARMELITE MONASTERY, ROBUCK ROAD

In August of 1877 the lease of Mount Dillon was assigned to the first prioress of the Carmelite community, Charlotte Dunne, by Sir Arthur A T Cunynghame.[3] In

---

1   *The Dublin Almanac and General Register of Ireland* for the year 1845.
2   *Thom's Directory* of 1850, 1857.
3   Archives of Carmelite monastery, Roebuck road, Dublin: item 4 of Schedule of Documents.

the following year, the nuns moved in, the first mass being said, in what had now become a monastery, on 15th of August of that year – the same date as the first mass had been said at the foundation in 1832 of the North William street monastery from which the nuns came to Mount Dillon. At that time religious orders were continuing to re-establish themselves throughout Ireland after the long bleak period following the dissolution of the monasteries at the time of the Reformation.

Carmelites had long been in Ireland, their first establishment being founded not later than 1270; they were introduced by St Simon Stock, who had become prior-general of the order in England some time after 1249-50. Ware says that the friary at Leighlinbridge was built before the end of the reign of Henry III (1272) and it would appear to be the first of the Irish houses. By the end of that century there were at least nine Carmelite friaries in Ireland. Up to that time these came under the English Province but after a long struggle a separate Irish Province was established at some date between 1303 and 1307.

The only medieval Carmelite friary, located in Dublin, was founded in 1278; it was built by Sir Robert Bagot on a site in the southern suburbs of the city on land which he bought from the Cistercian abbey of Baltinglass. In 1539 the friary was surrendered by the prior, William Kelly, at the time when monasteries were being dissolved. However, later in that century during the reign of queen Elizabeth the Calced friars returned to Dublin, first to Cork street. Later they returned to their ancient site now occupied by the modern Carmelite Priory in Whitefriar street. There, a link with pre-Reformation Dublin is to be found in the medieval statue of the Virgin Mary, known as Our Lady of Dublin.

There are, however, no records of the presence of Carmelite nuns in pre-Reformation Ireland, although the Carmelite sisterhood was canonically established in 1453 and soon spread throughout Europe. The first establishment in Ireland seems to have been in Loughrea around 1680; the first in Dublin, at a date before 1760, was located initially at Arran quay, later moving to St Joseph's in Ranelagh. From here other houses were established over time, the one at North William street being founded on August 15th 1832. Here the nuns, as so often had happened during penal time, ran an orphanage despite the fact that theirs was a contemplative religious order. The opportunity to follow their chosen way of life came with the move to Mount Dillon although there were still problems to be overcome especially in the relation to how they would support themselves; these, after some initial vicissitudes, were however soon overcome.[4]

---

4   Gwynn and Hadcock, *Medieval religious houses,* 281-84, 289, 310-11; James R Rushe, *Carmel in Ireland: a narrative of the Irish province of Teresian, or Discalced Carmelites (AD 1625-1896)* (Dublin & London 1903) 268-83; personal communication from Carmelite monastery, Roebuck road, Dublin.

The early prioresses had been professed at North William street; they were Charlotte Dunne (Sr Mary Joseph Magdalene de Pazzi of the Sacred Heart of Mary (1878-1903)), Emily (or Eliza) Mary Anne Joseph Sisk (Sr Mary Agnes Aloysius Magdalen of the Sacred Heart of Jesus (1904-09)).

At the time they moved to Mount Dillon, the property consisted of a large mansion – the one built in the last quarter of the 18th century for Thomas Dillon's father – set in a substantial expanse of land, 16 acres, 3 roods and 32 perches Irish measurement (equivalent to 27 acres, 1 rood and 31 perches statute measure). The document accompanying the sale described the property thus: 'The mansion-house, out-offices, gardens, and demesne lands, formerly called Mount Dillon, now called Mount Carmel, situate in the townland of Roebuck, and county of Dublin'. The property bounded Roebuck grove which was then unoccupied (previously called Roebuck house before Abraham Brewster changed its name during his occupancy). Both properties were linked together in the terms of sale with the purchaser of Mount Dillon bound to indemnify that of Roebuck grove against payment of the combined head-rent (£129-3s-8d) payable on the two properties; one of the early vicissitudes faced by the sisters. According to the monastery records (c.1915), the rent was paid to Major Richardson through his agent Mr Vernon (he was agent to the Pembroke Estates). Later, in 1954, the ground rent was bought by Mr Richardson. Given the similarity in name, these Richardsons may have some connection with the Richards family who were, according to Ball & Hamilton writing in 1895, in possession of the Roebuck estate which their ancestor, Solomon 'the celebrated Dublin surgeon' had purchased from lord Trimleston at an unspecified date, probably at the turn of the 18th and 19th centuries. The rateable valuation at the time the sisters moved in was £170; it had been £221 in 1847 but dropped to £119 from 1863 to 1869 before rising to £170 in 1870.[5]

By the 1960s the old house was found to be suffering from dry and wet rot and needed re-roofing. It was a major problem which had to be tackled. The decision was made that a new building was needed and, in order to fund the project, land was sold to St Kilian's German school. The old house was demolished in 1974 after the new purpose-built convent was constructed; its first sod was turned in late 1973. Later, at the request of archbishop McQuaid, some 4 acres, on the city side of monastery, was sold to the De La Salle order to build a primary school; they were refused permission to build a secondary school, so after some time they sold it on to Cert Ltd (the state run training body for the

5   Archives of the Carmelite monastery, Roebuck road, Dublin; Ball & Hamilton, *Parish of Taney*, 139, 181; *Thom's Directory* at various dates.

catering industry), who in turn, at a later date, sold it on to the institution which set up the Islamic centre which remains there to this day. The original entrance to the monastery was via the big brown gate (it has a cross on top) on the main road just past the Mosque. Its gate lodge was Mount Carmel cottage, but it was knocked down to allow for road widening and a new cottage was built in its lieu just inside the brown gate. The current gate lodge to the monastery was built when the entrance was shifted around the corner to its present location on Roebuck road.

In line with the wishes of one of the Carmelites' most revered saints, St Teresa of Avila, as found in her writings, the community is small with a family-like atmosphere; it consists today of nine sisters. Their daily life is centred on prayer both communal and solitary. However, there is also time for work, recreation, reading and study. The nuns make altar breads which they supply to churches in Dublin and throughout all of Ireland; this is their main source of support. There are gardens to be tended with their vegetables and flowers. Poultry are kept, cattle graze lazily as the two dogs and the donkey look on thus conjuring up a truly rural atmosphere only yards away from the busy city road outside the walls. A lake once existed in the monastery gardens but it was filled in before the sisters moved there. Two streamlets come into the grounds, join as one, before flowing out into UCD land at the back of the monastery. However, they turn back again before leaving finally, flowing on through UCD, under the Stillorgan dual carriageway, then through the land of St Joseph's home for the blind, then under the Merrion road and afterwards into the sea. On occasion they overflow, possibly taking on surface water from the Goatstown road.

The name of the house into which the nuns moved originally was changed to Mount Carmel. However, around 1926 a new name was adopted: Carmelite Monastery of the Immaculate Conception. Before the new parish of Clonskeagh was formed, with its church in Bird avenue, the chapel in the monastery was a chapel of ease for Donnybrook church. It was located in what had been the ballroom of the old house; a room of grand proportions such that, long before the sisters arrived, it is believed that it had been used on one occasion to hold a wedding. The nuns' choir was in the main body behind a grille facing the altar which was at the end of the room. To one side, there was space for local people who attended mass there. At mass times, this was always full with the crowd spilling out beyond the window at the side. People also went to mass in the convent at Mount Anville; it could be a long walk to go to one of three possible churches: Donnybrook, Milltown or Dundrum. It was apparent that there was a growing need for a new church and parish.

However, even to this day people still come in substantial numbers to mass at the monastery where it is currently held daily, Monday to Saturday. Indeed it is a particular feature of the monastery that, although the community is contemplative, people are welcome to attend. They are also welcome to Lauds (morning prayer) which begin at 7.00 am and may stay for mass immediately afterwards. Similarly, the community welcomes people to attend evening prayer held from 5 pm to 6 pm and Vespers which begin directly afterwards. As well as that people come to the monastery, or write to the community, asking for prayers for whatever needs they have; all are welcomed.

In the recent history of the monastery one event stands out clearly: the arrival there in the year 2000 of the relics of St Therese of Lisieux. This was a unique event and the community did not know what to expect in terms of local people calling to venerate the relics. In the event the size of the crowd that came, turned out to be enormous. Long before the casket containing the relics arrived at 1.30 pm on that Tuesday the grounds and every part of the area surrounding was packed to capacity. After it arrived and was in place in the chapel people kept coming and there were many there throughout the evening and all night. In fact, when the priest was about to begin mass at 7 a.m. he could hardly get to the altar as the people had overflowed into the sanctuary; many had come an hour beforehand to secure a place in the chapel. School children on their way to school came of their own volition and later that morning a number of patients from the Central Mental Hospital visited. The crowds continued to come until it was time for the casket to leave at 12 pm after its stay of just 22 hours at the monastery. Although it was a unique event, it merely highlighted the fact that the monastery, although it is contemplative, has a strong connection with the local Clonskeagh people. In fact, ever since the monastery was founded around 130 years ago local people have visited it and valued it. [6]

ISOLATION HOSPITAL, LATER FEVER HOSPITAL, LATER CLONSKEAGH HOSPITAL

At the end of the nineteenth century the mortality rate in Dublin was appallingly high; at 33.6 per thousand living, it was higher that the rate prevailing in other major cities in Europe and the United States. In fact it was almost as bad as that which then existed in Calcutta. This state of affairs gave rise to much recrimination and a variety of causes was put forward by concerned people as being at the root of the problem. The result was that an inquiry into the state of public health was set up with public meetings being held in City Hall during February

---

[6]   My thanks to Sr Teresa Whelan for her generous co-operation while researching material on both Mount Dillon and the Carmelite monastery.

and March 1900. Filthy and overcrowded tenements, poor connection of houses to the main sewers, badly regulated slaughter houses and refuse dumps close to homes and the foul condition of the Liffey were among the causes it highlighted. These, it was stated, weakened people's resistance to disease and their ability to overcome it when they fell under its hold. But, above all, there was the problem of infectious and communicable diseases; these accounted for approximately one third of all deaths in Dublin at this time. Diseases such as typhus, smallpox, scarlet fever, diphtheria, cholera, measles, typhoid fever and tuberculosis struck at different times. Already in 1889 the adoption by Dublin Corporation of the Infectious Disease (Notification) Act meant that sanitary officers could take action when the occurrence of a communicable disease was reported by a physician or by the family of the person with the disease. One of the actions that they could take was to isolate the person with the disease. This approach by Dublin Corporation was soon followed by the townships of Pembroke and Rathmines. The system, however, was not as effective as it might have been due to laxness by the physicians but, particularly, due to a profound fear among the poor of Dublin of being consigned to a fever hospital, perhaps because it seemed to them to be akin to being sent to the workhouse. Nevertheless, the system did contribute to tackling the problem but it also highlighted another problem: where to put these patients who had to be isolated. Dublin at this time had as many hospitals per head of population as other cities; however, it had a higher rate of infectious diseases which required specialized resources. In times of epidemics these came under great pressure. A smallpox outbreak in 1894-95 highlighted this lack of proper facilities. During this time a number of infected middle-class individuals were horrified to learn that they had to share the same wards as similarly infected paupers in convalescent sheds which were erected in the grounds of the South Dublin Union workhouse. But even without the pressure of an epidemic facilities were still required to house those who had to be isolated; some general hospitals did build a fever building alongside their main building although this was dangerous and not good practice. There was thus an acknowledged need for isolation hospitals to be built away from the existing hospitals and, indeed, away from the centres of population.[7]

It is against this background that steps were taken to construct an isolation hospital at Clonskeagh. It has already been observed that the Pembroke and Rathmines townships were quick to follow Dublin Corporation in adopting the Infectious Disease (Notification) Act of 1889. The Urban District Councils of

---

7   Joseph V. O'Brien, *"Dear dirty Dublin": a city in distress, 1899-1916* (Berkeley, Ca. 1982) 101-116.

both of these townships were later to set up joint boards to tackle various problems, prominent among which was a joint hospital board. With both councils equally represented on it, its main purpose was the construction of an isolation facility for patients suffering from smallpox; the location chosen was Clonskeagh, more precisely Vergemount house. The contractor employed to build it was Humphreys Ltd., Iron Buildings Works, Knightsbridge, Hyde Park, London S.W. In their specification for the facility, dated February 24th, 1902, the contractor states 'We propose to supply and erect in a substantial manner a Galvanized Corrugated Iron *hospital for 20 beds as per our design No. 3*' and '*Wards to be 50ft x 20ft*' (words in italics entered by hand, the rest is preprinted). Clonskeagh was chosen as it was outside the urban district and, because of this, it was thought that it would avoid the type of objections that were met when a facility for patients with advanced tuberculosis was proposed for Leeson park by the Royal Hospital for Incurables in Donnybrook.

However, objections there were; local residents objected. In this they were led by Mrs Boswell who owned the adjoining twelve houses in St James' terrace, located at the beginning of Clonskeagh road. She said she lived there (the directories of the time do not bear this out) and collected rent from her tenants in the other eleven houses. She claimed that if the isolation hospital went ahead she, her family, her tenants and, indeed, others living in the near neighbourhood would be in danger of being infected by 'aerial convection' emanating from the hospital. In order to prevent this she sought an injunction from the courts to stop the whole project from going ahead. In this she was initially successful; however it was unanimously set aside by the three judges in the court of appeal. In their judgement they found that there was no sound scientific foundation for the assertion that infection was carried by 'aerial convection'. They did, however, acknowledge the fear of infection that existed but pointed out the advances that had been made by way of vaccination. Their dismissal of the claims of Mrs Boswell and others meant that the construction of the hospital could proceed. With that the Pembroke and Rathmines Joint Hospital Board went ahead and built the hospital.[8] Later another controversy hit the hospital; this time it was totally different in nature. The hospital was funded by ratepayers and some nationalists among them complained that there were no Roman Catholics on the board despite the fact that most of the patients in the hospital were of that religious persuasion.[9]

---

8   Séamas Ó Maitiú, *Dublin's suburban towns 1834- 1930* (Dublin 2003) 182; W. N. Osborough, *Law and the emergence of modern Dublin: a litigation topography of the city* (Dublin 1996) 67-68.

9   Ó Maitiú, *Dublin's suburban towns*, 183.

The hospital continued in its role as an isolation hospital for a considerable time catering, not just for smallpox, which declined after the last attack in 1903, but for other infectious diseases such as diphtheria and scarlet fever as well. The underlying fear of the hospital can, perhaps, be seen in the name attributed to the horse-drawn vehicle which conveyed the patients to the hospital "The Sick Cab".[10] The first time the hospital appears in *Thom's Directory* is for the year 1904 and the entry is as follows: Conjoint Boards of Pembroke and Rathmines Urban Council (£20); *Isolation Hospital* – Lieut. Colonel F G Adye Curran, chairman Hospital Board – residence, 42 Upper Rathmines road; F Warren, esq., physician and surgeon, medical officer in charge – residence, 50 Mountpleasant place.

The £20 refers to the rateable valuation assigned to it, a very favourable valuation given that Vergemount house had been rated at £98. In the following year the entry was somewhat similar except that reference to the chairman was dropped and another name was added: R M Byrne, matron. This lasted until 1910 when Mrs Rice is given as matron. The matron's name is omitted from 1918 onwards as was that of the Conjoint Boards from 1931. In 1938 a new medical officer is listed Dr H E Redmond, LRCSI; he was succeeded in 1940 by Dr F N Elcock, LRCPI who remained in the position at least until the end of the 1950s. From 1960 onwards the name Isolation Hospital is dropped and Clonskeagh Hospital is used instead; at that point the name of the resident medical officer (if such a post still continued) is not given in the directories. Although the directories do not mention it, the title Fever Hospital was also used on occasions in other sources. However, with the advances in medicine the need for isolation and fever hospitals became less and less; from 1969 Clonskeagh hospital was used to treat psychiatric patients. Ten years later it changed again, this time it was turned to a facility mainly for geriatric patients.[11] Soon a new premise called St Broc's was built specifically for that purpose. This, together with some administrative offices for the Health Service Executive, is the main function it serves to this day.

MARISTS AT CASINO ON BIRD AVENUE, LATER MOUNT ST MARYS

In 1919 the Marists, realising that after 1925 no one would be allowed to teach in a secondary school who did not have a university degree or diploma in teaching, sought permission of the archbishop of Dublin to look for a house in Dublin

---

10 O Brien, *"Dear dirty Dublin"*, 115; J Nolan, *Changing faces* (Dublin 1982) 197.
11 Douglas Bennet, *The encyclopaedia of Dublin* (Dublin 2005) 47.

from which their novices would have access to the National University. On receiving that permission the search began; Casino in Bird avenue was visited in January 1920 and found to be suitable for their purposes. The following month it was purchased and the name changed to Mount St Mary's. The sale having been completed in May, Casino was taken over by two Marist priests in June. It was two more years before the first novices took up residence. When they did the house took on the name of Mount St Mary's House of Studies; the Rev Francis McVicar was superior and on the staff with him were Rev Thos W Conran, novice master and Rev Peter McKeown, his assistant.

The founder of the Marist Fathers (there are other branches of the Marists apart from the Fathers – Brothers, Nuns and laypeople) was Fr Jean Claude Colin (1790-1875), a native of a town in the Beaujolais region in France. Growing up in post-revolutionary France when there was strong opposition to the church, Colin along with some others made a pledge in 1816 to establish a Society of Mary (hence the name Marists). Initially, as a small group of priests, they preached missions in the rural areas of the diocese to which they belonged. Their success inspired their bishop to entrust the conduct of the local seminary to them. But it was to be the foreign missions where they made the most impact. In January 1836 the pope assigned the missions of Western Oceania (New Zealand, Tonga, Samoa, Fiji and other islands of the Pacific ocean) to the group and the following April the Society of Marist Fathers was canonically approved; later that year Fr Colin was elected the first Superior General and the first group of Marist Fathers set off for the South Pacific.

Their arrival in England in 1850, at the request of the archbishop of Westminster, was to minister to the large post-famine influx of Irish immigrants. This contact with the Irish and with Ireland led to an invitation to establish a boarding school in Dundalk in 1861 and a school in Dublin (Catholic University School) in 1867. This followed from the reputation they had, by that time, gained as successful educators in France. Other foundations and ministries followed but it was in their work as teachers at secondary level that initiated their move to set up a house of studies in Dublin and their arrival at Casino in 1920.

The first novices who took up residence in 1922 were sixteen in number and they took their profession in September 1923. They followed their courses at university while studying philosophy and scripture at Mount St Mary's. The students walked to and from the university every day. The impression given of the place by some of those involved in its early days is that of the healthiness of the surroundings; the words of the superior encapsulate this: 'the place is a perfect sanatorium'. This echoes the opinion of the doctors who, as we have seen, sent Isaac Butt to recover (unsuccessfully) in the clean country air of Clonskeagh more than forty years earlier; this reputation for healthiness was also a factor in the choice of Clonskeagh as the location of the Masonic Orphan Boys' school. Another impression was the beauty of the garden said to have been still preserved as it had been designed by Doctor Emmet, Robert's father. As well as that it was said that experts had pronounced the soil of the whole property to be the richest in the county Dublin.

However, not everything was so auspicious; there were financial troubles. The original price paid for Casino was £3,500 although this was reduced by £359 by an arbiter when it was discovered that the lease of nearly 4 acres of the property was shorter than had been stated. Contributions towards the purchase price were made by various Marist foundations in England as well as in Ireland but a substantial loan had also to be taken out. This together with loans for other purposes, such as providing proper accommodation, left the house in considerable debt. Extensions added in the 1920s were made possible by the acquisition of the interest held in property by Miss Fowler, Sir Arthur Meldon and Mrs Thompson; the latter had received the property from a descendant of George Frederick Moulds who had first leased Casino to Dr Emmet in the 18th century.

In the 1930s as well as being a house for students attending university, it became a novitiate; numbers in residence rose accordingly. Later, in 1949, full-time philosophy and theology classes were begun and continued for many years. In the 1950s Mount St Mary's remained the common scholasticate for both Irish and English students after the division of the Anglo-Irish province into two. In 1966 it became home to the English novices and for a time Mill Hill students came for their philosophy. This was provided later for all students at Milltown Institute. Between 1922 and 1970 two hundred priests had been trained at Mount St Mary's.

As well as training priests, the staff and priests there help the local community in Milltown and Clonskeagh; they celebrate mass, give retreats and generally help the local clergy in whatever way is needed. Many local activities, run by Residents Associations and others, have taken place on the Marist premises and the Marists feel themselves to be very much part of that community. One of the most significant contributions which they have made was the provision of a site for the church on Bird avenue. It was built on what was described as 'the lower field'. As a result, the old gate lodge on Bird avenue was taken down and a bungalow was built at what was originally a side entrance on Dundrum road; that now became the main entrance. Casino had always been listed in the directories, from the first time they covered the area in the 1830s, under the heading of Bird avenue. The entrance on Bird avenue and the driveway up to the house can be clearly seen on the first Ordnance Survey map of the area. A good description of this entrance, driveway and, indeed, of the general atmosphere of the grounds is given by an early student writing in the

1920/21 annual. Giving himself the pseudonym 'Bird of Passage', he writes: '"Mount St Mary's" claims an enhancing present, charming at all times, but especially beautiful in life-diffusing May and the leafy month of June. [It] ... commands a full and glorious view of the Dublin mountains and of Dublin bay. ... The main entrance, with its massive gates and stag-crowned piers, is by Bird avenue ...; and if ever [an] avenue deserved its name it is surely this ... On entering the impressive portals, the visitor is confronted with a magnificent and extensive property ... (going) up the winding avenue, a pretty view is shortly gained of the stately mansion ... (with) its waving fields, its shaded walks, its lordly trees, its pretty setting at the foot of the Dublin mountains'.[12]

LITTLE SISTERS OF THE POOR, ROEBUCK ROAD

According to their annals, the Little Sisters of the Poor opened their first Novitiate on the 23rd May 1941 in Clonsilla on a property that was leased to them for three years by Sir Christopher and Lady Nixon. A small number of residents moved in and plans were put in place to open what was to be their second Home for the elderly in Dublin. However, it soon became apparent that the house in Clonsilla was not suited to the Sisters' purpose and a search began for one that was more in keeping with their needs. In June 1942 the annals state that 'a very nice property was found at Roebuck road ... called "The Hermitage" comprising 17_ acres of land on which stood a fine solid three storied house, with basement and outhouses'. It is most likely that Sir Christopher Nixon, who had been raised at Roebuck grove, a mansion to the rear of The Hermitage, had some input into finding this property for the sisters. They accepted the terms of sale from Madame Mansergh, the famous opera singer whose stage name was Fanny Moody, and signed the Deeds of Sale on 30 July 1942. Madame Mansergh handed over the keys to them on 7 September of the same year. The rateable valuation of the property at the time was £146. Madame Mansergh moved to a more modest property at Trimleston lodge (it was rated £63-15s at the time) as the sisters moved in. Thus began a new era in the work of the Little Sisters of the Poor in Ireland.

The religious congregation to which they belong was founded by Jeanne Jugan, who was born in Cancale, Brittany in 1792. After its foundation in 1839 it soon spread throughout France and was canonically approved by pope Pius IX in 1854. True to the spirit of its foundress its aim is, according to its constitution,

---

12   Kerr, *Emmet's Casino,* 8-15 with additional material from the website of the Marist Fathers; Society of Mary in Ireland (last update: 14 September 2004).

to be 'at the service of the aged' and that includes those of all religions. In keeping with this aim, it adds an extra vow to those normally taken by members of religious orders – a vow of hospitality. By the middle of the 19th century it had around 100 foundations in France and in 1851 the first of those abroad was established in England. Plans were afoot at the time to move into other countries including Ireland. Given the difficulties that had to be overcome it took some time before it was possible to put these plans into action and it was not until 1868 that the first of its Irish foundation was established in county Waterford; at that time the foundress was still alive. Eventually there would be five houses in Ireland, one each in Cork and Waterford and three in Dublin where the first was founded in 1881. By the end of the twentieth century there were 280 foundations in six continents, one of which was that in Roebuck road.

After the purchase of The Hermitage it was planned that a second home for the elderly, modelled on that of St Patrick's Kilmainham, would be established there. It was also planned that the novices and postulants be transferred there from Clonsilla. The Superior at the time was Sister Norah Boland. Mr Byrne, architect, was commissioned to draw up plans for what would be known as St Brigid's Home for the aged to accommodate from 30 to 35 residents. The builders employed for the project were Messrs. O'Callaghan & Co. Some apartments were also built to receive the novices. By 26 May 1943 some buildings were ready for occupation and were blessed by archbishop McQuaid. Three new residents were received and two were transferred from Clonsilla. Two sisters moved in to look after them. Although the buildings were far from complete – there was no electricity on the property, no central heating and only a temporary chapel- the novices and postulants moved in on 25 June 1943; it would be more than a year before central heating was installed in October 1944. The original chapel was completed some weeks later; it was replaced by the present one in 1979. The purpose-built Novitiate and Retreat House, which still exists, was begun in January 1948 and completed in October of the following year.

In the year that archbishop McQuaid blessed the first part of the building in The Hermitage (1943) he expressed the wish that the Congregation would acquire the large property that was next door to them – Roebuck castle. It must have come on the market at that time; Mrs Westby had been living there since the death of her husband, Francis Vandeleur, around 1930. On 30 September 1943 the property was acquired; it had at that time a rateable valuation of £318. It would now become the second Home for the elderly in Dublin and residents were moved there from The Hermitage on 17 May 1944. The majority of the residential accommodation provided for them was in the North Wing of the castle; this was built in the 1950s. However, problems encountered there with Fire and Safety Regulations saw residents move back to The Hermitage at dates

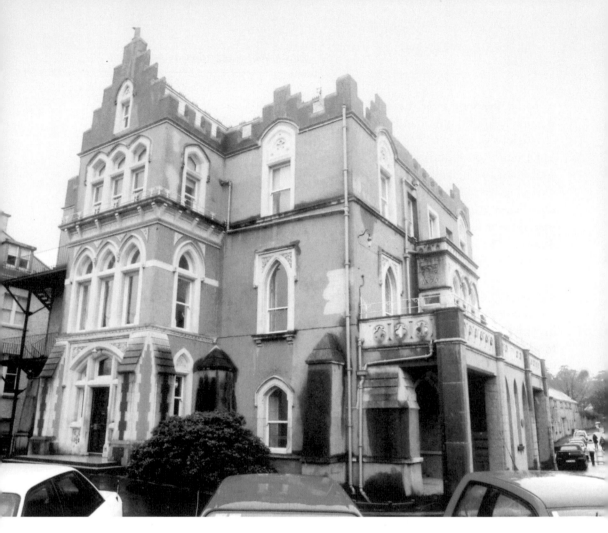

Roebuck castle today, now home to the Faculty of Law in UCD
(*Photographer: Matt Walsh*)

between 1952 and 1979. The building they vacated was subsequently demolished and a chapel was built there in its site in 1960. As well as that, residents' apartments at Roebuck castle "Holy Family Home" were also found to be no longer in conformity with Fire and Safety Regulations. The sisters now faced a big problem – a new Nursing Home was needed.

To finance this, their only asset – the land surrounding their properties – had to be sold. There was almost 35 acres of land there and initially they put the castle and 31.64 acres of land up for sale. In the event, 21 acres was initially sold to the Dublin construction firm, Dwyer Nolan Ltd. for a figure, believed by the newspapers of the time, to be £2.3 million. This company built a substantial number of houses on that land; the address adopted for them was 'Roebuck castle'.

Using the money from this sale, the sisters went ahead with the building of the new Home in the grounds of The Hermitage. The ground breaking ceremony took place on 11 May 1983 and, with the name of "The Holy Family Home" under which it had existed in Roebuck castle, it was blessed by Dr Joseph Carroll, auxiliary bishop of Dublin and officially opened on 29 December 1985. It had cost £9 million to build and became home for 79 elderly men and women. It had individual rooms with toilets en suite, two infirmaries, physiotherapy and occupational therapy rooms, a chapel, hair dressing, laundry, cafeteria and shopping facilities. There were plans for 12 independent living apartments to be built for elderly people who preferred to have their own private accommodation; this, however, had to be put on hold due to financial constraints. The remainder of the land, consisting of 10.5 acres approximately, together with Roebuck castle itself was then put up for sale; that is, the part that had not been sold originally. UCD bought this lot and paid around £750,000 for it (according to another source £620,000 was paid for the buildings and 10 acres in 1986); it now uses the premises left by the nuns for a variety of uses, the castle housing the Faculty of Law. The chapel became an assembly hall and the first honorary conferring ceremony at Belfield was held in it in July 1987.

The net result of the cost of building the new Home at the Hermitage and the money received from the sale of their only asset, the land and the castle, still left the Sisters with nearly £2.5 million of a debt. Despite this the Sisters carried on with their work which continues in Roebuck road to this day. With 80 single rooms, all fitted with full facilities, and a community of between 16 and 20 nuns and 60 members of staff it is a major provider of services to the elderly. It welcomes and gets voluntary support from the local community. This support, always there, has recently received formal church recognition when The Association of Jeanne Jugan was canonically approved in 1998. This is an association of lay men and women who choose to participate in the work of the sisters in a special way. They can contribute in a variety of practical ways but always in a manner that reflects the vision of the foundress, Jeanne Jugan.[13]

---

13 A variety of documents was provided by Sr Angela, Mother Superior, Holy Family Residence. These include items related to the sale of property, including Roebuck castle, to pay for the new residence. As well as that Sister Marie Aimée, of St Brigid's Novitiate, supplied information which was taken from the Congregation's annals in relation to the purchase and subsequent development of The Hermitage. For information relating to the purchase and subsequent use of the property sold by the nuns to UCD: McCartney, *UCD, a national idea*, 398.

MILLTOWN/CLONSKEAGH CREDIT UNION

In November 1966, a meeting of interested people in the Boys' school, St Columbanus road, was addressed by Miss Nora Herlihy, a pioneer of the Credit Union movement in Ireland. As a result, a small study group was set up and, quite soon afterwards, on Friday 30 December 1966, Milltown Credit Union came into being. Officers on the first committee were as follows: Pat O'Brien, president; Terry Jordan, secretary; Pat Cahill, vice-president; Tom Newman, treasurer. The committee also included Tom Byrne, Tom Carroll, Pat Hogarty and Frank Finn. The supervisory committee consisted of Tom Dolan, Sean O'Brien and Jimmy O'Farrell.

The first meetings were held in the local rent office by kind permission of Dave Storey, without whose co-operation the whole project might never have got off the ground. However, it was soon found necessary to move to a more spacious building and in this regard help was at hand from the parish priest who allowed the use of the Boys' school in St Columbanus road and, at a later date, also the Boys' school in Milltown (both Clonskeagh and Milltown were at this time part of Donnybrook parish). These facilities, which allowed better services to be given to members, both reflected and stimulated the growth of the business of the Union then being experienced.

Welcome as was the permission to use these facilities, it was nevertheless the intention that a premise belonging to the Credit Union itself be acquired. This was successfully achieved in November 1969 when new office premises were purchased. That was a start, although a major one, but much work had still to be done to make them suited to the purpose in mind. A lot of planning and rebuilding had to be undertaken to turn them into the substantial property that became available in the early 1970s. The result was a building worthy of its members where they could transact their business in the main office with some comfort and minimum delay. There were also several interview rooms provided where members could make loan applications and discuss their affairs in confidence with Credit Committee members or the manager who was also Loans Officer. Observing the building from the front, it is surprising to find that more space was provided downstairs for a boardroom, offices, kitchen and other uses. All this space was considered necessary as, in order that members could be provided with the best possible service with loans when they needed them, efficient accounting systems had to be put in place so that accounts would be processed with the utmost accuracy. As the number of members grew – there were 1600 in the early 1970s when the share capital was around £64,000 and continuing to grow – the most modern accounting equipment was purchased and put to use. This ensured that, along with the supervisory committee, members could invest their savings in the Credit Union with the utmost confidence.

It was readily acknowledged that the success of the early years would not have been so easily achieved had it not been for the help received from other Credit Unions, in particular those in Dundrum, Donnybrook, Ballyfermot, Raheny, Marino and many others. It also got help from the staff and Field Officers of the Credit Union League of Ireland. The early success was also much helped by a band of men and women on the board of directors who were dedicated to the Credit Union ideal. A group of young women also helped out in the early years; they showed up week in week out without fail. Their dedication inspired the education committee to formulate a policy for 'Youth participation in the Credit Union' which it was hoped would involve them in a separate democratic union, controlling their own affairs and providing for their own needs by practising the principles of self-help.

In 1970 the name of the Credit Union was changed to Milltown/Clonskea Credit Union Ltd. It then served the district in and around Clonskeagh, Milltown and part of Churchtown. Shortly thereafter the then treasurer, Tom Newman, was appointed full time general manager and Caroline Brangan joined the staff. The directors and committee members did not get salaries; their services were given voluntarily to the community. By that stage the Credit Union was well established and the description of its situation in 1971 was as follows:

Milltown/Clonskea Credit Union Limited
Registered Office – Dundrum Road, Windy Arbour, 14.
(Telephone and Office Hours details given)
Directors and Supervisors 1971
        Chairman – Thomas Byrne
        Vice-President – William Reddy
        Secretary – James Walsh
        Treasurer – John O'Connor
        Directors – Thomas Carroll, Christopher Gleeson, Michael Kavanagh, Gerard Hendrick, William Gill, Patrick Moran, James O'Farrell, Mrs Mason, Mrs Flynn, Arthur Staves, Ed. Armstrong.
        Supervisors – Laurence Gillick, Liam McGrath, Paul Twomey.
        General Manager – Thomas Newman.

A solid foundation had been laid for the success which the Credit Union is today. Further building work was later undertaken. Architects Deaton Lynch and builders M J Clarke & Sons combined to produce, in 1994, the premises that continue to serve the needs of the Credit Unit in carrying out its day to day business.[14]

ISLAMIC CULTURAL CENTRE OF IRELAND

In 1996 the Islamic Cultural Centre of Ireland (ICCI) was established in Clonskeagh, on a site that was once part of Mount Dillon later called Mount Carmel. It was constructed with the help of a generous contribution given by Sheikh Hamdan Bin Rashid Al Maktoum, deputy ruler of Dubai and minister of finance and industry of the United Arab Emirates (UAE). When completed, it was inaugurated on the 3rd Rajab 1417 H (14 November 1996) under the auspices of Mary Robinson, president of Ireland, and in the presence of Sheikh Hamdan Bin Rashid; others present at the opening included UAE officials as well as Arab, Muslim and Irish dignitaries.

In the years since its inception, the centre's activities and accomplishments have been many and diverse including services for Muslims as well as awareness of Islamic culture for non-Muslims. It has sought to strengthen the Muslim community's bond with their religion and traditions with particular emphasis being placed on the second generation. Opportunities have been provided for gaining religious knowledge and for preserving and sustaining Arabic, the language of the Quran. Traditions and morals, considered to be a part of every society which considers itself religious, are at the centre of the ICCI's programmes.

The centre is housed in a building which is considered to be an architectural masterpiece and an innovative model for the structure of Islamic centres in the West. Admired by Muslims and non-Muslims alike, it won the "Best Design of 1997", an Irish prize awarded for its aesthetics, its success in meeting the Muslim community's needs and its blending in with the surrounding environment. At its centre is the mosque, simply yet aesthetically designed, with accommodation for 800 men in addition to 200 women in a terrace. At each of its four corners there are buildings which provide particular services.

At the first corner one finds the schools and educational section. Here the Muslim national school is located. It is a full time school owned by the Muslim community and sponsored and funded by the Irish Department of Education. In 2001 there were 250 pupils on the rolls at the primary level. The premises

---

14   Information on the history of the Milltown/Clonskea Credit Union has been taken from a booklet on the Union published in the early 1970s. Access to this has been kindly made possible for me by Mr Noël Jones.

belong to the ICCI which also financially supports its Islamic education and Arabic language department. On this corner the Arab school is also located. It implements the Libyan curricula to help overseas students pursue their studies once they return home – all Arab countries officially recognize certificates issued by this school. Also at this corner are the Nurulhuda Quranic school and the language learning centre for adults. The former is totally dedicated to teaching the Quran and Arabic to youngsters and the Quran to adults. More than 130 students attend specialised classes for memorising the Quran while, during the summer, a variety of educational and entertainment programmes are offered. In the latter, structured courses in Arabic and English are provided according to the needs of those participating. The Arabic programme attracts Muslim converts and non-Muslims who wish to learn the language for business or other reasons. The English programme, in co-operation with the South Dublin Vocational Committee, provides language classes for non-native speakers.

The social services are located at the second corner. Situated here are the Centre's administration offices, the office of the General Secretariat of the European Council of Fatwa and Research and the library, with an admirable collection of thousands of valuable books, which provides references for researchers in both Arabic and English. There is also an audiovisual library which consists of a large variety of lectures, sermons and Islamic movies. Separate provision is made here for women with all the necessary facilities such as halls, study rooms and a nursery; it is here that they organise their activities and lectures in Arabic and English. On the ground floor at this corner there is a large shop and a spacious restaurant, both of which are frequented by both Muslims and non-Muslims. In this general area is located also a mortuary with all the appropriate equipment required to meet the highest level of health criteria.

The third corner has a well equipped multi-purpose hall, suitable for indoor football, basketball and volleyball; there have been many sports tournaments held here. The hall can also be used for events such as banquets, parties, confer- ences and daily Iftaar in Ramadan. There is also a fully-equipped gymnasium where men and women may separately carry out scheduled exercises. This corner also has a small seminar room with a capacity of seventy persons. The fourth and final corner has ten apartments, nine of which are rented to employees of ICCI and to others. The other has been converted into a guest-house for Muslims who are in Ireland for a short visit.

A wide variety of cultural activities are provided by ICCI; this includes publications, printed matter and Islamic awareness and cultural programmes. Among the publications are: a quarterly newsletter in English (occasionally in Arabic) covering news and activities of the Centre – it is distributed free of charge; books such as two in Arabic, the first including all Fatwas declared in the first three sessions of the European Council for Fatwa and Research, the second entitled 'The relation with the West: dialogue or conflict?', compiled by a group of Muslim thinkers and scholars, concludes that dialogue is the basis of such relations; the first book of Fatwas published in English, with the expectation (in 2001) that it would soon be published in German, French, Spanish and Albanian; a series of booklets (3 already published in 2001) entitled 'Islam is the way of life' to present a simplified explanation of Islam and religious duties for Muslims in a manner suitable for western life without any extremism or slackness; a calendar produced at the beginning of every Hijri year to link Muslim communities living in the West and their youth with religious events and ceremonies.

Concerned that a lack of Islamic education in the West and the possible loss by new Muslim generations of their Islamic identity has spurred the ICCI to give financial support to the existing Muslim national school and to the establishment of the Nurul Huda school. The latter began in the mosque with 50 students before being established as a school specialising in memorising the Quran; it is now the corner stone for teaching the Quran in Ireland. Each year, during Ramadan, ICCI holds a Quranic competition in which people who are fully or partially memorising the Quran participate according to their different age groups. Prizes are awarded during the yearly festivities of Eid-ul-Fitr. The ICCI also reaches out to Muslim students who attend non-Muslim schools; in consultation with the administrations of such schools, Muslim teachers are appointed to teach religion to these students.

Regular lectures and courses at the centre are the responsibility of the Imam; he gives two lectures a week and courses on various religious topics are also given. Occasional lectures are given by eminent scholars, lecturers and Islamic thinkers; these come from various countries such as Saudi Arabia, Egypt, Canada, USA, Britain, Sudan, Lebanon, Qatar, Iraq, Denmark, Palestine, Kuwait, Yemen, UAE and Pakistan.

An important aspect of the Centre is that it is the permanent headquarters of the European Council for Fatwa and Research; it is financially supported by Al Maktoum Foundation. The Council has prominent and elite scholars among its members most of whom are from Europe. It convenes twice a year and has on many occasions met on the ICCI's premises. The Council tackles many issues related to Muslims in the West through discussions, research, analysis and composing study papers in order to formulate appropriate solutions to these issues based upon pertinent jurisprudential laws while taking into consideration the western context.

ICCI also provides Islamic awareness courses and debates designed to highlight the truth about Islam and refute the doubts raised by its opponents. It organises conferences, gatherings and dialogues locally on such subjects as the environment and medicine; at a European level, on multiculturalism, identity and citizenship as well as on leadership and management skills. Another role of ICCI is in preparing Imams and sponsoring students of Islamic disciplines; it is the official examination centre of the European college of Islamic Studies (France) branch of the European Institute for Humanities. Free lectures are provided by ICCI for students of this college and there are a number of students (both male and female) on its rolls. The ICCI pays particular attention to the youth, arranging exchange visits with youth associations of different European countries, providing good facilities to occupy and entertain them and organising a variety of activities both at the Centre and outside.

Finally, in order to promote integration and cooperation with Irish society ICCI has exchanged several mutual visits between its representatives and government bodies of the Republic of Ireland. The president of Ireland, Mrs McAleese, the former president, Mrs Robinson, the taoiseach, the ministers of foreign affairs and of education, TDs, party leaders and other prominent government figures have visited the Centre.[15]

---

15   *Islamic Cultural Centre of Ireland, an Islamic cultural landmark in the western world. Five years of benevolence 1996-2001: a concise illustration of the ICCI's main activities and achievements during the foregoing period* (December 2002) passim. Every effort has been made to accurately reproduce, in an abbreviated form, the contents of this booklet.

17

Industry, quarrying and transport

U P T O T H E P R E S E N T D A Y there is considerable industrial activity in the neighbourhood of Clonskeagh even if what is there now is more akin to commerce rather than to what is traditionally thought of as industry. This is particularly so since the closure of the Smurfit cardboard works located in the area where in years gone by the lower of the two mills in Clonskeagh was to be found. A number of business parks have been constructed around the general Clonskeagh area in recent years. It is not, however, the purpose of the exercise being undertaken here to plot the progress of this activity. Instead, its focus is on the older industry in the area. Unfortunately, much of the detail surrounding this has been very difficult to unearth but what has been recovered is included in what follows. It is therefore merely an introduction with much left to be covered in any future examination of the subject.

MILLS AT CLONSKEAGH IN MEDIEVAL TIMES

The reference to wheat being grown in the manor of Rathbo in the year 1305 that can be seen when the sheriff of Dublin seized '50 crannocs, the crop of 40 acres of wheat'[1] and the Fleetwood Survey of the Cromwellian period which reported that the townland of Rabuck contained 400 acres (12 in meadow, 360 arable, 28 in pasture and no waste) have another aspect to them that is of interest. An important part of a feudal manor in the medieval period was the mill for grinding corn which the lord owned. His tenants were compelled to use this mill and in this way the lord increased his revenue. For example, the same Fleetwood Survey tells us that there was one mill in the townland of Rabuck, obviously on the Dodder at Clonskeagh 'in use worth, in Anno 1640, ten poundes'.

The mill which was a meeting point also provided opportunity for certain

---

1   Mills, *Calendar of the Justiciary Rolls... Edward I*, i(ii) 165.

legal matters pertaining to the manor to be dealt with; matters relating to land tenure especially but others as well. Some manors, for instance, held what was called a *court leet;* this acted as a court of law where routine matters of a local nature, but not necessarily directly related to the running of the manor, were processed such as public order and, in earlier times, even capital offences. We know from the inquisition of 1575 that lord Trimleston had a mill at Clonskeagh at that time but there is no evidence available for an earlier one; it seems, however, most likely that one did exist. The technology of mills was known in Ireland long before the Normans arrived in the latter half of the twelfth century; there is good evidence from as early as the 8th century that both horizontal and vertical mills were in use in Ireland. The horizontal, which was technologically simpler, was most common; it was particularly suited to fast flowing rivers of relatively small size. Unlike the vertical mill it did not require gears to transfer the power retrieved from the flowing water to the place where that power was put to use; such use was most commonly the grinding of corn. The structure associated with it was straightforward. It consisted of a two story building with the water wheel in the lower one lying flat in or close to the river into which the water was channelled. As the wheel rotated a shaft firmly attached to it also rotated; in the second floor immediately above it the shaft was attached to a grinding stone. As well as this moving stone there was a fixed stone; the movement of one against the other ground the corn.[2]

We can only speculate as to whether there was such a mill at Clonskeagh before king Henry II granted the land to Thomas de St Michael in the latter part of the 12th century; if there was not we can be almost sure that one would have been constructed soon after the land was granted. The river Dodder was particularly suited to such an enterprise. In a deed recording the granting of the manor of Rath by Nicholas de Hynteberge to Sir Robert Bagod around the year 1280 reference is made to 'a site of a mill, where a mill stands, with the duct of the water of the Dodder to the mill, thence descending to the sea'. The location of this mill is not clear from reading the deed but it was somewhere near Donnybrook.[3]

An interesting observation from the inquisition of 1575 is that it refers to a mill in the singular. We know from the evidence associated with the perambulation of the city of Dublin in the mid 1700s that there were two mills at Clonskeagh at that time, one at the south west of the bridge, the other at the

---

2   John Bradley, 'Mills and milling', Seán Duffy (ed) *Medieval Ireland: an encyclopedia* (New York 2005) 337-38.
3   Pembroke Estate Office, *Calendar of ancient deeds and muniments,* 5.

north east of it. The mill on the south west was on the territory of the manor of Rathbo; the other, however, came within the jurisdiction of the city authorities. The latter could have been there for a very long time but we have no evidence whatever concerning any early history that may be associated with it. The mill on the south-west side of the bridge was there in 1575 and most likely also from an early period of the feudal manor of Rabo. We have already noted the fact that medieval manorial mills within the feudal system often had court proceedings associated with them. Here, then, is a possible separate court to that referred to in the map found in 1835 in the Grand Jury room of Dublin. In describing the boundaries of Dublin an asterisk was put beside places where it says 'a court is called'; one such asterisk is put, as we have seen in Chapter 2 above, beside Clonskeagh lane which was on the north-west of the bridge. It is possible, then, that courts were anciently held on either side of the river close to the bridge.

MILLS AT CLONSKEAGH FROM THE LATE 18TH CENTURY ONWARDS

All the observations with regard to mills at Clonskeagh made above, it need hardly be explained, are about the period before the use of mills was turned into an enterprise of industrial size by Henry Jackson in the latter part of the 18th century. At a time, probably before Henry Jackson set up his iron works at Clonskeagh, there was a report of a mill being swept away in the vicinity. This report was carried in the *Dublin Evening Post* and it stated that, on the 25 November 1786, the weir of John Carbery's paper mill at Clonskeagh 'is entirely swept away by the floods'. He had rebuilt the weir two months previously at great expense and was now as a result 'drove to the verge of ruin'. He nevertheless appears to have remained in business as a papermaker since his initials are found, possibly as watermarks, on works published in the 1790s and as late as 1806. [4] Whether the paper used in these publications was made at his mill in Clonskeagh or not has not been discovered but it does seem to be most likely since repairing the weir, expensive though it may have been, would have been less costly than moving his whole papermaking operation to some other location on the Dodder, the original cause of his woes in 1786. If it is the case that he was still operating a papermaking mill at Clonskeagh into the early years of the 19th century, then it would have been downstream of the bridge since it is known that Henry Jackson had been operating a mill upstream of the same bridge since at least the last decade of the 18th century.

One of the earliest descriptions of Henry Jackson's mills at Clonskeagh, after

---

4   Pollard, *Members of the Dublin book trade*, 84-85.

he was arrested during the 1798 rising, is that given by lieutenant Archer who carried out a survey of county Dublin for the Dublin Society (the forerunner of the RDS) in 1800. Under the general heading of 'State of mills of every kind', we find the following: 'Clonskeagh – Two iron-work wheels; Jackson and White. Three iron-work wheels; Mr Stokes and company'.[5] This would suggest that at that time there were two separate works in operation using mills and that Henry Jackson, who had not as yet been exiled to America, still had some form of arrangement with the person who brought the White element into the name of his company. Some years later we get more detail about Jackson's mills. It is found in the work of D'Alton, writing in 1838, where he says: 'Above the latter [i.e. Messrs. Wright and Stanley's factory which was downstream of the bridge] are iron mills, erected originally on a very great scale by a Mr Jackson, at an expense of £2,000, having two powerful water-wheels twelve feet in diameter by seven wide, one twelve by five, and a fourth twelve by three, each possessing a head and fall of sixteen feet and upwards, with all befitting apparatus of hammers, shears, cylinders, rollers, etc., and complete ranges of workshops. The whole interest in this concern was sold by auction in 1834 and is now the property of Mr M'Casky, who employs about 10 persons'.[6] We know that by that time Jackson had long ago left Ireland (he settled in Baltimore in 1805) but who were and what happened to Messrs White and Stokes has not been discovered.

Evidence from maps of the area around the period under discussion is minimal. Rocque's map of c. 1760 makes no reference to a mill at Clonskeagh although there is a clear indication of a building immediately on the south west side of the bridge in the location in which we know that Jackson's mill existed some decades later. The next map, Taylor's of 1816, shows two iron mills, one upstream of the bridge and the other downstream. Interestingly, it also shows a pathway starting at a point just beyond the bridge, where the mill was located, and proceeding the whole distance as far as the Dundrum road close to where the latter crosses the Dodder at the ford in Milltown. This seems almost certainly to be the pathway (or a later version of it) which caused the owner of *The Dublin Journal* to issue such a stern warning some 27 years previously. Writing in his edition of 25 July 1789 he made this call to action 'The path-way, which for time immemorial remained open from Milltown to Clonskeagh, through the lands of Roebuck [i.e. south of the river], has been recently stopped up, and intersected with fences and barred gates. If the freeholders of the county respect themselves, they will investigate this matter, and check, in the outset, an

---

5   Archer, *Statistical survey of the county Dublin*, 206.
6   D'Alton, *History of the county of Dublin*, 808.

encroachment which may, in a short time, be extended not only throughout the vicinity of the metropolis, but throughout the whole county, and drive the foot passenger from the usage of the foot paths into the sludge of the high roads'. While this call to action tells us a good deal about the relative merits of footpaths and main roads from the point of view of walkers, it also tells us that, in blocking access by people, some activity was being planned for this area. We know from the first Ordnance Survey map of 1837 that there had been a major development in the area in previous years in that a large pool or head race had been provided there for use by the mills in the iron works at the bridge. Neither of the maps (Taylor of 1816 and Duncan of 1821) shows this pool but the absence of an item from a source is not proof that it did not exist. It seems highly unlikely that a mill of the size that Jackson operated at the end of the 19th century could have satisfactorily operated without having a head of water of some substance to power his mills (according to D'Alton it had a head of sixteen feet, a not inconsiderable head contrived from the river Dodder). That being the case, it is quite possible that it was Jackson who had blocked the way as the first step to making a pool there which would, some time later, feed into his mills. But if he did, then he may have provided another pathway, a little further away from the river and the pool, for the walkers and this is what Taylor recorded in his map of 1816.

We have already noted D'Alton's statement in 1838 that Mr M'Caskey had bought Jackson's iron works at auction in 1834 and, quite fortuitously, that is the year in which Clonskeagh is listed for the first time in the directories. The result is that, using them, we can trace subsequent owners of those works. As we have noted when discussing The Hermitage on Roebuck road, William M'Caskey, the man who had bought the works in 1834 died that same year. Prior to this purchase he was described in 1830 as being an 'iron manufacturer' with an address at 22 Church street. He was succeeded in his ownership of the Clonskeagh works by Thomas M'Caskey, possibly his brother. It is not clear, however, if he succeeded him immediately since there is no mention in the directories of any owner of the mills for the years 1835 to 1838 inclusive. However, during those missing years, Thomas M'Caskey is entered in the *Post Office Annual Directory and Calendar* for 1836 as: T. M'Caskey, ironmonger and Sheffield warehouse, 8 Kennedy lane. This shows that he was in the iron business during these years and it is possible that the works at Clonskeagh were allowed to lie fallow for a few years since, as we already noted, there were only 10 persons employed when William M'Caskey owned the business in 1834. As well as that it does seem strange that D'Alton, writing in 1838, did not mention that Thomas M'Caskey was, at that time, the owner (if, indeed he was) but confined himself to a reference to what had happened 4 years previously when the plant was bought by William M'Caskey. Thomas M'Caskey was certainly in possession of the mills from 1839 to 1841 (there was no entry for 1842); this was a relatively short time and gives some strength to the proposition that the mills may not have been in operation for some years before we know that he took them over.

There were momentuous changes in 1843 but first it is clear from both the directories and the first Ordnance Survey map of 1837 that there was a stuff factory downstream of the bridge, before the weir and on the city side of the Dodder, run by Thomas Maiben Baird (1834-39) and J Baird (1840-42), most likely powered by the mill there. Then in 1843 both the M'Caskeys and the Bairds bow out and the following are listed for that year: Thomas Portis 'spade, shovel and edge tool manufacturer' and John Rochford & Son, 'Clonskea forge mills and 38 City quay'. Both works were apparently sold separately to two different operators. The question then to be asked is this: which of the two were sold to each person? The answer is found, helpfully, in the notes made by Sir Richard Griffith who carried out a survey of valuations in the area sometime around 1850. As part of his methodology, he organised his findings according to civil parish and townland and it is here we find the answer. Under the heading of Roebuck townland he recorded that John Rochford was the owner of iron-mills, a house, offices and a garden as well as land measuring 5 acres 3 roods 26 perches, all valued at £132.[7] The answer to our question is found in the fact that Rochford's mills were in the townland of Roebuck which immediately identifies them as being on the south side of the river. That means that he owned the upstream iron-works which, in turn, tells us that the Portis mills were downstream and on the city side of the river. A further, although incidental, piece of information we get from the Griffith Valuation is that there were four people with the name Portis who had property in Clonskeagh c. 1850: Hannah, John, Mary and Thomas Portis.

In 1847, while Thomas Portis is still in possession of his works they are recorded as having a rateable valuation of £60. Portis continued to operate the iron mills until 1852 and, in the following year, we find Mrs Portis listed as the proprietor; it is, however, the last year that a Portis would be thus listed. And very significantly, the next year (1854) sees the first entry of a name that was to become almost synonymous with the iron mills at Clonskeagh – Thomas Henshaw. It is quite clear that he had bought the business hitherto owned by the Portis family since, like them, he is described in that year's entry as ' spade, shovel and edge tool manufacturer'. To confirm this, the Rochford mills are recorded in the same year; the entry for them now reads: 'John Rochford & Son,

7   William E Hogg, *The millers and the mills of Ireland of about 1850* (Dublin 2000) 191.

manufacturer of anchors etc Clonskea iron mills'. He had been joined in his business for a very short time by James Dodd, brassfounder; however, he only appears on one occasion in the directories, in 1847. Another curious item is found in the directories in the late 1840s and early 1850s. It is reported in the general description of Clonskeagh that as well as 'two hammer-smith iron works' being there, there was also a 'marble saw mill'. No mention is made of this in the listing of mill owners that follows underneath that general description nor is there any mention of the source of the marble or the use to which it was put when sawn. It was, apparently, a short lived enterprise that did not survive but which of the two mill owners was the entrepreneur has not been discovered. In the 1862 directory it is noted that John had been succeeded by Henry Hugh Rochford. However, it would appear that the actual transaction of ownership was registered in the previous year. This is most likely to be the legal transaction recorded in the Memorial of Deeds at the Registry of Deeds, Dublin in 1861 where Henry Rochford is recorded as being the owner of a mill at Clonskeagh.[8] Henry Hugh seems to have expanded the business which is described in 1863 as: 'spade, shovel, scrap, iron shafting, railway, and draining tool manufacturer, Clonskeagh iron works'. However, that may not have been a success as he is seen to remain as proprietor for only another 3 to 4 years. His last listing is 1866 and in the following year a very noticeable change can be detected with regard to both mills at Clonskeagh for in that year (1867) there is only one iron-works reported.

It is: 'Thomas Henshaw & Co., spade, shovel, scrap, iron shafting, railway, and draining tool manufacturer, Clonskeagh iron works'. It will be immediately noted that, although the name is Thomas Henshaw & Co., the description of the works is the exact same as that which Henry Hugh Rochford had used as recently as 1863. Henshaw had bought the upstream mill as a going concern from the Rochfords. As well as that the entry contains a new title for Henshaws; it is now Thomas Henshaw & Co. where previously it was merely Thomas Henshaw. However this had not been brought about by the purchase of Rochford's business as it is apparent from an advertisement some years earlier, in the 1858 Directory, that the status of the business had already been changed to Thomas Henshaw & Co. The latter was now the proprietor of both sets of mills at Clonskeagh and this is confirmed by an advertisement that appeared in the directory in the same year (1867). Under the section of the advertisement which is concerned with Henshaw's business in Christchurch place and Kennedy's lane

---

8   Idem, *The millers and the mills of Ireland: a database list (1700-1900)* (Dublin 2000) unpaginated but arranged alphabetically according to townland; see Clonskeagh.

THOMAS HENSHAW AND CO.,
(Successors to LUKE BUTLER,
5, CHRISTCHURCH PLACE, AND 16, KENNEDY'S-LANE),
Wholesale Furnishing and Builders' Ironmongers; also Manufacturing General Ironmongery and Tool Warehouse,
81, MIDDLE ABBEY-STREET,
SPADE, SHOVEL, AND TOOL WORKS. CLONSKEAGH,
Beg to call attention to their extensive Stock of Hardware, in all its different branches, which they are prepared to supply on the most moderate terms. Iron Wire for Fencing, and Galvanized Wire Netting, at reduced prices.
Agents for the Sale of THOMAS PERRY and SONS' Patent Fire-resisting WROUGHT IRON SAFES, with drill-proof doors and powder-proof Locks. They are the best safeguards in the world against fire and thieves. On the 30th July, 1857, the above were PUBLICLY TESTED at BELFAST, in the presence of many influential gentlemen, and their superiority in resisting prolonged intensity of heat, and in baffling all attempts to effect access by drilling instruments, was placed beyond doubt. STRENGTH and QUALITY CONSIDERED, THEY ARE CHEAPER THAN ANY OTHER MADE. NO MERCHANT SHOULD BE WITHOUT ONE.
The above in Stock at 5, CHRISTCHURCH-PLACE, and 81, ABBEY-STREET.

THOMAS HENSHAW & CO.,
Wholesale Furnishing & Builders' Ironmongers & General Hardware Merchants,
5, CHRISTCHURCH-PLACE, AND 15 & 16, KENNEDY'S-LANE,
Beg to call attention to their extensive, varied, and well-selected Stock of Ironmongery, in all its different branches. It consists of Parlour, Drawing-room, and Bed-room Grates; Kitchen Ranges, Cottage Ranges, Sash Weights; Iron Rim, Mortice, and Stock Locks; Hinges of all descriptions; Wrought and Cut Nails; Eave Gutters, Down Pipes and Fittings, Metal Skylights, Ventilating Bricks; Cast-iron Chimney-pieces, with and without Grates; Rabbit Traps, Fox Traps, Galvanized Wire Netting, Fencing Wire, Sheet and Perforated Zinc, Sink Traps, Furnace Doors and Frames, Hot Air and Plain Stoves.
ALSO
MANUFACTURING and GENERAL IRONMONGERS and TOOL WAREHOUSE,
81, MIDDLE ABBEY-STREET
RAILWAY, MINING, DRAINING, QUARRY, EDGE TOOL, SCRAPT IRON, CHAIN, SPADE AND SHOVEL WORKS,
UPPER AND LOWER MILLS, CLONSKEAGH.
Letters addressed to **5, CHRISTCHURCH-PLACE,** Dublin.

(Top) Advertisement for Henshaws, dated 1858, at a time when they owned the lower mill only; (Below) Advertisement for Henshaws, dated 1867, the year they are first reported as owners of both upper and lower mills

and its warehouse in Middle Abbey street, all of which were in the city, the following is found: 'Railway, mining, draining, quarry, edge tool, scrapt iron, chain, spade and shovel works – Upper and Lower Mills, Clonskeagh'. There was little change in the directory entries in subsequent years. The rateable valuation dropped to £50 in 1878; the downstream mills alone had a valuation of £60 in 1847. It would be unwise to draw too much of a conclusion from this drop until a proper study of changes in valuation throughout the 19th century has been carried out. In any case the rate jumped again; this time to £80 in 1915 during the Great War. It is possible that both the £50 and the £80 valuations just described referred to one of the works only since in 1918 two separate valuations are given, £47 and £80, and it is quite likely that these refer to the two separate works. If that is the case, the £80 would most likely refer to the upstream mills. In 1894 a legal transaction was recorded in the Memorials of Deeds at Registry of Deeds, Dublin whereby the Hibernian Bank became the proprietors of a mill weir and mill race at Clonskeagh.[9] The significance of this is that it reminds us that mill weirs and mill races, being expensive infrastructures essential to mills, were valuable assets. In this case, it would appear that the weir and race in question must have been the property of Henshaws prior to the legal transaction. Why they were sold, if that is what the legal transaction entailed, is not apparent.

Around 1918 the Henshaw company structure was changed; it became a limited company. The next change in the entries came in 1933 when the listing said simply 'Clonskeagh iron works (£47 & £80)'; why the name Henshaws was dropped is not clear but what is clear is that change was now taking place. When it began has not been discovered but from 1940 onwards there are entries in the directories of the name of the manager of the lower mills, R S Hamilton. In 1946 we find that he is the manager of Industrial Appliance and Mill Engineering Co., Red Mills. However, this company does not appear to have lasted for a substantial length of time; it is listed for the last time in 1949. Then after a few years with no entry we find the following in the same location in the directory for the year 1953: Jefferson Smurfit and Sons, Ltd., card box manufacturers. In 1960 we note that its address is given as 66-67 Clonskeagh road and its rateable valuation £650. That rose to £750 in 1965 and £875 in 1969. In that year there was another item entered immediately below it: 'Clonskeagh Board Mills Ltd' most likely part of the Smurfit operation. In 1974 it was trading under the title: Smurfit Paper Mills Ltd. A new era had dawned but, as would become clear in the early years of the 21st century, that dawn would in time fade as the site was fated to lose its industrial heritage and become residential. As for the upper mills they continued to be listed until the end of the 1950s. Soon thereafter they too disappeared along with the mill pool and the site was turned into a linear park of great beauty and tranquillity. The owner of *The Dublin Journal* who had written so passionately in 1789 about the blocking off of the pathway on the south side of the Dodder between Clonskeagh and Milltown to facilitate, as we have argued, the work needed to put the mill pool or head-race in place, would be very pleased with the eventual outcome.

---

9   Ibid.

Finally, a word about the house associated with the mill. We have seen that in the notes prepared for the Griffith Survey of the Clonskeagh area (c. 1850) it was said that the then miller John Rochford was the owner of a house, offices and a garden as well as iron-mills. There is, however, no reference to this house in the directories; that is, until 1952 when we find that John Thompson is listed in the Clonskeagh section with an address 'Mill House'. He is initially recorded as being a grocer but from 1960 a newsagent and tobacconist. It is not clear whether the house in question is the house originally associated with the iron-works or just a modern name which uses a local feature as an element in its makeup.

MILLS IN WINDY ARBOUR — SILK, PAPER, STARCH, BARK, SAW, FLOUR MILLS

It is often forgotten that Dublin was once famous for its silk industry. Although a great many of those employed in the industry lived and worked in the Coombe, Pimlico, Spitalfields, Weavers square and surrounding areas, a number of people in the Windy Arbour area were also once similarly employed. It is said that most of the inhabitants were skilled at silk weaving under the management of Mr Sweeny. It is also said that the industry flourished there[10] but, as will be seen, this may be an exaggeration. The particular location was chosen, no doubt, because of the availability of clean water supplied by the river flowing through the area on its way to the Dodder.

The silk trade was introduced into Ireland from France by the Huguenots. There is evidence that in 1682 a number of Huguenots, including a silk weaver, were admitted to the franchise of the city; in subsequent years many more were admitted. By 1727 raw silk to the value of £38,697 per annum was being turned into finished product and the number employed is so doing was considerable. Silk was also being combined with other material such as cotton and worsted wool to make products like tabinet or poplin. However, the industry faced many difficulties from imported (or smuggled) silk and stuff made with silk. The Irish parliament in College green sought to protect the fledgling industry by imposing a duty on imported product. Although it continued to be increased, the duty never managed to stem the inward flow. French imports, in particular, were the greatest problem and these were sometimes re-labeled in Britain thereby exempting them from the duty. The result was a dramatic drop in the number of looms, 800 in 1730 to 50 in 1763. In an effort to stimulate industry at this time

10   W St Joyce, *The neighbourhood of Dublin*, 180.

parliament gave £8000 to the Dublin Society (later the RDS); it prioritised the silk industry, setting up a Silk Warehouse in Parliament street in 1764. It gave a boost to the industry leading to a period of prosperity but it was short-lived.

By 1784 half of Dublin's looms were unemployed and the Silk Warehouse was closed by an act of parliament in 1786, deemed a failure. The Dublin Society had spent more than £28,000 on the industry, more than on anything else. After the Act of Union, when many of the aristocratic class had departed to London, the silk trade was almost totally annihilated. It was the 'free trade' within the United Kingdom, of which Ireland was now a part, that was mainly responsible for this. Despite silk weavers voluntarily reducing their wages the decline continued. There was dreadful poverty among the silk weavers. Finally, in 1840 the old Corporation of Weavers ceased to exist. The only thing that was salvaged was poplin; it was then used mainly in the making of neckwear, the poplin tie.[11]

The location of the Silk Mill in Windy Arbour can be seen in the Ordnance Survey map of 1837 where it is entitled 'Idle Silk Mill'; (incidentally, those who prepared the map refer to Windy Arbour as 'Sandy Arbour'). It is approximately a little more than a mile from the end of Bird avenue as one goes towards Dundrum. Also indicated on the map are some buildings and a head race with a pond, obviously constructed to provide power for the mills. In the printed version of the first Ordnance Map of the area, published in 1843, this mill has got a new name 'Starch Mill'. Prior to the mill being used for the production of silk, it had for many years been used for making paper. This is clearly shown in a number of maps of the area. The Rocque map of 1760, Taylor's of 1816 and Duncan's of 1821 all indicate that there was a paper mill there. That would suggest that it was transformed into a silk mill at some time between 1821 and 1837, a most unpropitious time as we have seen. Perhaps this is the reason why it was so short lived. The pond and the mill were already in place and the ability to weave silk but the market had collapsed. This evidence would appear to suggest that the statement by Joyce that the inhabitants of Windy Arbour were once 'extensively engaged in the silk industry' was somewhat of an exaggeration.

A word of caution is necessary. Due to the scarcity of evidence and the fact that maps may have marked only the principal mill (assuming that there was more than one mill there at the time any of the maps were being drawn) it is possible that the succession of uses to which the mill was put, as described above, may not be accurate. There may have been some smaller mills in operation. That

---

11   J. J. Webb, *Industrial Dublin since 1698 and the silk industry in Dublin* (Dublin 1913) 126-79; Joyce, *The neighbourhood of Dublin*, 180; *Centenary of Holy Cross church, Dundrum*, 31.

this is so is suggested by the entry in *Thom's Directory* for 1846 that Bartholomew Wall and Son operated a bark mill there that year. This is only three years after the published version of the first Ordnance Survey map marked only a starch mill in the area. To add to the difficulty in interpretation, this bark mill is found only once (1846) in the directories and there is no mention of him to be found in another source dated only a few years later c. 1850. Around that time, according to the notes made in preparation for Griffith's Valuation for county Dublin, there were two mills in Windy Arbour. The information in these notes relates to an area under the heading of Clonskeagh and subheading of Farran-boley; that can only apply to Windy Arbour, it being the only part of Farran-boley which has a river, a necessary prerequisite for a [water]mill. The first of these mills is a saw mill owned by John Lee. The acreage of the property is not given but it is stated that he had an office attached to the mill and the whole property was given a rateable valuation of £20. The second mill found in the notes is described, somewhat incongruously, as a 'flour and saw mill' and was owned by James Henderson. The acreage of the property is not given here either but it was said to have 'offices' attached – perhaps a different office for flour and for saw milling – and was also given a rateable valuation of £20. We can get some perspective on the size of these milling operations when we compare this valuation with that given to John Rochford's iron works at Clonskeagh bridge in the same source; its valuation was £132.[12] What happened to the bark mill or the starch mill that had been recorded there only a few years earlier? One possible answer can be suggested by the description of the mill owned by James Henderson as described by the notes prepared for Griffith's Valuation. Although we described 'a flour and a saw mill' as being somewhat incongruous there may, in fact, be nothing incongruous about it if we remember that the mill supplied power; what use the power was put to depended upon the business opportunities that were available at the time. The technology involved would have been quite simple and it would not have been very difficult to adapt from one use to another. Something of this nature seems to have happened in the late 1840s at Clonskeagh when it is recorded that there was a marble saw mills there while also noting the presence of the two iron mills upstream and downstream of the bridge. As regards the starch mills, it may be noted here that Hogg says it was located at Millmount terrace and a survey carried out by him in 2002 recorded that nothing of it then remained.

Before entering the Dodder, the river flowing through Windy Arbour is now channeled underground; however, its actual point of entry is easily visible if one

---

12 Hogg, *The millers and the mills of Ireland of about 1850*, 191.

walks along the pathway in the linear park from Milltown bridge, past the Packhorse Bridge, until the rear of the Shanganagh Apartments are in view across the river, well before one arrives at the newly refurbished Nine Arches Railway bridge. The origin of this river, the Slang (Slann), is said to be in the Three Rock Mountain and on its way it is augmented by an overflow from the Little Dargle river. It flows in the vicinity of Sandyford road, near Ballaly, and then through Dundrum before passing through Windy Arbour on its way to the Dodder. In times past, water was taken from the river, well upstream, to power two mills near the Packhorse Bridge in Milltown.[13]

OTHER INDUSTRIAL ACTIVITY IN CLONSKEAGH AS FOUND IN THE DIRECTORIES

A variety of industries have been recorded in the directories, some of which seem to have had short lives. In most cases, nothing further than the entry in the directory has been discovered. The year of the directory entry and the rateable valuation (where available) is given and an entry may be repeated where something of substance is seen to have changed from that which had previously been given. Directories examined from c.1834 up to and including the third quarter of the 20th century. The following list is merely indicative; it does not aspire to be in any way comprehensive.

> *Stuff factory:*
> Thomas Maiben Baird (1834-39); J Baird (1840-42). This factory is clearly marked on the first Ordnance Survey map, surveyed in 1837, corrected and published in 1843. It is located downstream of the bridge before the weir and on the city side of the Dodder.
> *Rope manufacturer:*
> John Sharp (1872).
> *Printing works and publishers:*
> Brown & Nolan, Ltd., printing works, Richview, Beech Hill road (1937); do. *(£1075)*(1938-40); Brown & Nolan, Ltd, The Richview Press, Ltd., publishers and general colour printers *(£1075)*(1941-60); do. *(£1683-10s)*(1962/3); do. *(£2,450)* (1974). Security Printing Ltd – there are two separate entries for this in the same directory (1974): i) Clonskeagh road (between nos. 67 & 73, beside Smurfits in directory; there may be some connection there); ii) Beech hill road.

---

13 Ordnance Survey Map 1837 in the National Archives of Ireland (ref. E 295. P. 1); Hogg, *The millers and the mills of Ireland: a database list,* unpaginated but organised alphabetically by townland; see under 'Windy Arbour'; Clair L. Sweeney, *The rivers of Dublin* (Dublin 1991) 66.

Thomas De La Rue & Co. Ltd., Beech hill road (c. 1974). Norman Waugh Ltd., printers' suppliers, 113 Clonskeagh road (c. 1969).

Manufacture of cotton and other textile products.

Eirecot Cotton Company, Ltd., manufacturers of absorbent cotton, Terminus Mills- sec^y. W Briscoe (1941); do. *(£150)*(1942-47). This appears for the first time in 1941, the year immediately following the last entry of the Tram depôt. The factory was located in the old tram depôt building which had also been the tram terminus; hence the element 'Terminus' in the title. In 1948 its business expanded; as well as absorbent cotton, it then manufactured wadding and absorbent surgical hose. It continued, with W Briscoe as secretary until 1958 when it was joined with another cotton manufacturing company which also operated at the Terminus Mills: Clonskea Cotton Co Ltd., manufacturers of sanitary towels (1943-57). From 1958 the company was entered as 'Eircot & Clonskeagh Cotton Company, Ltd., manufacturers of absorbent cotton wool, wadding, and surgical hose, sanitary towels. Terminus Mills. Sec^y W Briscoe'; *£150*(1958-60). Its rateable valuation had risen to £350 in 1963. However, the next time we find it (1965) the title had changed to: Robinson-Eirecot Cotton Co Ltd. *(£350)*. It was still trading under this name in 1974.

Donegal Design Ltd., Friarsland Mill, Roebuck road *(£50)*(c. 1965 – c. 1974).

Manufacture of Jams and Jellies.

Chivers and Sons (Ireland), Ltd., jams and jellies manufacturers, Beech hill road (1953-57); do. Beech Hill factory (1958-60); do. makers of table jellies, preserves etc., Beech Hill factory (1962/3-69). Chivers had already been in existence before it moved to its new factory at Clonskeagh in 1953. Later, in 1970, it moved to its present factory at Coolock.

Roebuck Jam Co. Ltd., Clonskea, Co. Dublin. This is the jam making industry set up by Charlotte Despard and Maud Gonne MacBride in 1924. It was closed down c. 1930.

Bakery equipment suppliers.

Foley, Duffy & Co., Ltd., bakery and general engineers, suppliers of bread, confectionery, automatic plant, bread slicers and wrappers, Clonskeagh (1953-55).

Electrical works.

Philips Electrical (Ireland) Ltd. *(£88)*(1955 – 1974 & later), Newstead house, Clonskeagh road; Philips Radio Manufacturing Co Ltd. (c.1969 – 1974 & later); Philips Electrologica Ireland Ltd., Electronic Data Processing (c.1974). Powerpak Ltd., car batteries, 105 Clonskeagh road *(£45)*(1969 – c. 1974). Peter Dand & Co. Ltd., radio distributors *(£45)*(1969 –c. 1974).

Round box manufacturers.

Wood, Rozelaar & Wilkes (Ireland), Ltd., Round Box Manufacturers, Clonskeagh road (on the south side of the bridge) (1955).

Finance company.

Sterling Mercantile Finance Co. Ltd, Newstead house (1956-c. 1969).

Building and building materials and equipment.

Gypsum Industries Ltd., Building Materials and Systems (1965-9), Wynnstay,

Clonskeagh road; do. (also) Manufacturers of Plaster, Plasterboard and Wood Wool (c. 1974 & later). John Jones Ltd., building contractors, Beech hill road (c. 1974). Concast Ltd., Beech hill road (c. 1974). Jones Group Ltd., holding company, Beech hill road (c. 1974). H A O'Neill, Ltd., heat & ventilating contractors, Beech hill road (c. 1974). Runtalrad Ltd., radiator manufacturers, Beech hill road (c. 1974). Climate Engineering Ltd., air conditioning contractors, Beech hill road (c. 1974). Irish Sprinkler & Fire Protection Ltd., Beech hill road (c. 1974). Leinster Homes Ltd., building contractors, Clonskeagh road (c. 1974).
P V Doyle Holdings Ltd., Clonskeagh road (c. 1974).
Industrial Stapling Machines:
Stapling Ltd., Industrial Stapling Machines, Strapping Tapes etc (1969). This was located on Clonskeagh road beside the Smurfit company. In 1974 it was still in the same location but then entitled: Wilson – Stapling Ltd., Industrial Stapling Machines, Strapping Tapes etc, Industrial Packaging Specialists.
Miscellaneous industries:
Roebuck Statue Factory (1953-8). Woodcraft Products Ltd (1953-58). Light Concrete Ltd (1953-58) – each entered under the non-specific heading of Roebuck.
Dublin Shipping Ltd., ship agents, Beech hill road (c. 1974). Celtic Coasters Ltd., Beech hill road (c. 1974).

QUARRYING IN THE CLONSKEAGH AREA

Whether quarrying of stone in an area is possible and, if so, the amount of stone is totally dependant on its natural geology. It would appear that at least some parts of the Clonskeagh area did have suitable geology to allow quarrying to take place. However, the history of the activity is somewhat spasmodic; references to it are sparse. Between October 1654 and November 1655 the Civil Survey of Ireland carried out its work in county Dublin. As a result, the report that followed described the 'Halfe-Barony of Rathdowne' in which Clonskeagh, south of the Dodder, is located, *inter alia,* as follows: 'The soyle thereof for the most part is dry and hott, haveing noe Woods, Boggs, Mines or Quarries theron'. Despite this suggestion that there were no quarries in Clonskeagh, many years prior to the Civil Survey, in the early 1300s, it was said that the stone buildings associated with the manor of Baggotrath, including its castle, were constructed with material quarried in Clonskeagh. Later, in 1772, Doctor Rutty had some essays printed which set out a natural history of the county of Dublin. It contains the following: '§37 Bluish grey compact limestone, with yellowish white calcareous spar, and yellow blende from the quarries near Milltown. §38 Ditto, ditto with veins of white calcareous spar, from the great quarries near Clonskeagh bridge.' Looking at the remains of these quarries today it is important to note his use of the word 'great' when referring to them. The reason for this is that the quarries have to be viewed within the context of the time and Dr Rutty gives us that context. To the modern eye these quarries may seem small but when in use during the 18th century they were obviously of substantial proportions. Sixty five years after Dr Rutty composed his essays, in 1837, the first Ordnance Survey indicated on its map of the area a quarry located on the opposite side of the road which leads to Donnybrook (i.e. Beech hill road and Beaver row) close to the second weir downstream from Clonskeagh bridge. The remains of this quarry can be seen to this day, especially at the entrance to a relatively new scheme of houses called Donnybrook court. The same Ordnance Survey map also marked another quarry further down the road to Donnybrook. It was located at the rear of the houses on Beaver Row stretching towards the site where Dublin Bus now has its depôt. It was, most likely, the other side of the same rock formation which was quarried further up the road towards Clonskeagh.[14]

Quarrying is, as we have said, dependant on the natural geology of an area. Another item similarly related is the botany found there; for that reason, it is considered convenient to insert the following item in this place. Writing in 1838, D'Alton suggests that a botanist would find the following growing in the general Roebuck/Clonskeagh area (Latin and English names): 'meum foeniculum, fennel; geranium molle, soft crane's bill; trifolium medium, zig-zag trefoil, a clover of great value for permanent pasture; picris echoides, bristly ox-tongue; carduus marianus, milk thistle and in boggy places between it and Lough Bray grows andromeda polifolia, wild rosemary, an elegant little shrub, which rises from six or eight inches to a foot in height, erect and branched.'[15]

PUBLIC TRANSPORT

When discussing the emergence of Clonskeagh as a residential area, the growth of public transport resulting from the increasing demand for a service between the city and Clonskeagh was used as an indication that the level of housing in the area was expanding and the place was becoming popular as a location in which to live. Initially the transport available was, in a sense, private in that it consisted of coaches, noddies and jaunting cars that could be hired. However,

---

14 Simington, *Civil Survey A.D. 1654-56: Vol. vii, County Dublin*, 259; Ball, *Historical sketch of the Pembroke Township*, 15; Dutton, *Observations on Mr Archer's statistical survey of the county of Dublin*, 79; Ordnance Survey Map of 1837 in the National Archives of Ireland (ref. E. 261. 1).

15 D'Alton, *History of the county Dublin*, 810.

with the intervention of the Carriage Office in Dublin castle which controlled the prices that could be charged for the carriage of persons and luggage as well as for the time spent waiting for a fare during a set-down, it could be said that transport had become public. Clonskeagh had first been added to the list of destinations over which the Carriage Office exercised control in 1794; Roebuck followed in 1831. There were other means of transport in operation in Clonskeagh some years after the Carriage Office had incorporated it into its schedule. There were coaches passing daily through it on their way to Enniskerry and Dundrum from the early 1820s and, although the advertisements do not say so, it seems likely that they would have served people living in the Clonskeagh and Roebuck areas as well as Enniskerry and Dundrum. By 1848 there were three of them passing through Clonskeagh daily and the name 'omnibus' (i.e. 'for all' in Latin) rather than coach then given to them certainly confirms their public nature. The introduction of omnibuses had been facilitated by a new Police Act in 1848 against strong opposition by the jarveys who till then had a monopoly on the provision of transport.[16] By 1858 these three omnibuses were reported to be plying several times daily to Clonskeagh from Dublin. This notice appeared each year in the directories until 1873. In the next year's directory this notice is dropped and a new one is noted for the first time: 'The tram-cars ply to Donnybrook from Nelson's pillar daily'. The terminus of the Donnybrook tram was where Dublin Bus now has its depôt, at the end of Beaver row which, of course, is on the road from Clonskeagh to Donnybrook. It would appear that these tram-cars had superseded the omnibuses; all of them were horse drawn. In 1882 the entry in the directory changed once more. This time the reference to the tram-car plying to Donnybrook is dropped. Instead it reported 'The tram-cars ply to Clonskeagh from College-green'.

The era of the tram had arrived in Clonskeagh although, as will shortly be shown, the actual date on which the first tram arrived there was in 1879. It was only seven years since the first horse-tram had begun commercial operation in Dublin on 1 February 1872. It had been operated by the Dublin Tramway Company between College green and Garville avenue, Rathgar. Exactly a year later, this company put its fourth tramline into operation, this time travelling to Donnybrook.[17] This tram-car service, although not going directly to Clonskeagh, was apparently used by people there to the extent that, as we have

16 Michael Corcoran, *Through streets broad and narrow: a history of Dublin trams* (Leicester 2000) 8.

17 James Scannell, 'From horse drawn trams to LUAS: a look at public transport in Dublin from the 1870's (*sic*) to the present time' in *Dublin Historical Record*, vol.59 no.1 (2006) 5-18: 6.

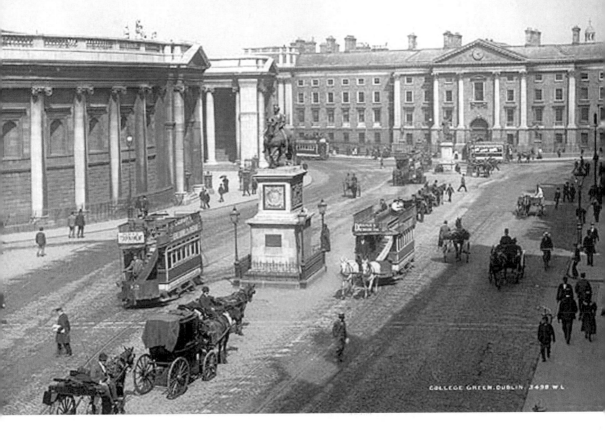

College green as it would have appeared when it was the city terminus for early Clonskeagh horse-drawn trams

seen, it put the omnibuses, which had served them for approximately the previous fifteen years, out of business. This is not surprising as, according to a report in the *Freeman's Journal* of 18 May 1896 and cited by Johnston 'Almost from the first, tram cars caught on in Dublin, and ... their popularity has steadily increased'.[18]

After the first tram company started operation others soon followed. One of these operated initially on the north side of the city only but in 1876 was authorised to extend one of its lines across Essex (now Grattan) bridge and on through Parliament street, Dame street into a new terminus in College green. The section from the College green terminus through Dame street became an

18   Denis Johnston, 'The Dublin trams', *Dublin Historical Record*, vol.12 no.4 (1951) 99-113: 105.

important part of an agreement that was soon reached between it and yet another company, the Dublin Central Tramway Company which had been set up under an act of 1878.

The chairman of this company was James Fitzgerald Lombard, who had amassed great wealth in the drapery business in Dublin; he was also the father-in-law of William Martin Murphy, then a successful building contractor specializing in tramways and railways. On 3 September 1878 he was engaged to equip the lines for this new company and on completion became one of its directors. It operated three routes and all of them started at College green terminus. The terminus here and the track along Dame street as far as the junction with South Great George's street it shared with the North Dublin Tramway Company but it then proceeded on its own tracks up Georges street, Aungier street and Camden street. At that point it divided into two, one proceeding into Harrington street, up South Circular road and ultimately on to Rathfarnham while the other turned into the now built-over Charlotte street, on through Charlemont steet, Ranelagh road and on to the Ranelagh Triangle (or Angle) where it divided again. Here one veered right going on ultimately up Palmerston road to its terminus at Palmerston park while the other went straight on to Clonskeagh.[19]

As well as laying down the tracks, work had also to be carried out on the Ranelagh side of the bridge over the canal; the characteristically hump-backed bridge was too difficult to negotiate for the two horses which drew the trams. The slope had to be made gentler and to this day one can observe the effects of this by noting the front of the houses on the left hand side of Ranelagh road immediately before the bridge; these houses were already built at the time this work was carried out. As one approaches the bridge it is quite noticeable that the gardens and footpaths to the front door get gradually higher reflecting the rise in the road that was brought about to overcome the problem encountered by the horse-drawn trams. A so-called 'tip-horse' was used to assist the two horses, which were yoked to the tram, to pull it up the steep gradient at the other side of the bridge.[20]

Of the three routes operated by the Dublin Central Tramway Company, the one to Clonskeagh was the only one to be serviced by single-decked trams. Although regarded as a branch line it was the first of the three to be put into public service. This was on 17 March 1879 and, although the weather on that day was very poor, the new service drew a positive comment on the following day from *The Irish Times*, a paper not known for its positive views on horse-trams.[21]

---

19 Corcoran, *Through streets broad and narrow,* 16-18.
20 Johnston, 'Dublin trams', III.
21 Corcoran, *Through streets broad and narrow,* 18-19; Johnston, 'Dublin trams', 107.

This has been cited by Corcoran in his book and, because it is particularly appropriate to a work that is concerned with Clonskeagh it is repeated here:

'The new line that was opened to Clonskea by the Central Tramways Company inaugurated the opening under the most favourable circumstances. The district has hitherto been accessible only by tortuous and embarrassing modes, although the residents include a large body of commercial gentlemen, but now a ready approach to the great business portion of the city is afforded. The citizens on the other hand are placed in the enjoyment of an additional 'lung' by the facility afforded of visiting a most salubrious and picturesque locality. The cars of the company have been built in Birkenhead and are designed to carry eighteen and twenty passengers inside and four – two each side of the driver – outside. The fittings are well designed and the seats are divided by brass rails to prevent any disputes between querulous passengers as to the accommodation for each'.

The reference here to 'a large body of commercial gentlemen' is a reminder that the tramway entrepreneurs only chose routes where there were people of some means living; they openly showed disdain for the less fashionable areas. The report also confirms the perception, which we have already encountered on a number of occasions, that Clonskeagh was a healthy place to live or to visit. [22]

The terminus at Clonskeagh was at Vergemount; *Thom's Directory* notes the presence of the Dublin Central Tramways depôt there for the first time in 1881. It has not been discovered what had previously been located in the space where this depôt was erected but it seems that there was not anything of great significance there since nothing of note is missing when a comparison is made between the entries in the directories before and after they list its presence. To have brought the tram further than Vergemount, had it been thought desirable so to do, would have presented some but not insurmountable difficulties with the very sharp right hand bend that immediately followed and the bridge over the Dodder soon afterwards. The depôt at Vergemount would have housed at different times many of the company's 200 horses; some of its 30 vehicles would also have been left there overnight. [23]

The company co-operated from its foundation, as we have seen, with the North Dublin Tramway Company. The advantages of co-operation in other ways led to the amalgamation of the three existing companies on 1 January 1881 under a name that was to become famous, the Dublin United Tramway Company (DUTC). Lombard and his son-in-law William Martin Murphy were

---

22 Corcoran, *Through streets broad and narrow,* 18-19.
23 Scannell, 'From horse drawn trams to LUAS', 7.

two of its seven directors whose annual fees were £1,500.[24] Despite the amalgamation, the directories continued to describe the depôt at Vergemount as the Dublin Central Tramway depôt until 1883, then Dublin Tramway depôt in 1884 before finally changing it to Dublin United Tramway depôt in 1885, a name it was to retain until trams ceased to operate on the route in 1939. It was assigned a rateable valuation of £115 in 1905; that rose to £121 in 1915 and remained at that until the end of its existence as a tram depôt. The first foreman named in the directories was James Kearns; he was listed as such in 1887-88. He may have been there longer than that since the next mention of a foreman is in 1896 when John Ryan is named and continued to be listed in that capacity until 1931. Writing in 1951 about John Ryan, then 95 years old and living in Sallymount avenue in Ranelagh, Johnston had apparently received first hand information from him about trams and his involvement with them. He said that from 1886 he was in charge of 154 horses in the Vergemount depôt. He had also been given special bonuses on occasions; one such happened in Westmoreland street when he prevented the two horses from bolting after becoming detached from the tram. At this time the city terminus of the Clonskeagh tram had been moved beyond O'Connell bridge up as far as Nelson's Pillar (it had been moved c. 1884, as a reference in *Thom's Directory* would suggest) where it was to remain for the remainder of its life. During the horse-tram era the first tram in the mornings left the Vergemount depôt at 8.00 am and the last tram from Nelson's Pillar departed at 10.22 pm, the earliest last tram of all; the fare was 3 pence single.

Although the first horse-tram went into commercial operation in Dublin in 1872, it was not long before thoughts were turning to other methods of traction other than the horse, thoughts driven mainly by economic factors. Electric traction soon became the most favoured alternative especially after a successful method of connecting electric power from a stationery source to individual moving trams was devised in America in the late 1880s. By the mid-1890s the Dublin Southern District Tramways Company which operated between Haddington road and Kingstown (now Dún Laoghaire) had successfully introduced electric trams and were attempting to extend them into the city where DUTC held sway. The latter, already contemplating the introduction of similar trams, was spurred into action. After much activity, the details of which need not detain us, DUTC had purchased the other line and electrified its own trams. The precise date on which the last horse-tram left the Vergemount depôt has not been discovered but it was probably on some day in 1899 or 1900. The last such tram to operate anywhere in Dublin was 14 January 1901 but this had

---

24   Corcoran, *Through streets broad and narrow,* 19.

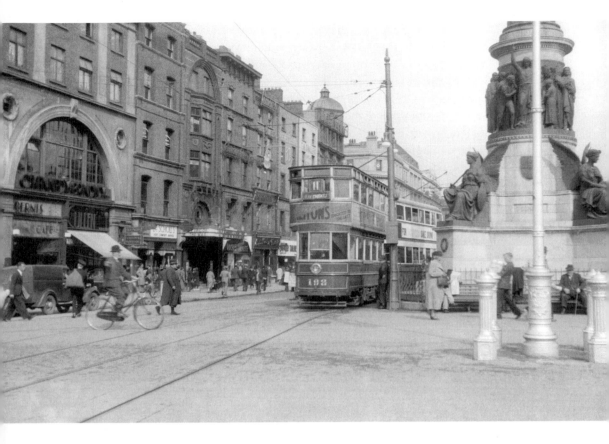

Clonskeagh tram leaves O'Connell street, 23 August 1938 (*Photographer: H B Priestley.*
Copyright: the National Tramway Museum)

got an artificial reprieve because of the difficulty presented to electric trams by the railway bridge in Bath avenue.[25]

In spite of the forebodings held by many, the electrification of the trams was a resounding success especially for the company's profits. The advent of electrical traction allowed for larger trams to be used. The depôt at Vergemount was able to hold 23 of these according to a 1910 publication. Initially, electric tram destinations were to be indicated by number with 5 being allocated to the Nelson's Pillar to Clonskeagh line. However, a different system was put into place during 1903 when instead of numbers the destination was indicated written in white letters on a black

25   Johnston, 'The Dublin trams', 110-111; Corcoran, *Through streets broad and narrow*, 31-6, 49; Scannell, 'From horse drawn trams to LUAS', 8-9.

background using a scroll lit from behind and with glass in front. As well as these each individual destination was given a specific symbol which was mounted on top of the destination box containing the scroll. All these symbols were made up of coloured squares, triangles and other shapes; the one assigned to Clonskeagh could be described as two overlapping yellow discs or two yellow impacted circles. However, the life-span of these coloured symbols was relatively short. In the Spring of 1918 they were replaced by numbers and in April of that year it was announced that the number 11 would be carried on the cars providing the Clonskeagh service, which by this time was operated via Leeson street.

The honeymoon DUTC enjoyed with the success of the electrification process did not last long however. The company was soon deeply involved in a bitter industrial dispute, long since known as the 1913 Lockout. After this came the Great War of 1914-18, the 1916 rising and the war of independence, followed by the civil war – all of which negatively impacted on the DUTC. Serious as these problems were they were nothing in comparison to what followed. This was the arrival on the scene of the bus with their flexibility in operation and low capital cost. From the early 1920s more and more privately run bus companies started to compete with the trams. By the mid 1920s, with the ever-increasing quality of buses making their competition a major problem, DUTC began operating their own bus service which they tried to integrate with their existing tram routes. In 1927 the Leyland Titan double-decked bus arrived on the market; this would in retrospect be seen as ringing the death knell for the whole tramway system. A further complication was the increasing number of privately owned motor cars competing for road space with the trams. The end was in sight in 1936 when DUTC ceased building new tram cars. This was soon followed by an announcement on 1 March 1938 that its policy was to ultimately replace all the tramcars with buses.

Two tram routes were abandoned to buses in 1938 but the major closures came in 1939. May 1st of that year saw the end of the northern section of the no. 11 route, Clonskeagh to Whitehall (this section had opened some years previously and had its terminus beside the Whitehall Garda station, built in 1934). The much older southern counterpart, from Nelson's Pillar to Clonskeagh, was abandoned to buses two months later, on 1 July. Also abandoned was the depôt at Vergemount. Buses carrying the number 11 now served the route from Vergemount to Mobhi road on the north side of the Liffey serving also Drumcondra road and Home Farm road. In time, as demand for its service grew with the building of new houses in the area, the Clonskeagh destination of the number 11 would move away from Vergemount outwards through the rest of Clonskeagh and beyond.[26]

---

26 Johnston, 'The Dublin trams', 100; Corcoran, *Through streets broad and narrow,* 62-3, 80, 88, 95, 103, 115, 121; Scannell, 'From horse drawn trams to LUAS', 9, 11.

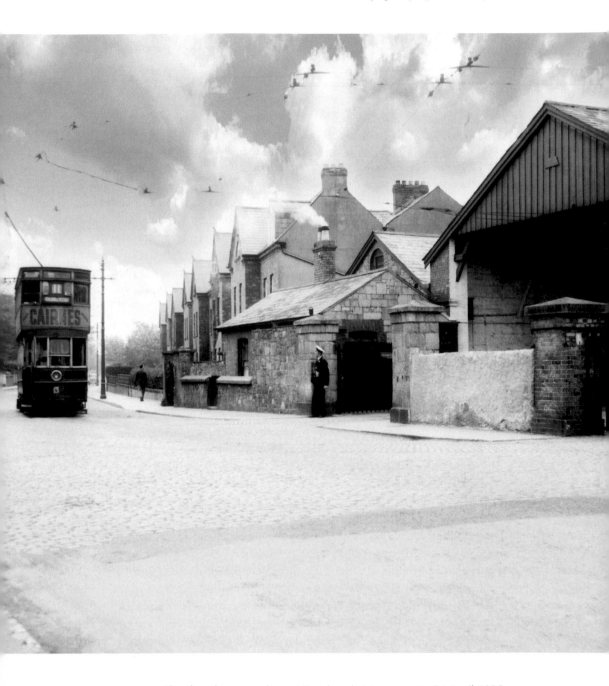

Clonskeagh tram arrives at Terminus in Vergemount, 24 April 1938
(*Photographer: W A Camwell. Copyright: the National Tramway Museum*)

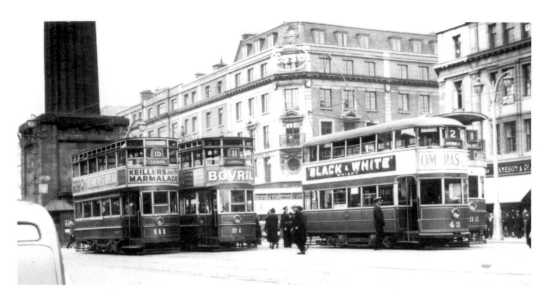

'In the heart of the Hibernian metropolis ...': Clonskeagh tram (number 11, in the middle) seen with others, before Nelson's Pillar (*Photograph: W A Camwell*)

The era of the Clonskeagh tram lasted just over 60 years (from 17 March 1879 to 1 July 1939) before passing into history but its memory lives on not least in the writings of James Joyce as he recorded in his work, *Ulysses*. In this Joyce, while telling of events on 16 June 1904, describes well the busy scene involving trams before (i.e. on the south side of) Nelson Pillar. A key figure there was the despatcher or timekeeper, as Joyce called him; it is likely that on that day it was captain Delayney who was on duty. As the trams had not as yet had individual destination numbers assigned to them the despatcher or timekeeper used the destination of a tram when he called out his order to it. The sounds he made when calling each tram would have been very familiar to Dubliners of the time.[27] All of this was captured by Joyce when he wrote: 'In the heart of the Hibernian metropolis: before Nelson's Pillar trams slowed, shunted, changed trolley, started for Kingstown and Dalkey, Clonskeagh, Rathgar and Terenure ... . The hoarse Dublin United Tramway Company's timekeeper bawled them off – Rathgar and Terenure! – Come on, Sandymount green. Right and left parallel clanging ringing a double-decker and a single-deck moved from their rail heads, swerved to the down line, glided parallel. – Start, Palmerston park.'[28]

27   Johnston, 'The Dublin trams', 101.
28   James Joyce, *Ulysses,* (Paris 1922; Picador edition London 1997) 112.

18

Culture – some contributions

THERE WERE MANY CONTRIBUTIONS made, down the years, to the cultural life of Ireland by people living in Clonskeagh some of whom are not very well known today. In what follows an attempt is made to illustrate a few examples of these while accepting that the list is not in any way complete.

WILLIAM MANWARING

Information on the first of these, William Manwaring, is somewhat sketchy but since it was announced in the *Public Gazetteer* that he died on 17 July 1763 'at his lodgings in Clonskeagh near Dublin' it seems that he should be included notwithstanding the paucity of the sources. It is not known when or where he was born; the first information on him is dated 1738 when he is said to be conducting his business at Corelli's Head, College green. According to the *Dublin Journal* he imported from Holland and London on 22 April of that year the best and newest music. Although described as a music seller, he was probably closer to what would today be described as an impressario. Two years later he took subscriptions for a work on musical technique and had an edition of certain favourite songs printed which he then put on sale in his business premises. Later, he sold tickets for the first performance on the musical glasses (i.e. the harmonica, an instrument of 18th century origin in which sounds are produced by application of moist fingers to drinking glasses or glass bowls). In 1743 he commenced publication of the *Monthly Masque, or an entertainment of musick* and continued to do so until his death. In 1747 he published *Collections of select minuets* with 'Eileen-a-roon' included. Later he took subscriptions for Scarlatti's *Lessons for the harpsichord* and settings of *English ballad songs* by S Murphy. He also produced a large book for the organist at St Patrick's cathedral. Around 1758 he had printed for him *Minuets for his majesty's birthday 1758* as performed at Dublin castle. In fact, it would appear that he was active in the music business up to the last year, at least, before his death in 1763 in Clonskeagh. It has not been possible to find out where he lodged in Clonskeagh or with whom. No one of the name Manwaring is found living in Clonskeagh in the directories but they, of course, become available long after he had died.[1]

JAMES HENTHORN TODD

It was not only through political activity that efforts were made in the nineteenth century to assert Ireland's right to take her place among the nations of the earth, to borrow a phrase from the concluding words of Emmet's speech from the dock. There were also efforts made in the cultural, literary and associated fields to establish a clear Irish identity now that Ireland was part of the United Kingdom. Central to this was, of course, the Irish language. Even at the time of the Union in 1801 the language and Gaelic culture in general were in dire straits. A variety of reasons, including the setting up of the primary school system on a national scale in 1831, contributed to a continued decline in the usage of the language. By 1851 the proportion of people who could speak Irish was merely 25%; those who could speak only Irish was 5%. These figures had reduced to 15% and 2% respectively by 1871.[2] Efforts to counteract this decline made thereafter, in particular, by *Conradh na Gaeilge* (the Gaelic League), founded by Douglas Hyde in 1893, as well as the related Gaelic sporting organisation, the Gaelic Athletic Association, founded by Michael Cusack in 1884, are well known. But what is, perhaps, not so well known is that there were very important contributions made much earlier on in the century by outstanding men of learning; doing pioneering work in the area of Irish language, antiquities and literature, searching out and preserving ancient Irish manuscripts, translating and publishing them.[3] These were serious high-minded people to whom much is owed by the Irish people. Among them were some residents of Clonskeagh; one in particular was the Rev James Henthorn Todd who lived for a number of years in Vergemount house, located where the Clonskeagh hospital now is.

He was born in April 1805; his father was professor of anatomy and surgery in the Royal College of Surgeons and the family home was at 5 Kildare street, the site where subsequently the Kildare Street Club was located. Although his father traced his ancestry to Scotland, on his mother's side Oliver Goldsmith can be found in the family lineage. The school he attended was particularly noted

---

1   Pollard, *A dictionary of members of the Dublin book trade 1550-1800*, 399; Ian Crofton (ed), *Concise dictionary of music* (3rd ed. William Collins & Sons, 1986) 212.

2   Macdonagh, 'Introduction: Ireland and the Union, 1801-70', in Vaughan (ed), *A new history of Ireland*, lx.

3   Comerford, 'Ireland 1850-70: post-famine and mid-Victorian', in Vaughan, *A new history of Ireland*, 393; Flanagan, 'Literature in English, 1801-91', in ibid: 502.

for its teaching of languages which included Latin, Greek, Hebrew, French, German and Italian. Such a foundation would be of particular value to him in his subsequent life's work. He entered Trinity College in 1820 and graduated in 1824 with an honours degree in science. However, less than two years later tragedy struck leaving him to care for his widowed mother and fourteen younger siblings; he was then twenty-one years old. This duty he took seriously; his male siblings were particularly successful, gaining positions of some note in their chosen careers while one of his sisters married Rev John Clarke Crosthwaite of Vergemount house in 1833. As well as that he was supportive of his mother and took her to live with him some years later when he moved into Vergemount house; he, however, remained unmarried.

From an early stage in his working life he showed himself to be very energetic in matters of a Celtic nature, in particular manuscripts containing material of great interest to scholars of Irish history. At the core of this activity was the Library of Trinity College, Dublin. And it was not just the manuscripts which the library already held that interested him; he also sought out, with assiduity, manuscripts of Irish interest that existed in England and elsewhere in Europe with a view either to purchase or to copy them for the library. Of particular note among these is the *Book of Dimma*, an ancient Irish manuscript book of the gospels, which he bought for £150 and Geoffrey Keating's *Foras feasa ar Eirinn* ('Compendium of wisdom about Ireland' or more simply 'History of Ireland') bought for 50 guineas. This latter is of note as it was written as part of an effort made by Irish Franciscans in Louvain in the seventeenth century to try and prevent knowledge of Irish history disappearing, in the aftermath of the collapse of Gaelic learning that followed Kinsale and the Flight of the Earls. As for the library's own stock of manuscripts, he sought and got permission from the board of the college to employ the famous John O'Donovan (the man perhaps best known for his edition and translation between 1848 and 1851, in seven volumes, of the Annals of the Four Masters, the manuscript of which had been the product of work done by the aforementioned Franciscans) to catalogue the Irish manuscripts in the library. It was Todd who gave, what is possibly the most famous manuscript in the possession of the college, the *Book of Kells*, the attention it properly deserved; some time previous to his tenure of office it had suffered badly at the hands of a binder, something that would never be allowed to happen from his time onwards.[4]

---

4   Simms, 'James Henthorn Todd', 5-13; Bernadette Cunningham, *The world of Geoffrey Keating* (Dublin 2004) 3.

Todd's involvement in the preservation of ancient Irish manuscripts took a further step forward in the winter of 1840/41 with the foundation of *The Irish Archæological Society*. The Society was founded, according to Todd, only after careful preparation and consultation when its greatest problem was in overcoming suspicion and mistrust.[5] This, it need hardly be recalled, was a time when two, to a large extent, mutually opposed political views prevailed as to how Ireland should be governed; by a government in Westminster or by one in Dublin. This problem for the Society was explained by Todd thus: 'In Ireland, where every thing is unhappily viewed, more or less, through the medium of party, it seemed to the public difficult to conceive how any Society could be formed without a leaning to one side or the other, and many persons very naturally held back until the real character of the Society should more fully develop itself.'[6] Only partially successful in its first year, to the great credit of the Society, and in particular to Todd himself, the problem was largely overcome in the following years. This can be clearly seen in a letter written by a friend to his brother Charles, with the *Irish Archæological Society* in mind: "He brought and kept together men who never before could be induced to act on any common ground for the benefit of Ireland ...for the first time the Regius Professor of Divinity and of Hebrew in Dublin may be seen acting together with the President of Maynooth, with one Roman Catholic gentleman joint secretary with your brother and another their assistant secretary ...".[7] It was most likely due to his efforts that the formidable Catholic archbishop of Tuam, Dr John MacHale, joined the society in 1842.[8]

During Dr Todd's long years as secretary a substantial number of works were published under the auspices of the Society. One of these was the product of his brother-in-law, Rev J C Crosthwaite. In 1844 he edited the *Book of Obits and Martyrology* of Christ Church cathedral from a manuscript held at Trinity College, Dublin, a work to which reference is made by historians to this day. This work includes a very substantial introduction by Dr Todd, (then also vice-president of the Royal Irish Academy) extending to 103 printed pages.[9] In 1848

---

5   John O'Donovan (ed. & tr.), *The banquet of Dun na n-Gedh and the battle of Magh Rath, an ancient historical tale*, Irish Archæological Society (Dublin 1842) 2.

6   Ibid. 1-2.

7   Simms, 'James Henthorn Todd', 16-17.

8   O'Donovan, *The banquet of Dun na nGedh*, 16.

9   John Clarke Crosthwaite, *The Book of Obits and Martyrology of the Cathedral Church of the Holy Trinity, commonly called Christ Church, Dublin*, Irish Archæological Society, (Dublin 1844) with an Introduction by James Henthorn Todd, DD, VPRIA.

Dr Todd edited and translated *Leabhar breathnach annso sis*.[10]

There were controversies during his tenure at the Society, of course. Some believed that the Society was too élite; membership was fairly expensive and it included a quite considerable number of dukes, marquises, earls and viscounts. The result was that a new society, entitled *The Celtic Society*, was founded in 1845, with much the same aims but lower membership fees. However, it soon ran into difficulties. One of the reasons for this was a perception among some of its members that the Society would do more for the perpetuation of Irish as a living language rather than merely publish Irish manuscripts of interest to scholars only. In fact it singularly failed to meet either of these objectives and membership fell away. In 1854 it was taken over by the *Archæological Society*, the very body which it had originally been set up to challenge; Dr Todd was involved in this event also.[11]

Dr Todd's association with Clonskeagh was, as already noted, through his brother-in-law, Rev John Clarke Crosthwaite. But he had other connections with it too. A member of the *Archæological Society* at its foundation in 1841, Rev Joseph H Singer, DD, MRIA, SFTCD lived in Clonskeagh, at the Roebuck end, for a number of years (c1836-1847). Around this time he gave the Donnellan Lectures in Trinity College (1835, 1837) and was appointed Professor of Modern History there in 1840. Later, after leaving Clonskeagh, he became rector of Raymochy in the diocese of Raphoe (1850), archdeacon of Raphoe (1851-2) and bishop of Meath until his death (1852-66).[12]

Another Clonskeagh connection was the lord chancellor Francis Blackburne, whom we have already met. The connection here is within a different context, although for Dr Todd, at least, on familiar ground; it was concerned with the Ancient Laws of Ireland, more commonly known as the Brehon Laws. Going back to ancient times in Ireland, these laws were still being used in parts of Ireland until the seventeenth century. The Elizabethan wars and the subsequent Flight of the Earls in 1607, however, saw them fall out of use, except for a few isolated areas, as the skilled practitioners no longer had patrons. Furthermore,

---

10 James Henthorn Todd (ed. & tr.), *Leabhar breathnach annso sis: the Irish version of Historia Brittonum of Nennius*, Irish Archæological Society (Dublin 1848).

11 Robert Somerville-Woodward, 'The Celtic Society', *Pages: Arts Postgraduate Research in progress*, Faculty of Arts, University College Dublin, vol. 5, 1998, 177-186; see note 64.

12 Irish Archæological Society, *Tracts relating to Ireland* (Dublin 1841) vol. 1, p12; Leslie & Wallace, *Clergy of Dublin and Glendalough*, 1056; *Pettigrew & Oulton Street Directory* for 1836; *Dublin Almanac* for years 1837 to 1847 inclusive.

English law was taking over. From then onwards interest in these ancient laws was merely antiquarian. Of particular importance in this regard was Dubhaltach Mac Firbhisigh (anglicized as Duald Mac Firbis). He was in a key position between the ancient system of the law schools where would-be practitioners were trained to a high degree and a later interest in Irish antiquity that was to be found among English speakers. He was, in fact, employed by one such person, Sir James Ware, who was a keen collector of ancient manuscripts; he was, however, killed by a soldier in 1670. Many of these manuscripts would later be of particular interest to the members of the *Irish Archæological Society*. Some members of this Society were very keen that the ancient laws contained in these and other manuscripts be edited and translated and thus made readily available to people without expertise in the Irish language. The task would be formidable (and expensive) as the language used in them was very complex, often being both archaic and technical while using abbreviations which were sometimes difficult to decipher. Various suggestions were made as to how the task should be tackled. Interest was not limited to Ireland; English and German scholars became involved too. In fact, some German scholars wrote to queen Victoria's husband, prince Albert, who was himself a German, urging that the project go ahead. Eventually, the United Kingdom government gave a grant of £5000 to facilitate the setting up and the maintenance of a 'Commission for the publication of the Ancient Laws of Ireland' and a further £500 a year to pay for the work involved in preparing and printing the laws. Twelve Commissioners were appointed, among whom were Dr Todd and the lord chancellor, Francis Blackburne. When work began, the task proved to be even more difficult than anticipated and was bedeviled by the government's reluctance to continue the payment promised for ongoing work. Although, when eventually finished and published in six volumes, the work contained many defects these were as much the product of the adverse conditions under which the two workers, John O'Donovan and Eugene (Eoin) O'Curry, toiled. Modern scholars, while noting these defects, are nevertheless very generous in their praise of much of their work.[13]

Another project which Dr Todd was involved in was the founding of St Columba's College, now at Rathfarnham. The background to the setting up of this college was a desire to provide an Irish based education, where the language would be cherished and in its foundation year 1843 Todd commissioned John O'Donovan to prepare an Irish grammar for its senior students. Although first located at a site chosen by Todd at Stockallen, near Navan, it soon afterwards

---

13   Boyne, *John O'Donovan*, 96-105; Fergus Kelly, *A guide to early Irish law*, School of Celtic Studies: Early Irish Law Series, Volume III (Dublin 1988, repr. 1995) 260-63.

moved to Holly Park, its present site at Rathfarnham. While he was living in Clonskeagh in 1851 he is on record as being principal of the college. He supervised the building of its new premises and was generally the driving force behind its initial success. He eventually moved to live near the College as did his mother who died at their house, Silveracre, off Grange road, Rathfarnham, in 1862. There, Dr Todd died some seven years later but not before he had completed the publication of yet one more scholarly work of importance to students of Irish history and antiquity, *Cogadh Gaedhel re Gallaibh: The war of the Gaedhil with the Gaill.* This work had been commissioned by the Master of the Rolls and is part of the famous Rolls Series. This truly illustrious man, whom archdeacon Cotton once described in 1850 as 'the *sine qua non* of every literary enterprise in Dublin' is commemorated in St Patrick's Cathedral, of which he had been Treasurer since 1848, by a high cross ornamented with Celtic designs.[14]

ROBERT ALEXANDER STEWART MACALISTER

Not long after the death of Dr Todd a person was born in Dublin in 1870 who would also, in time, contribute substantially to our understanding of the ancient history of Ireland. Like Dr Todd he too would come to live in Clonskeagh for a period of time. He was Robert Alexander Stewart Macalister; he lived during the second decade of the twentieth century in 5 Connaught place, now re-numbered 9 Clonskeagh road. Born, as we have said, in Dublin in 1870 he was the son of a professor of anatomy at Trinity College. His father later transferred to the chair in Cambridge. After early studies in Germany, he graduated with an MA from Cambridge and was soon honoured by LittD from Universities of Cambridge, Dublin and Wales and by the LL.D from Glasgow. At the outset, he went on an archaeological expedition to Palestine where he took charge of excavations. He published many reports but also continued to write on Irish antiquities. His brillance was already apparent in his early work as he laid a firm foundation for his later pursuits in the archaelogical, historical, mythological and philosophical fields.

It was archaeology however, in particular that of his native land, that he was most interested in. When the Dublin Commission, set up under the Irish Universities Act (1908), advertised a single chair in Celtic archaeology and early Irish history at UCD he applied for the post; so too did Eoin MacNeill. Because of his work in the Middle East, Macalister had at this stage gained an international reputation with professors of archaeology in many prestigious universities

---

14 Simms, 'James Henthorn Todd', 17-22; *Dublin Almanac* for 1843, 1844, 1845, 1847; *Thom's Directory* for 1846 to 1856 inclusive.

praising his work. Recognising his ability but also that of MacNeill, the Commission decided to divide the subject into two chairs and Macalister was appointed Professor of Celtic Archaeology with MacNeill taking up the early Irish history post. Some years later when MacNeill was under arrest after the 1916 rising Macalister took over some of his duties at UCD and offered the extra money that he got for so doing to MacNeill's wife.

As professor, Macalister was at the centre of all achaeological activity that was taking place in Ireland. From an early period he was a member of the Royal Society of Antiquaries of Ireland and it did not take him long before he advanced to Fellowship. From 1910 until 1918, while he lived in Clonskeagh, he edited the Society's Journal with distinction and in 1924 was honoured by election as President. His scientific work earned him membership of the Royal Irish Academy in 1910, the year after he was appointed professor at UCD. Subsequently he became the first of UCD's professors to be elected president of the Academy in 1926. Throughout the years he continued to contribute important papers to its *Proceedings*; in fact, hardly a volume appeared during his active years that did not contain a contribution from him. Among the areas that received his attention and remain important to scholars are: the early settlements near Dingle; the memorial slabs at Clonmacnoise; the monuments of Tara; the high crosses at Monasterboice. His early publications include *Ireland in Pre-Celtic Times*, *Archaeology of Ireland* and *Archaeology of Palestine*. But he is best remembered, perhaps, for his great work, published in two volumes, *Corpus Inscriptionum Insularum Celticarum*; it replaced his earlier *Studies in Irish Epigraphy* and it still remains a source-book of immense value for the scattered earliest records of the country.

While his academic work was considered to be to the forefront of his contemporaries, it was not his only area of activity. Anything that touched on the interests of archaeology saw him involved. A good example of this was the introduction of up-to-date legislation for the protection of our ancient monuments in 1930, a measure that was largely the result of his tireless efforts. He became Chairman of the National Monuments Advisory Council in that year and continued to press for a full-scale archaeological survey of the country. The standards of excavation have become much more sophisticated than those which existed in the time Dr Macalister was professor at UCD but it was he who established the base on which those advances could be made. He remained as professor at UCD until retirement in 1943. He died in Cambridge in 1950.[15]

---

15   Royal Irish Academy: Minutes of Proceedings: Session 1950-51 in *Proceedings of the Royal Irish Academy* 54 (1950-51) 10-12; McCartney, *UCD, a national idea*, 27-9, 67-8, 104.

MICHAEL SEYMOUR DUDLEY WESTROPP

Another resident of Clonskeagh who made a major contribution to the cultural life of Ireland was Michael Seymour Dudley Westropp; he has left us a lasting legacy in his fine work on Irish glass. After publishing widely on the subject in learned journals such as the *Journal of the Royal Society of Antiquaries of Ireland* and the *Proceedings of the Royal Irish Academy* (he was a member of that Academy from 1910), the first edition of his main work, *Irish glass: a history of glass making in Ireland from the sixteenth century,* first appeared in October 1920 while he was living in Clonskeagh. This work has remained since that time 'the standard book on the history of glass-making in Ireland from the sixteenth century to the end of the nineteenth century' and has recently (1978) been re-issued in a revised edition. He was responsible for bringing a professional approach to the subject; prior to his work, the subject had been the exclusive domain of amateurs.

Born at Rookhurst, Monkstown, Co Cork on 2 April, 1868 his first career was that of a military man; he joined the Cork Militia and gained his first commission as 2nd lieutenant in the Royal Irish Rifles at the age of twenty. He did not remain long in the military, however, resigning his commission ten years later. In 1899 he joined the National Museum of Ireland and went to live in Clonskeagh around ten years later in 1908. In 1930 he was promoted Keeper of the Art Division of the Museum. While in the Museum, a relatively new collection of glass, silver and ceramics was assembled, mainly due to his endeavours. His interests were not confined to glass, however; he was also keenly involved in entomology, gathering together a wide collection of butterflies and moths, so much so that a specific species of moth carries his name – *Muralis var. Westroppi.* In 1936 he retired from his position at the National Museum but continued to live at no. 10 St James's terrace, Clonskeagh until his death, aged 86, on 24 December 1954. He had lived there since 1908.[16]

MÁIRTÍN Ó CADHAIN

During the 1950s Máirtín Ó Cadhain, then at the heighth of his career, lived in Clonskeagh at no. 13 Ardnabel road, later renamed and renumbered as no. 2 Beechmount drive. Born in 1906 in the Cois Fhairrge Gaeltacht of county Galway he got his first education locally and gained a scholarship to Teachers'

---

16 Mary Boydell (rev. ed), *Irish glass: a history of glass making in Ireland from the sixteenth century by M S Dudley-Westropp, MRIA* (Dublin 1978) iii-iv; see also some articles in *Proceedings of the Royal Irish Academy C* 29 (1911-12) and *Journal of the Royal Society of Antiquaries of Ireland* 47 (1917) & 57 (1927).

Training College in Dublin. Afterwards he returned to teach in his native place but soon became disillusioned by what he saw of the government's approach to education. He joined the IRA in the 1930s, the result of which was dismissal from his teaching post. He afterwards made a precarious living from occasional teaching appointments and from labouring work. The arrival of the second world-war saw him interned in the Curragh camp with many other IRA members. Here he put his skills to good use teaching fellow internees Irish language, culture and literature. His skills were such that many of his pupils afterwards retained a love of the language for the remainder of their lives. But it was not just teaching that occupied him there, he also read widely not just in Irish but also in English, German, French and some Russian. He also began to develop his own peculiar style of writing, particularly in short stories.

Released after the war he did various jobs until he was employed in 1949 in the translation department attached to the Dáil. Despite this he continued his fight on economic and cultural issues. To quote Eoghan Ó Tuairisc on this aspect of his struggle 'As a freelance journalist he shaped a vitriolic style, using the most shattering idioms of the living Irish speech laced with phrases from seventeenth century literature and new coinages from the thinking of Darwin, Einstein and Freud ... attacking the dehumanising of life and the castration of culture with a blistering invective and a scurrility unsurpassed since Swift'. None of this violence and aggression, however, is found in his creative writing. In that he sought to make the Irish language responsive to the thinking and feeling of modern life. His ability and skill in the language was recognized by Trinity College which appointed him a lecturer in modern Irish in 1956. Later, in 1969, he was appointed to the chair of Irish and was made a fellow of the college in the following year.

His first collection of short stories appeared in 1939 and was followed by others of the same genre. However, in 1949 his major work, by which he is perhaps best known, *Cré na Cille,* was published. A facinating work, it is set in a graveyard where those already buried carry out conversations with one another with particular interest paid to the latest person who has just joined them. The intrigues and petty jealousies of a small rural population are the centre piece of these conversations. It was translated into a number of European languages as part of an effort made by UNESCO to promote masterpieces written in the world's lesser-known languages.

Other works followed, one of which, *An tSráith ar Lár* published in 1967, won him the first ever prize awarded by the Irish-American Institute of St Paul, Minnesota; it amounted to £2,000. He also had the unique honour of being the first writer, who wrote only in Irish, to be elected to the Irish Academy of Letters.

He died in Dublin on 18 October 1970 leaving behind him a variety of unpublished work which almost equalled in size the amount he had published during his life.[17]

TOM NISBET

It was not just in the area of literature, history and archaeology that contributions were made to the cultural life of Ireland by residents of Clonskeagh, a substantial one was made in the visual arts as well. This was the result of the work of the painter Tom Nisbet who lived in Bird avenue from the 1950s onwards. Born in Belfast c. 1910, he soon moved to Dublin where the attended the Metropolitan School of Art; this would later become the National College of Art and Design. In his early life, he worked as a scene painter at the Theatre Royal after which he opened the Grafton Gallery in Harry street. Many artists exhibited there; these included Arthur Armstrong, Bea Orpen and Colin Middleton. Tom Nesbit is, perhaps, best remembered for his watercolours in which he depicted various scenes in Dublin and its surroundings. He was a member of the Royal Hibernian Academy for many years and exhibited there for the first time in 1936. After that his work was displayed at every Academy exhibition, even to the extent of having seven watercolours at the 2001 exhibition, the last year of his long life. He died 12 May 2001 at the age of 91.[18]

ANTHONY T LUCAS

Bird avenue was home to another man who was actively involved in the cultural life of Ireland for a number of years – Anthony T Lucas. He served as the Director of the National Museum of Ireland from 1954 to 1976, the longest period to date that anyone has held that position. Born in Clonsilla, Dublin, the son of an Austrian butler father (who was interned by the British during the First World War) and a county Meath mother his first experience of work was as a primary teacher. It was during this phase of his life that he took up residence at Cois Coille in Bird avenue around 1937. He pursued further studies leading to a degree, on foot of which he joined the museum around 1948 in the Folklife section. When there he progressed so rapidly that he had become the Director within a relatively short number of years.

A substantial scholar, with exacting standards, he concentrated mainly on folklife and archaeology with particular emphasis on the written sources with the

---

17 Boylan, *Dictionary of Irish biography,* 247; Máirtín Ó Cadhain, *The road to Brightcity: short stories translated by Eoghan Ó Tuarisc* (Swords, Co Dublin 1981) 7-9.
18 Miriam Stewart (ed), *Arts Ireland,* 39 (May 2001).

result that some would consider him to have been the finest social historian in Ireland since Eugene (Eoin) O'Curry. He made considerable contributions to international conferences and published very many academic papers of great substance and standard. A list of these has been compiled by Etienne Rynne; it makes impressive reading. With the exception of 1948 he published every single year from 1946/47 right up to his retirement from the museum in 1976; in most years he had multiple publications.[19] These were highly influential not least among some of his staff at the museum. One such work, published in 1973 by Gill and Macmillian in agreement with UNESCO was entitled: *Treasures of Ireland: Irish pagan and early christian art.* Later in life, in 1989, he published *Cattle in ancient Ireland.*

As well as publishing, he was an energetic general secretary of the Royal Society of Antiquaries of Ireland between 1946 and 1969 and for the next four years its president.[20] A conservative in the manner in which he ran the museum he was, nevertheless, responsible for the inspired choice of a young 25 year old archaeologist to conduct the very successful excavations at Wood quay – Dr Pat Wallace – now his esteemed successor. On retirement, the well-known folklorist, Caoimhín Ó Danachair edited a *festschrift* in his honour under the auspices of the Royal Society of Antiquaries of Ireland.[21]

---

19 Caoimhín Ó Danachair, *Folk and farm: essays in honour of A T Lucas,* Royal Society of Antiquaries of Ireland (Dublin 1976) 9-14.
20 Ibid. Forward by the President of the Royal Society of Antiquaries of Ireland in 1976, Henry A Wheeler.
21 My thanks to the current Director of the National Museum of Ireland, Dr Pat Wallace, for providing me with much of the information on which this is based.

19

Sport

FIRST ALL-IRELAND FOOTBALL CHAMPIONSHIP

GIVEN THAT THE FIRST All-Ireland football championship was played in Clonskeagh on 29 April 1888, it seems appropriate that a full report of the proceedings should be given here. This is taken from the *Freeman's Journal* where it was published on the following day, Monday 30 April, 1888. In that paper the report was as follows:

Gaelic Athletic Association
> Great Championship Meeting at Clonskeagh
> The Limerick Commercials win All Ireland Football Championship

To say that the Gaelic Championship Meeting at Clonskeagh on yesterday was of absorbing interest not only to Gaels of Dublin but to those of every county where the Gaelic Athletic Association holds sway, is only echoing the sentiments of every supporter of our National pastimes. This was due to the importance of the matches set down for decision and the great issue which depended on the result of the same. The mere fact of the final tie for 1887 football Championship, notwithstanding that it is a year behind its time, being one of the items in the programme was sufficient to surround the meeting with an importance which was nothing short of national. It is not necessary to go into here the causes which prevented last year's championship being decided before this. They are well known to everyone and were simply the outcome of the disorganised and regrettable conditions in which the Association was for a large portion of the last year. However, last year's storms and troubles have long passed away and with the conclusion of the 1887 Championship, the remembrance of an unpleasant past is completely obliterated. The two teams – the Limerick Commercials and the Dundalk Young Irelands – which fought out the final tie on yesterday, are ones who have made their names famous by their brilliant achievements. In the Inter-County Championships the Limerick men were successful in defeating the champions of Meath, Kilkenny and Tipperary, while the Dundalk men headed the list against Wexford and Waterford.

Coming to the match, it must be said that it was a splendid exhibition of skill, science, speed and stamina; that it was a model in every way, the feeling between the combatants being of the friendliest nature; and that it was won fair and square, without fluke or fortune, by the Commercials. As regards the three matches played in the Dublin County Championships, two of them [i.e Kickham's (hurling) & Feach M'Hugh's (football)] were of great importance as the winners are bound to have a good "look in" for their respective championships. Fortunately the meeting was favoured with glorious weather, which added greatly to the comfort of the players, and to the three or four thousand spectators who were present. Though the gathering was by no means a small one, still it would have been much larger were it not for the short notice and small publicity given to the fact that the final tie of last year's football championship would take place. This was not the fault of the Dublin County Committee, who were only informed of the fact at practically the last moment and consequently they were unable to give the teams a reception which they otherwise would have done. In consequence of the meeting of the Central Council of the GAA taking place tomorrow, there were several of that body present including Messrs. Maurice Davin (president), R J Freeman (treasurer), J Cullinan, Alderman Mangan, T O'Riordan, W Prendergast (hon. sec.) and J Cullen (record sec.). The various arrangements were most successfully carried out under the supervision of the County Dublin Committee – Messrs. J P Cox, W Burke, T Power, J Drea, P P Sutton, C Greaves, J Bagnall and J Fitzpatrick. The following are the details.

C J Kickham's V Michael Davitt's
(Hurling)
   [detail report; result – Kickhams 1-2; Davitt's 1-0; referee J P Cox]

Feach M'Hugh's V Dunleary
(Football)
   [detail report; result – Feach M'Hugh's 1-2; Dunleary 0-2]

Brian Boru's V St Patrick's
(Hurling – a replay)
   [detail report; result – Brian Boru's 2-1; St Patrick's 0-1]

Limerick Commercial's V Dundalk Young Irelands
(Final tie 1887 Football Championship)
Notwithstanding that this championship is a year out of date, still the mere fact that it was a final tie of an All Ireland championship and that the competing teams were of the high standing of the Limerick Commercials and the Dundalk Young Irelands, was sufficient to invest it with the greatest interest and importance. At 2.30 ^{pm} the teams lined up, Mr John Cullinan, MCC, GAA (Bansha) acting as referee which position he filled with great judgement and tact and with scrupulous exactness. The Young Irelands winning the toss, took the wind. Play was started by Limerick Commercials but the Dundalk men getting possession made a brilliant run down the right wing and caused the former to

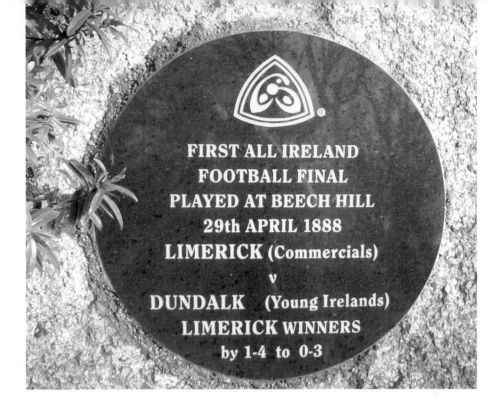

Plaque commemorating first All-Ireland football final played at Beechhill

defend in which they were successful for five minutes when the Northerns scored a point, quickly followed by two more. A burst now by Limerick ended in a point which concluded the scoring for the first half during the remainder of which the play was very fast. The second half was not very old when the Commercials, playing with great dash, began to press Dundalk sorely and eleven minutes after the change of sides Limerick ... placed a goal to their credit. The Dundalk men rallied, broke through the Commercials who saved what looked like an inevitable goal. Nothing interesting occurred until the conclusion when Mr Cullinan declared the Limerick men the winners and the champions of Ireland by 1-4 to 3 points for Dundalk. The hand play, punting and general knackiness of the Dundalk men, of whom Louth can be proud, could hardly be excelled but they were unable to withstand the fast determined charging of the boys from Garryowen. [Names of players on both teams are then given].

CLONSKEAGH'S BENBURB FOOTBALL CLUB: ITS CLAIM TO HAVE HOSTED THE FIRST COUNTY DUBLIN HURLING AND FOOTBALL FINALS

What is perhaps less well known is that only three weeks later, on Whit Sunday and Monday, a major festival of sport under the auspices of the Gaelic Athletic Association took place in the grounds of the Benburb football club. This included the final ties of the hurling and football championships of the county Dublin. Such championships were relatively new since county committees of the GAA were first introduced only two years previously. The Benburb grounds were described in the newspaper report of the event as being in Donnybrook but the Benburb club is known to have been based in Clonskeagh. Although it is not immediately clear from the newspaper reports as to whether the two events (the first All-Ireland football final and this major sports festival which included the two county finals) took place at the same venue, it is almost certain that they did; it is highly unlikely that two separate venues capable of hosting such important events would have been in such close proximity to one another. Because of this it is felt to be also appropriate to reproduce the newspaper reports surrounding it.

Two days after the All-Ireland final, a report appeared in the *Freeman's Journal* on 1 May 1888 informing its readers that programmes were just then available for 'the Gaelic Carnival at Donnybrook on Whit Sunday and Monday'. As well as the two county finals, an array of different sports including running, long and high jumping, weight throwing, raising and striking the hurling ball and football place kicking was expected to take place on Whit Sunday. It was anticipated that the following day, Whit Monday, would be the big day. More athletic events, open to all amateurs, as well as a hurling and football match were on the programme. It was also planned to have miscellaneous amusements such as dancing, merry-go-rounds, velocipedes, circuses, swings and similar items. The report summed it up as 'a tempting programme'. It stated that in the previous year 'fully 20,000 people attended and thoroughly enjoyed themselves'. This report concluded by announcing that entries for the various events would close on the following Sunday week; they would be received by Mr P B Kirwan, of the *Sports* office in Middle Abbey street. This was but one of the reports of the upcoming event.

Two years previously, in 1886 (the year the GAA introduced county executive committees), there was a Whitsuntide sports festival held, under GAA auspices, at the Abattoir grounds on the North Circular road, lent for the occasion by the Corporation. Among the wide variety of sporting events that took place hurling and football were included. However, there is no reference made to anything resembling county finals being held there (*Freeman's Journal* 12 & 14 June 1886). In the following year, the Whitsuntide event reported as being 'framed by the county Dublin executive' took place 'by kind permission of Lord French, in Elm Park, Merrion'. It did not include county finals but did include a hurling and a football match; these, however, were the result of invitations sent out to teams in advance to take part. Two hurling teams entered and played on Whit Sunday morning; four football teams entered and there was a play-off first, one of which took place on Whit Sunday evening while the other, having been played before the week-end event, allowed the winners of these two to play the final tie on

Whit Monday; nowhere in the reports were these called 'county championships'. (*Freeman's Journal* 3 & 12 May 1887).

The fact that these two Whitsuntide events did not include county finals and that which was staged at the Benburb club grounds in 1888 did, would suggest that the latter can claim that it played host to the first county Dublin hurling and football championships held at a Whitsuntide festival. It is not clear whether there were any county finals played elsewhere at other times of the year in 1886 or 1887. If not, then the finals played in the Benburb club grounds in 1888 can claim to be the first such games played. That together with the first All-Ireland championship played there three weeks previously would be truly a remarkable record for a club to hold.

On Whit Monday, 21 May 1888, a report of the previous day's events appeared in the *Freeman's Journal.* An excerpt from this goes as follows:

> Gaelic Carnival at Donnybrook
> [the report begins by giving the names of the judges]
> Yesterday the annual Whitsuntide Athletic Carnival of the Gaelic Athletic Association was commenced at Donnybrook on the grounds of the Benburb Football Club. The weather was simply charming and the attendance very large, not much less than 6000 being present at mid-day when the sport was at its best. The programme was made up of a series of events confined to members of affiliated clubs in Dublin in addition to a hurling and football tie for the championship of the county. It is a matter for regret that a more suitable ground is not available for the occasion. During the progress of an exciting event it is only a natural impulse on the part of spectators to crowd in on the field of play and nothing but the stoutest of barriers can avail to keep them back. This was manifest from time to time yesterday but the people if eager were most good-humoured and were always amenable to even a hinted remonstrance from any of the authorised officials. ...
>
> Football
> County Dublin Championship
> The Feagh M'Hugh F C beat Kickham's F C by 2-6 to 1-5. The match all through was most spiritedly contested ....
>
> Hurling
> County Dublin Championship
> The Kickham H C beat the Metropolitan H C by 2-2 to 7 points. This was a splendid match ....
>
> [following on from the reports of these finals, the results of the field sports were given in detail].

The rest of the Whitsuntide festival continued on that same Monday on which the report, from which the above is excerpted, appeared in the *Freeman's Journal*. As regards the grounds, they are now believed to have been in Beechhill which is between Clonskeagh and Donnybrook (there is a plaque erected beside the entrance to the houses and apartments which are now located in Beechhill). The exact location, according to a book published in 1982, was in the 'open space bounded by Smurfit's headquarters and Richview' and the club had its premises in a location behind O'Shea's public house. According to the same source, nearly all the members of the Benburb club worked in Henshaw's mills beside the bridge and because of that they were dubbed with the nickname 'The Dirty Shirts'. Referred to as 'The Clonskeagh Benburbs' the colour of their football jerseys was green and had Henshaw's trademark, the Red Hand of Ulster, emblazoned on them.[1] Be that as it may, there is a more direct connection between the Red Hand and the title of the club 'Benburb'. This title commemorated one of the most important battles won by the native Irish during the wars of 1641 to 1652 – the battle of Benburb fought in 1646. The successful prosecution of the battle, considered to be the most spectacular military success by native forces against Anglo-Scots opposition, has been attributed to the skill of Owen Roe O'Neill who had been a highly experienced military commander on the Continent. The Red Hand had its origins in the coat of arms of Owen Roe's family, the O'Neills, although it would later be adopted as a symbol of Ulster.[2] To associate it with the battle of Benburb and the title 'Benburb' would, therefore, have been quite natural. It would appear that the club continued to function at some level until 1972 when 'through the good offices of John Sheridan' it joined up with the Kilmacud Crokes GAA club.[3]

It is of some interest to note the names of the people who owned Beechhill around that time we are discussing: the 1880s. *Thom's Directory* for 1882 gives Herbert H Murray, esq., treasury remembrancer & deputy paymaster-general, Treasury, Dublin castle as residing in Beechhill; its rateable valuation was £100. In the following year, however, another person, Thomas Ingham Dixon, railway contractor, took up residence. In 1887 he is listed as simply a 'contractor' with an office at 7 Anglesea street; later in 1899 it would be in 74 Dame street. While

---

1   Nolan, *Changing faces*, 194, 196.
2   Articles on the Battle of Benburb and the Red Hand of Ulster in Brian Lalor (ed), *The encyclopaedia of Ireland* (Dublin 2003) 88, 918; the contributors are John McCavitt and Jonathan Bardon respectively.
3   Information on the joining of the Benburb club with Kilmacud Crokes is carried on the latter's website.

living in Beechhill he is known to have been an active businessman. In 1884 he won a contract from the Board of Works for the construction of a pier between Carnsore Point and Greenore Point and another contract from the Board engaged him, between 1884 and 1886, in repairing and extending the pier, raising the groin and deepening the harbour at Check Point, Waterford harbour (*National Archives*: OPW 8/59 &75). Earlier in his career he had, among other things, built the Birr and Portumna Railway. This particular contract gave rise to a famous story about 'The Lost Railway'. It would appear that during its building, work was suspended because of a dispute between the Railway Company and the Board of Works. Taking advantage of the suspension in work, local people descended on the unfinished line and helped themselves to the rails and sleepers which they put to various farm and domestic uses; all that was left were the cuttings, embankments and bridges. Eventually, of course, work got underway again and the railway line was commissioned five years later. However, it did not last long; work had originally begun in 1863 and by 1878 the line was derelict.[4] The last entry in the directories for Thomas Ingham Dixon at Beechhill is in 1902. After that he apparently went to live in Surrey, England where he died in 1904. Although it is not certain that it was in his grounds that the sporting events took place it is a strong possibility. For that reason, it might prove to be of some interest to a researcher in GAA history to follow up and find out more about this particular man; more research is also needed on the claim made above in relation to the first county Dublin football and hurling finals.

OTHER SPORTS

As regards other sports in the area, the sporting activities of the Masonic Orphan Boys' School has been described in the chapter on schools; reference has also been made there to the promotion of sports in St Gall's national school in Milltown. One other item worthy of comment is the Palmerston Rugby Club. It had its grounds just off Prospect lane, Milltown road. Although this may not now appear to be located in Clonskeagh it was so described when the club first acquired the grounds in 1925. The grounds, it should be noted, bordered on those of Vergemount house (Clonskeagh hospital) and are behind St James's terrace. As well as that, the civil parish boundary which can be traced up from the Dodder river along the back of the grounds of Clonskeagh hospital proceeds through Prospect lane before turning right at Milltown road thus enclosing

---

4 *Midland Tribune* 6 February 1904; Offaly Historical & Archaeological Society website.

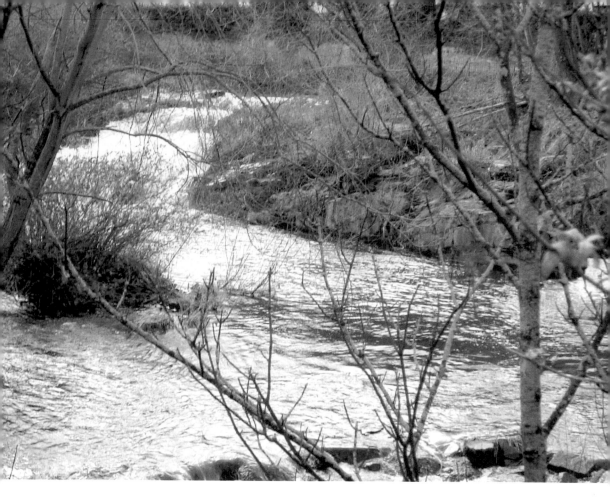

Dodder waterfall, below Clonskeagh bridge

within the civil parish the Palmerston rugby club grounds. In 1973 the club purchased 16 acres of land in Kilternan and played their first match there in 1980. They merged with the De La Salle club in 1985, the first two Irish rugby clubs to merge. There are apartment blocks and houses now on the land once occupied by the club off Prospect lane. Apart from activities on the field at the old grounds, the club's pavilion was once a very popular venue for social occasions, in particular dances. The only reminder now of the one-time presence of the club in the area is the name given to some of the new buildings e.g. Palmerston grove.

Bibliography

PRIMARY SOURCES

Agnew, Jean (ed), *The Drennan – McTier letters: 1776-1793* (Dublin 1998)

Copy of Will and four Codicils of John Richard Corballis: National Archives of Ireland, small private collections 999/658 13

Documents relating, *inter alia*, to deeds of title: Archives of the Carmelite monastery, Roebuck road

Dowden, W S (ed), *The letters of Thomas Moore* (2vols, Oxford 1964)

_____ (ed), *The Journal of Thomas Moore* (6vols, Newark 1983-91)

Eustace, P Beryl (ed), *Registry of Deeds, Dublin: Abstracts of Wills*, Irish Manuscripts Commission (3 vols, Dublin 1954-84)

First Ordnance Survey Map of Donnybrook (1837): National Archives OS/105 E 261

First Ordnance Survey Map of Taney parish (1837): National Archives OS/105 E 295

First Report of the Commissioners appointed to inquire into the corporations in Ireland, presented to both Houses of Parliament by command of His Majesty, House of Commons 1835 Volume 27

Gilbert, John T (ed), *Calendar of ancient records of Dublin in the possession of the Municipal Corporation of that city* (Dublin 1889) Volume1

_____ (ed), *Chartularies of St Mary's Abbey* (2 vols, London 1894)

Gilbert, Lady (ed), *Calendar of ancient records of Dublin in the possession of the Municipal Corporation of that city* (Dublin 1911) Volume 15

Griffith, Margaret C (ed), *Calendar of Inquisitions formerly in the Office of the Chief Remembrancer of the Exchequer prepared from the MSS of the Irish Record Commission*, Irish Manuscript Commission (Dublin 1991)

Herity, Michael (ed), *Ordnance Survey letters: Dublin* (Dublin 2001)

List of the documents associated with the Title to Roebuck house drawn up by Seán MacBride.

Mills, James (ed), *Calendar of the Justiciary Rolls or proceedings in the court of the Justiciar of Ireland preserved in the Public Record Office of Ireland: Edward I* (Dublin 1914) Volume 1

Morris, James (ed), *Calendar of the Patent and Close Rolls of Chancery in Ireland, of the reigns of Henry VIII, Edward VI, Mary, and Elizabeth* (2 vols, Dublin 1861-62)

O'Byrne, Eileen (ed), *The Convert Rolls*, Irish Manuscripts Commission (Dublin 1981)

O'Connell, Maurice R (ed), *The correspondence of Daniel O'Connell* (8vols, Dublin 1977-80)

Ordnance Survey map drawn for *Thom's Directory* of 1875: Gilbert Collection, Dublin City Library and Archive

Papers of John Woulfe Flanagan: National Archives of Ireland, Private Sources 1189/14/9; 1189/2/7; 1189/16/4 &10; 1189/17/9

Parker, Charles Stuart (ed), *Sir Robert Peel from his private papers* (3vols, London 1891-99)

Pembroke Estate Office, *Calendar of ancient deeds and muniments preserved in the Pembroke Estate Office, Dublin* (Dublin 1891)

Pembroke Estate Papers: National Archives of Ireland, Private Sources 97/46/ 4/31 (Survey by Captain Martin, RE in 1866)

Pender, Séamus (ed), *A census of Ireland circa 1659 with supplementary material from the Poll Money Ordinances (1660-1661),* Coimisiún Láimhscríbhinní na h-Éireann (Dublin 1939)

Report of the Masonic Orphan Boys' School of Ireland, Adelaide Hall, Merrion for the year 1884 (Dublin 1885); ditto for years 1885 to 1887, each published in the subsequent year

RETURN to an Address of the Honourable The House of Commons, dated 13 March 1890: *Ordered by* The House of Commons *to be printed,* 8 *April* 1891

RETURN to Two Orders of the Honourable The House of Commons, dated 4 May 1876 and 9 March 1877: *Ordered by* The House of Commons, *to be printed* 1 *March* 1878

Royal Irish Academy: Minutes of Proceedings: Session 1950-51 in *Proceedings of the Royal Irish Academy* 54 (1950-51)

Sheehy, Maurice P (ed), *Pontificia Hibernica: medieval papal chancery documents concerning Ireland* (2 vols, Dublin 1962)

Simington Robert C (ed), *The Civil Survey A.D. 1654-56: Vol. VII County of Dublin,* Irish Manuscript Commission (Dublin 1945)

Sweetman, H S & Handcock, G F (ed), *Calendar of documents relating to Ireland preserved in Her Majesty's Public Record Office: 1302-1307* (London 1886)

Virginia Military Institute Archives [http://www.vmi.edu/archives] January 2006

White, Newport B (ed), *Extents of Irish monastic possessions 1540-1541* (Dublin 1943).

DIRECTORIES

Pettigrew and Oulton (1834-1847) i) *The Dublin Almanac and General Register of Ireland;* ii) *The Dublin Directory*

Pigott & Co's Directory and Guide (1824)

The Complete Catholic Directory, Almanac, and Registry for the year of Our Lord 1847

The Gentleman's and Citizen's Almanack (compiled by Samuel Watson to 1794; by John Watson Stewart to 1822; by the late John Watson Stewart to 1839)

The Post Office Annual Directory (from 1833); *General Post-Office Directory for Dublin and its vicinity* (1839)

Thom's Directory (1844-2004)

Wilson's Dublin Directory (1770-1837)

NEWSPAPERS

Dublin Evening Post

Freeman's Journal

Irish Catholic Chronicle

Irish Independent

The Dublin Journal

The Nation

SECONDARY SOURCES

Aked, Charles, *Complete list of English horological patents up to 1853* (Ashford, Kent 1975)

Akenson, Donald H, 'Pre-university education, 1782-1870' in Vaughan, *New history of Ireland*, 523-37

_____ *The Irish education experiment: the National System of Education in the nineteenth century* (London & Toronto 1970)

Allen & Townsend, *Catalogue of the late Lady Redmond's well-known collection of antique furniture and fine art property at St Anne's, Clonskeagh road, Clonskeagh to be sold by Public Auction on Monday June 9th 1941 and following 3 days at 12 Noon prompt*

Anon., 'Engineers in the Zulu War 1879' [http://www.remuseum.org.uk/campaign/rem_zuluwar79.htm] > website of the British army's Royal Engineers

Archer, Joseph, *Statistical survey of the county Dublin, with observations on the means of improvement; drawn up for the consideration, and by order of The Dublin Society* (Dublin 1801)

Ashton, T S, *The Industrial Revolution 1760-1830* (Oxford 1968)

B[ush], J, *Hibernia curiosa: a letter from a gentleman in Dublin to his friend at Dover in Kent, giving a general view of the manners, customs, dispositions, etc., of the inhabitants of Ireland, collected in a tour through Ireland in 1764* (2nd ed, London 1782)

Baillie, G H, *Watchmakers and clockmakers of the world*, Volume 1 (London 1929, 3rd ed. repr. 1996)

Ball, F Elrington, *The judges in Ireland, 1221- 1921* (2vols, London 1926)

_____ & Hamilton, Everard, *The parish of Taney: a history of Dundrum, near Dublin, and its neighbourhood* (Dublin 1895)

_____ *A history of the county Dublin*, Volume 2 (Dublin 1903)

_____ *The vicinity of the International Exhibition Dublin: an historical sketch of the Pembroke Township* (Dublin 1907)

Barnwall, Stephen B, 'The Barnewall family during the sixteenth and seventeenth centuries', *The Irish Genealogist* 3 (1963)

Barry, P C, 'The Holy See and the Irish National Schools', *Irish Ecclesiastical Record*, 5th ser., 92 (1959) 90-105

Beckett, Ian F W, 'Women and patronage in the late Victorian army', in *History* 85 (2000) 463-480

Beckett, J C, *The making of modern Ireland: 1603-1923* (London 1981)

Bence-Jones, Mark, *A guide to Irish country houses* (London 1988)

Bennet, Douglas, *The encyclopaedia of Dublin* (Dublin 2005)

Bieler, Ludwig (ed) *The patrician texts in the book of Armagh*, Scriptores Latini Hiberniae Volume 10 (Dublin 2000)

Blackburne, Edward, *Life of the Right Hon. Francis Blackburne, late Lord Chancellor of Ireland* (London 1874)

Blair, John & Sharpe, Richard (ed), *Pastoral care before the parish* (Leicester 1992)

Boase, Frederic (ed), *Modern English biography* (3vols Truro 1891-97)

Book of Honour Committee, *Dublin City & County Book of Honour* (Dublin 2004)

Boydell, Mary (rev. ed), *Irish glass: a history of glass making in Ireland from the sixteenth century by M S Dudley-Westropp, MRIA* (Dublin 1978)

Boylan, Henry, *A dictionary of Irish biography* (3rd ed, Dublin 1998)

Boyne, Patricia, *John O'Donovan (1806-1861): a biography*, Studies in Irish Archaeology and History (Kilkenny 1987)

Bradley, John, 'Mills and milling', Seán Duffy (ed) *Medieval Ireland: an encyclopedia* (New York 2005) 337-38

British Association for the Advancement of Science [http://www.net/the-ba/AbouttheBA/HistoryoftheBA/_BriefHistory2.htm] July 2006

Burns, J F, *Shop window to the world* (Dublin 1966)

Bushnell, T A, *"Royal Mail": a centenary history of the Royal Mail Line, 1839-1939* (London 1939)

Byrne, Francis J, *Irish kings and high kings* (Dublin 2001)

Cameron, Sir Charles A, *History of the Royal College of Surgeons in Ireland* (2nd ed, Dublin 1916)

Cardozo, Nancy, *Maud Gonne* (New York 1990)

Casey, James, *The Irish law officers: roles and responsibilities of the Attorney General and the Director of Public Prosecutions* (Dublin 1996)

Clarke, Aidan, *The Old English in Ireland, 1625-42* (Dublin 2000)

Clarke, Frances, "Son of a Water Drinker_ and 'Anti-Everythingarian_' in *History Ireland* 15/3 (2007)

Clarke, Howard B, 'Conversion, church and cathedral: the diocese of Dublin to 1152' in Kelly & Keogh *History of the Catholic diocese of Dublin*, 19-50

Cloncurry, Valentine, *Personal recollections of the life and times, with extracts from correspondence of Valentine Lord Cloncurry* (Dublin 1849)

Cockayne, G E, (ed. H White, R S Lea), *The complete peerage or a history of the house of lords and all its members from the earliest times* (London 1959)

Comerford, R V, 'Ireland 1850-70: post-famine and mid-Victorian', in Vaughan, *A new history of Ireland*, 372-395

Connolly, Philomena, *Medieval Record Sources* (Dublin 2002)

Cook, David R, *Lancastrians and Yorkists: the Wars of the Roses* (Harlow 1991)

Coolahan, John, *Irish education: history and structure*, Institute of Public Administration, Dublin (Dublin 1981)

Corcoran, Michael, *Through streets broad and narrow: a history of Dublin trams* (Leicester 2000)

Cosgrove, Art. *Late medieval Ireland, 1370-1541*, (Dublin 1981)

Costello, Peter & Farmer, Tony, *The very heart of the city: the story of Denis Guiney and Clerys* (Dublin 1992)

Counihan, H E, 'In Memoriam: Dr Dorothy Stopford Price' in *Journal of the Irish Medical Association* 34 (1954)

Coyle, E A, 'County Dublin Elections (1790)', *Dublin Historical Record*, 44/2 (1991) 13-24

Craig, Maurice, *Dublin: 1660-1860* (London 1992)

Crofton, Ian (ed), *Concise dictionary of music* (3rd ed. William Collins & Sons, 1986)

Crosthwaite, John Clarke, *The Book of Obits and Martyrology of the Cathedral Church of the Holy Trinity, commonly called Christ Church, Dublin*, Irish Archæological Society (Dublin 1844) with an Introduction by James Henthorn Todd, DD, VPRIA

_____ *Modern hagiology: an examination of the nature and tendency of some legendary and devotional works lately published under the sanction of the Rev J H Newman, the Rev Dr Pusey, and the Rev F Oakley* (2vols, London 1846)

Cullen, L M, *Princes and pirates; the Dublin Chamber of Commerce 1783-1983* (Dublin 1983)

Cunningham, Bernadette, *The world of Geoffrey Keating* (Dublin 2004)

Curran, Joseph M, *The birth of the Irish Free State: 1921-1923* (Alabama 1980)

Curran, William Henry, *Sketches of the Irish bar with essays, literary and political* (2vols, London 1855)

_____ *The life of the Right Honourable John Philpot Curran, late Master of the Rolls* (2vols, London 1817)

D'Alton, John, *Illustrations, historical and genealogical, of king James's Irish Army List (1689)* (Dublin 1885 repr 1997)

_____ *The history of the county of Dublin* (Dublin 1838)

Daly, Mary, 'The county in Irish history', in Mary Daly (ed), *County and Town: one hundred years of local government in Ireland,* Lectures on the occasion of the 100th anniversary of the Local Government Ireland Act, 1898 (Dublin 2001)

de Courcy, J W, *The Liffey in Dublin* (Dublin 1996)

Dickson, David (ed), *The gorgeous mask: Dublin 1700-1850* (Dublin 1987)

_____ & English, Richard, 'The La Touche dynasty', in Dickson, *The gorgeous mask,* 17-29

_____ 'Paine and Ireland' in Dickson, Keogh & Whelan, *The United Irishmen,* 133-50

_____ Keogh, Dáire & Whelan, Kevin (ed), *The United Irishmen: republicanism, radicalism and rebellion* (Dublin 1993)

_____ *New foundations: Ireland 1660-1800* (Dublin 1987)

Doherty, Gillian M, 'The Synod of Thurles, 1850' [http://multitext.ucc.ie/d/The_Synod_of_Thurles_1850] May, 2006

Donnelly, N, *History of Dublin parishes* (2vols, Dublin 1912)

Donnelly, William, *General alphabetical index to the townlands and towns, parishes, and baronies of Ireland* (Dublin 1861 repr. 1984)

Dudley Edwards, Ruth, *Newspapermen: Hugh Cudlipp, Cecil Harmsworth King and the glory days of Fleet street* (London 2003)

Dutton, Hely, *Observations on Mr Archer's statistical survey of the county of Dublin* (Dublin 1802)

Ellis, Stephen G, *Tudor Ireland: crown, community and the conflict of cultures 1470-1603* (Harlow 1985)

Enright, Séamus, 'Women and Catholic life in Dublin, 1766-1852' in Kelly & Keogh, *History of the Catholic diocese of Dublin,* 268-93

Etchingham, Colmán, *Church organisation in Ireland: AD 650 to 1000* (Maynooth 1999)

Fagan, Patrick, *The second city: portrait of Dublin 1700-1760* (Dublin 1986)

Farrar, Henry, *Irish marriages: being an index to the marriages in Walker's Hibernian Magazine 1771 to 1812* (London 1890)

Feiling, Keith, *A history of England* (London 1966)

Ferguson, Kenneth, *King's Inns barristers: 1868-2004* (Dublin 2005)

FitzPatrick, Elizabeth & Gillespie, Raymond (ed), *The parish in medieval and early modern Ireland* (Dublin 2006).

Fitzpatrick, S A Ossory, *Dublin: a historical and topographical account of the city* (Dublin 1907)

Fitzpatrick, William John, *History of Dublin Catholic cemeteries* (Dublin 1900)

_____ *"The Sham Squire" and the informers of 1798* (Dublin 1866)

_____ *The life, times, and contemporaries of Lord Cloncurry* (Dublin 1855)

Flanagan, Thomas, 'Literature in English, 1801-91', in Vaughan, *A new history of Ireland*, 482-522

Gardiner, Juliet & Wenborn, Neil (ed), *The History Today companion to British history* (London 1995)

Garvin, Tom, *1922: the birth of Irish democracy* (Dublin 1996)

Gaughan, J Anthony, (ed), *Memoirs of Senator Joseph Connolly (1885-1961): a founder of modern Ireland* (Dublin 1996)

Geoghegan, Patrick M, *Robert Emmet: a life* (2nd ed, Dublin 2004)

_____ *The Irish Act of Union* (Dublin 2001)

Gibbs, Vicary (ed), *The complete peerage of England Scotland Ireland Great Britain and the United Kingdom* (vol xii, 1959)

Green, Hope, 'Tribal flag gives rare glimpse of Afghan past' in *B.U. Bridge* (Boston University community's weekly paper) vol. 5, no. 10, 19 October 2001

Gwynn, Aubrey, 'Origins of the see of Dublin', in Gerard O'Brien (ed), *The Irish church in the eleventh and twelfth centuries* (Dublin 1992) 50-67

_____ & Hadcock, R Neville (ed), *Medieval religious houses: Ireland* (Dublin 1988)

Gwynn, Denis, *Daniel O'Connell* (Oxford 1947)

Hall, F G, *The Bank of Ireland: 1783- 1946* (Dublin 1949)

Harris, Walter, *The history and antiquities of the city of Dublin, from the earliest accounts; compiled from authentick memoirs, offices of record, manuscript collections and other unexceptional vouchers* (Dublin 1766)

Hill, Jaqueline, 'The politics of Dublin Corporation: 1760-92' in Dickson, Keogh & Whelan, *The United Irishmen*, 88-101

Hogan, Gerard, 'Hugh Kennedy, the Childers Habeas Corpus application and the return to the Four Courts' in Caroline Costello (ed), *The Four Courts: 200 years. Essays to commemorate the bicentenary of the Four Courts* (Dublin 1996) 177-219

Hogg, William E, *The millers and the mills of Ireland of about 1850* (Dublin 2000)

_____ *The millers and the mills of Ireland: a database list (1700-1900)* (Dublin 2000)

Holland, Martin, 'The election of Daniel O'Connell as Lord Mayor of Dublin, 1841' (unpublished essay)

_____ 'Dublin and the Reform of the Irish Church in the Eleventh and Twelfth Centuries', *Peritia* 14 (2000) 111-60

_____ 'The twelfth-century reform and Inis Pátraic', in Ailbhe MacShamhráin (ed), *The Island of St Patrick: church and ruling dynasties in Fingal and Meath, 400-1148* (Dublin 2004)

Holy Cross Centenary Committee, *Centenary of Holy Cross Church, Dundrum* (Dublin 1978)

Hopkinson, Michael, 'From treaty to civil war, 1921-2' in J R Hill (ed) *A new history of Ireland* VII 'Ireland, 1921-84' (Oxford 2003) 1-61

Horgan, John, *Noël Browne: passionate outsider* (Dublin 2000)

Inglis, B, *The freedom of the press in Ireland: 1784 –1841* (London 1954)

Irish Archæological Society, *Tracts relating to Ireland* (Dublin 1841)

Islamic Cultural Centre of Ireland, an Islamic cultural landmark in the western world. Five years of benevolence 1996-2001: a concise illustration of the ICCI's main activities and achievements during the foregoing period (December 2002)

Johnston, Denis, 'The Dublin trams', *Dublin Historical Record,* vol.12 no.4 (1951) 99-113

Jones, Thomas, *Whitehall diary* (ed) Keith Middlemas (3vols. London 1969 -71)

Jordan, Anthony J, *Seán MacBride* (Dublin 1993)

Joyce, James, *Ulysses,* (Paris 1922; Picador edition London 1997)

Joyce, P. W., *The origin and history of Irish names of places* (Dublin 1869 repr. 1995)

Joyce, W St John, *The neighourhood of Dublin* (Dublin 1912)

Keen, Maurice H, *England in the later Middle Ages: a political history* (London 1986)

Kelly, Fergus, *A guide to early Irish law,* School of Celtic Studies: Early Irish Law Series, Volume III (Dublin 1988, repr. 1995)

_____ *Early Irish farming: a study based mainly on the law-texts of the 7th and 8th centuried AD,* Early Irish Law Series Volume IV, School of Celtic Studies, Dublin Institute of Advanced Studies (Dublin 2000)

Kelly, James & Keogh, Dáire (ed), *History of the Catholic diocese of Dublin* (Dublin 2000)

Kerr, Donal (ed), *Emmet's Casino and the Marists at Milltown* (Dublin 1970)

_____ *Peel, priests and politics: Sir Robert Peel's administration and the Roman Catholic church in Ireland, 1841-1846* (Oxford 1982)

_____ 'Dublin's forgotten archbishop: Daniel Murray, 1786-1852' in Kelly & Keogh, *History of the Catholic diocese of Dublin,* 247-67

Kerr, Ian, *John Henry Newman: a biography* (Oxford 1988)

Kilian: Mönch aus Irland – aller Franken Patron – 689-1989 Katalog der Sonder-Ausstellung zur 1300-Jahr-Feier des Kiliansmartyriums, 1 Juli 1989 – 1 Oktober 1989.

King, Cecil H, *Strictly personal: some memoirs of Cecil H King* (London 1969)

Kingston, John et al, *Parish of the Sacred Heart, Donnybrook* (Dublin 1966)

Kotsonouris, Mary, *The winding up of the Dáil Courts: 1922-1925* (Dublin 2004)

Lalor, Brian (ed), *The encyclopaedia of Ireland* (Dublin 2003)

Lawlor, Caitriona, 'Seán MacBride and Amnesty International' in *Village Magazine.*

_____ *Seán MacBride: That day's struggle, a memoir 1904-1951* (Dublin 2005)

Lee, Joseph, *The modernisation of Irish society 1848-1918* (Dublin 1973)

Lee, Sidney (ed), *Dictionary of National Biography* (London 1909) Volume 21

Leslie, J B (compiled) & Wallace, W J R (rev. ed. & updated), *Clergy of Dublin and Glendalough: biographical succession lists* (Dublin 2001)

Lewis, Samuel, *A topographical dictionary of Ireland* (2vols, London 1837)

Lydon, James, *The lordship of Ireland in the Middle Ages* (Dublin 2003)

_____ *The making of Ireland from ancient times to the present* (London 1998)

Lyng, Tom, *Castlecomer connections: exploring history, geography and social evolution in North Kilkenny environs* (Castlecomer 1984)

Lyons, F S L, *Ireland since the famine* (London 1989)

Lyons, J B, *Brief lives of Irish doctors* (Dublin 1978)

M. B. 'The Dublin public and the stage' in *Souvenir of the twenty-fifth anniversary of the opening of the Gaiety Theatre 27th November 1871* (Dublin 1896) 19-32

MacDonagh, Oliver, *The Emancipist Daniel O'Connell 1830-47* (London 1989)

_____ 'Introduction: Ireland and the Union, 1801-70', in Vaughan, *A new history of Ireland*, xlvii-lxv

_____ 'Ideas and institutions, 1830-45' in Vaughan, *A new history of Ireland*, 193-217

Mac Thomáis, E, 'Dublin 1798', *Dublin Historical Record*, 51/2 (1998) 117-33

MacShamhráin, Ailbhe, 'The emergence of the metropolitan see of Dublin, 1111-1216' in Kelly & Keogh *History of the Catholic diocese of Dublin*, 51-71

_____ 'The Monasticon Hibernicum project: the diocese of Dublin', Seán Duffy (ed), *Medieval Dublin VI: proceedings of the Friends of Medieval Dublin Symposium 2004* (Dublin 2005) 114-143

Madden, R R, *The history of Irish periodical literature* (2 vols, London 1867)

_____ *The life and times of Robert Emmet Esq* (Dublin 1847)

Mansergh, Nicholas, *The Irish Free State: its government and politics* (London 1934)

Maxwell, Constantia, *Dublin under the Georges* (Dublin 1997)

Mayes, Charles R, 'The early Stuarts and the Irish peerage', *The English Historical Record* 73(1958) 227-251

McCartney, Donal, *UCD, a national idea: the history of University College, Dublin* (Dublin 1999)

McDowell, R B, *Historical essays: 1938-2001* (Dublin 2003)

_____ *Ireland in the age of imperialism and revolution 1760-1801* (Oxford 1979)

_____ *The Irish administration:1801-1914* (London 1964)

McMahon, Deirdre, 'The Chief Justice and the Governor General controversy in 1932', *Irish Jurist* 17 (1982) 145-67

Meagher, William, *Notices on the life and character of his Grace, Most Rev Daniel Murray, late archbishop of Dublin as contained in the commemorative oration pronounced in the Church of the Conception, Dublin on the occasion of his Grace's Month's Mind* (Dublin 1853)

Meenan, F O C, *Cecilia street: the Catholic University School of Medicine 1855-1931* (Dublin 1987)

Mills, James, 'The Norman settlement in Leinster – The Cantreds near Dublin', *Journal of the Royal Society of Antiquaries of Ireland,* 24 (1894) 161-75

Mooney Tighearnan & White, Fiona, 'The Gentry's Winter Season' in Dickson (ed), *The gorgeous mask,* 1-16

Morrissey, Thomas J, *Towards a National University, William Delany SJ (1835-1924): an era of initiative in Irish education* (Dublin 1983)

Mulvihill, Margaret, *Charlotte Despard: a biography* (London 1989)

Munter, Robert, *A dictionary of the print trade in Ireland 1550-1775* (New York 1988)

Murphy, John A, *Ireland in the twentieth century* (Dublin 1975)

Murray, Jim, *Classic Irish whiskey* (London 1997)

Musgrave, Sir Richard, *Memoirs of the Irish rebellion of 1798* (repr. Fort Wayne 1995)

Nolan, J, *Changing faces* (Dublin 1982)

Ó Cadhain, Máirtín, *The road to Brightcity: short stories translated by Eoghan Ó Tuarisc* (Swords, Co Dublin 1981)

Ó Cróinín, Dáibhí, 'Armagh, Book of', Seán Duffy (ed), *Medieval Ireland: an encyclopedia* (New York & London 2005)

_____ Review article on Etchingham, *Church organisation* in *Peritia* 15 (2001) 413-20

Ó Cuív, Brian, *Aspects of Irish personal names,* Institute of Advanced Studies (Dublin 1986)

Ó Maitiú, Séamas, *Dublin's suburban towns 1834- 1930* (Dublin 2003)

Ó Tuathaigh, Gearóid, *Ireland before the famine 1798 – 1848* (Dublin 1972)

O'Brien, Joseph V, *"Dear dirty Dublin": a city in distress, 1899-1916* (Berkeley, Ca. 1982)

O'Byrne, Emmett, *War, politics and the Irish of Leinster: 1156-1606* (Dublin 2003)

Ó Danachair, Caoimhín, *Folk and farm: essays in honour of A T Lucas,* Royal Society of Antiquaries of Ireland (Dublin 1976)

O'Donovan, John (ed. & tr.), *The banquet of Dun na n-Gedh and the battle of Magh Rath, an ancient historical tale,* Irish Archæological Society (Dublin 1842)

O'Dwyer, Peter, O. Carm., 'The history of Gort Muire: 1944-1994' abridged for

the Irish Carmelites' website [http://www.carmelites.ie/Ireland/Gort%
20Muire/gmhistory.htm]

O'Ferrall, Fergus, *Daniel O'Connell* (Dublin 1981)

O'Halpin, Eunan, 'Politics and the state', J R Hill (ed), *A new history of Ireland,*
VII Ireland, 1921-84 (Oxford 2003) 86-126

O'Riordan, Tomás, 'Cullen, "Letter on the Catholic University to Dr Tobias
Kirby"   [http://multitext.ucc.ie/d/Cullen_Letter_on_the_Catholic_
University_to_Dr_Tobias_Kirby] May, 2006

Osborough, W N, *Law and the emergence of modern Dublin: a litigation
topography of the city* (Dublin 1996)

Otway-Ruthven, A J, 'The mediaeval church lands of co. Dublin', in J A Watt, J
B Morrall & F X Martin (ed), *Medieval studies presented to Aubrey Gwynn
SJ* (Dublin 1961) 54-73

_____ *A history of medieval Ireland* (2nd ed, London 1980)

Pakenham, Thomas, *The year of liberty: the bloody story of the great Irish Rebellion
of 1798* (London 1969)

Papanikitas, Andrew N, '*Droch Fhola*: medical influences in Bram Stoker's
Dracula, a tale of biological evil' in *Guy's, King's & St Thomas's Hospitals
Medical and Dental Schools Gazette,* October 2002 and reproduced on the
Gazette website: http://www.gktgazette.com/2002/oct/features.asp

Parkinson, Danny, 'The Corballis/Corbally families of Co Dublin', *Irish Family
History: Journal of the Irish Family History Society,* 8 (1992) 84-94

_____ 'The Corballis-Corbally Families of Co. Dublin', *Dublin Historical Record*
45/2 (1992) 91-100

Parkinson, R E, *History of the Grand Lodge of Free and Accepted Masons of Ireland*
(2vols, Dublin 1957)

Pollard, M, *A dictionary of members of the Dublin book trade, 1550-1800, based on
the records of the Guild of St Luke the Evangelist, Dublin* (London 2000)

Rafter, Kevin, *Martin Mansergh, a biography* (Dublin 2000)

_____ *The Clann: the story of Clann na Poblachta* (Cork 1996)

Rawlings, A L, *The science of clocks and watches,* British Horological Institute
(Upton 1993)

Redmond, Joseph, 'The schools of Donnybrook' in Kingston, *Parish of the Sacred
Heart, Donnybrook,* 47-51

Reynolds, J J, *Footprints of Emmet* (Dublin 1903)

Richter, Michael, 'Columbanus (c. 540-615)', Seán Duffy (ed), *Medieval Ireland:
an encyclopedia* (New York & London 2005)

Roche, Desmond, *Local government in Ireland,* Institute of Public Administration
(Dublin 1982)

Ronan, Myles V, 'Archbishop Bukeley's Visitation of Dublin, 1630', *Archivium
Hibernicum* 8(1941) 56-98

_____ 'History of the Diocese', *Reportorium Novum: Dublin diocesan historical record*, 1 (1955) 27-44

Royal Irish Academy, *Dictionary of the Irish language* (Dublin 1913-76)

Rushe, James R, *Carmel in Ireland: a narrative of the Irish province of Teresian, or Discalced Carmelites (AD 1625-1896)* (Dublin & London 1903)

Ryan, John, 'Pre-Norman Dublin' in Howard Clarke (ed), *Medieval Dublin: the making of a metropolis* (Dublin 1990)

Scannell, James, 'From horse drawn trams to LUAS: a look at public transport in Dublin from the 1870's (*sic*) to the present time' in *Dublin Historical Record,* 59/1(2006) 5-18

Sharpe, Richard, 'Some problems concerning the organization of the church in early medieval Ireland' *Peritia* 3 (1984) 230-70

Shiel, R L, *Sketches of the Irish bar* (2vols, New York 1854)

Simms, G O, 'James Henthorn Todd', *Hermathena: a Dublin University review,* 109 (1969) 5-23

Smith, Cornelius F, 'In the beginning: 1837 – 1875' in Cornelius F Smith & Bernard Share, *Whigs on the Green* (Dublin 1990) 36-59

Smyth, Alfred P, *Celtic Leinster: towards an historical geography of early Irish civilization A.D. 500-1600* (Blackrock, Co. Dublin 1982)

Smyth, James, 'Dublin's political underground in the 1790s', in Gerard O'Brien (ed), *Parliament, politics and people: essays in eighteenth-century Irish history* (Dublin 1989) 129-48

Somerville-Woodward, Robert, 'The Celtic Society', *Pages: Arts Postgraduate Research in progress,* Faculty of Arts, University College Dublin, vol. 5, 1998, 177-186

Souvenir, *Blessing and dedication of the Church of the Immaculate Virgin Mary of the Miraculous Medal, Clonskeagh: Feast of the Nativity of Our Lady 8th September, 1957* (Brown & Nolan, Richview press, Clonskeagh, Co. Dublin 1957)

St Kilian's school chronicle with added material from the school principal, Mr Rolf Fenner

Stephen, L & Lea, S (ed), *Dictonary of National Biography* (London 1908) Volume 5

Stewart, Miriam (ed), *Arts Ireland,* 39 (May 2001)

Stuart, William Gailland, *Watch and clockmakers in Ireland* (Dublin 2000)

Sweeney, Clair L, *The rivers of Dublin* (Dublin 1991)

Sweeney, Maxwell, 'The Gaiety story' in *Gaiety Theatre 75th anniversary 1871-1946* (Dublin 1946)

Tindall, George Brown, *America: a narrative history* (2nd ed, New York & London 1988) Volume 1

Todd, James Henthorn (ed. & tr.), *Leabhar breathnach annso sis: the Irish version of Historia Brittonum of Nennius*, Irish Archæological Society (Dublin 1848)

Towey, Thomas, 'Hugh Kennedy and the constitutional development of the Irish Free State, 1922-1923' *Irish Jurist* 12 (1977) 355-70

Townend, Peter (ed), *Burke's genealogical and heraldic history of the Peerage, Baronetage and Knightage* (104th ed, London 1967)

Unknown, *Dublin 18th century printers: list and index* (c. 1930)

Vaughan, W E (ed), *A new history of Ireland* V *Ireland under the Union, I 1801-70* (Oxford 1989)

Wall, Maureen, 'The Catholic merchants, manufacturers and traders of Dublin 1778-1782', *Repertorium Novum* 2/2 (1960) 298-323

Walsh, William J, 'The law in its relations to religious interests: IX. The Board of Charitable Donations and Bequests in Ireland', *Irish Ecclesiastical Record*, 3rd ser., 16 (1895) 875-94

Ward, Alan J, *The Irish constitutional tradition: responsible government and modern Ireland 1782-1992* (Dublin 1994)

Ward, John, 'McCormack on Brighton pier' in *The Record Collector*, 37 (1992) 62-9 reproduced on the McCormack Society website [http://www.mccormacksociety.co.uk/]

Ward, Margaret, *Maud Gonne: a life* (London 1993)

Webb, Alfred, *A compendium of Irish biography comprising sketches of distinguished Irishmen and of eminent persons connected with Ireland by office or by their writing* (Dublin 1878)

Webb, J J, *Industrial Dublin since 1698 and the silk industry in Dublin* (Dublin 1913)

White, Eric Walter, *A history of English opera* (London 1983)

White, Terence de Vere, *The road of excess* (Dublin 1945)

_____ *Tom Moore, the Irish poet* (London 1977)

Whittaker, T K, 'Origins and consolidation, 1783-1826', in F. S. L. Lyons (ed), *Bicentenary essays: Bank of Ireland 1783-1983* (Dublin 1983) 11-29

Wilson, David A, *United Irishmen, United States: immigrant radicals in the early republic* (Dublin 1998)

Wilson, W J R, *Faithful to our Trust: a history of the Erasmus Smith Trust and The High School, Dublin* (Dublin 2004)

Woolf, Alex, 'Amlaib Cuarán and the Gael, 941-81', in Seán Duffy (ed), *Medieval Dublin III: proceedings of the Friends of Medieval Dublin Symposium 2001* (Dublin 2002) 34-43

Wright, G N, *An historical guide to ancient and modern Dublin* (2 vols, London 1821)

Young, John, *They fell like stones: battles and casualties of the Zulu war, 1879* (London 1991)

Index